The Healing Power of Herbs

revised and expanded 2nd edition

The Healing Power of Herbs

revised and expanded 2nd edition

The Enlightened Person's Guide to the Wonders of Medicinal Plants

Michael T. Murray, N.D.

Prima Publishing

P Prima™ is a trademark of Prima Publishing, a division of Prima Communications, Inc. Prima Publishing™ is a trademark of Prima Communications, Inc.

WARNING—DISCLAIMER
Prima Publishing has designed this book to provide information in regard to the subject matter covered. It is sold with the understanding that the publisher and the author are not liable for the misconception or misuse of information provided. Every effort has been made to make this book as complete and as accurate as possible. The purpose of this book is to educate. The author and Prima Publishing shall have neither liability nor responsibility to any person or entity with respect to any loss, damage, or injury caused or alleged to be caused directly or indirectly by the information contained in this book. The information presented herein is in no way intended as a substitute for medical counseling.

Library of Congress Cataloging-in-Publication Data

Murray, Michael T.
    The healing power of herbs : the enlightened person's guide to the wonders of medicinal plants / Michael T. Murray. — Rev. & expanded 2nd ed.
        p.   cm.
    Includes index.
    ISBN 1-55958-700-8
    1. Herbs—Therapeutic use—Encyclopedias.   I. Title.
RM666.H33M865   1995
615'.321—dc20   94-39025
                                                                            CIP

97 98 99 AA 10

Printed in the United States of America

How to Order:

Single copies may be ordered from Prima Publishing, P.O. Box 1260BK, Rocklin, CA 95677; telephone (916) 632-4400. Quantity discounts are also available. On your letterhead, include information concerning the intended use of the books and the number of books you wish to purchase.

Dedication

To my wife, Gina—I am truly thankful that we are sharing our lives.

Our child, Alexa Michelle, who has taught me so much about life.

My parents, Cliff and Patty Murray, and my grandmother, Pauline Shier, for a strong foundation and a lifetime of good memories.

Contents

Section I   Introduction

Section II   Materia Medica

Section III   Recommended Herbs for Some Specific Health Conditions

Foreword to the Second Edition

Herbal medicine may seem a little strange to people grounded in established Western medical practices. However, 80 percent of the world's population depend on plants to treat many common ailments. In addition, 30 percent of modern conventional drugs are derived from a plant source. Herbal medicine is not so strange, after all.

For example, the herb *Ginkgo biloba* is the most popular prescription drug in Germany and France. This plant has been shown to help alleviate senility, short-term memory loss, and ringing in the ears. *Ginkgo biloba* was prescribed more than five million times in Germany during 1988. That same year in Germany, the sale of herbs exceeded $5 billion.

Saw palmetto berry is another good example. The oil of this berry has been used effectively to treat BPH (benign prostatic hyperplasia) in Europe. In France alone, sales of this oil extract have exceeded $300 million annually.

Herbs have been used safely and effectively for at least 5,000 years. However, the Western medical system does not encourage the use or scientific validation of herbal therapy, so the mainstream public knows relatively little about it. When you consider that herbs are free of most of the side effects associated with synthetic drugs, this omission doesn't make much sense.

The United States government established a drug regulatory process to determine drug toxicity. These regulations require 10 to 12 years of research, at a cost of approximately $300 million per drug. Once the research is approved, the drug company holds the patent rights and drug prices are set to recover this expense.

Today, if common herbs are to be approved as medicines, they, too, are subject to this lengthy and costly approval process. However, patents can not be granted for plants or other natural compounds. Therefore, no private enterprise can justify the cost. So even though private enterprise can manufacture and distribute herbal products, it cannot legally tell consumers what these herbal products do.

How can we find out about the therapeutic value of herbs? By doing our own research. *The Healing Power of Herbs,* by Michael T. Murray, N.D., is an easy-to-read book for all ages and educational backgrounds. It provides a comprehensive overview of the history and use of herbal medicine. It cites extensive research on the safety and effectiveness of herbs for most of today's illnesses. It lists herbs that can be used to treat dozens of self-limiting, self-diagnosable health complaints. The interested reader can easily find chapters on the appropriate herbal treatments for arthritis, colds, flu, cough, allergies, and many other minor but annoying conditions.

In addition, Dr. Murray cites references to the scientific studies conducted worldwide. This long list will help the serious student of herbal medicine continue his/her research.

Through his prolific writings and research, Dr. Murray is the person most responsible for introducing herbal extracts and herbal standardization to the American consumer. I believe Dr. Murray will continue to lead the renaissance for herbal medicine in this country.

Those who wish to be in the forefront of herbal knowledge will truly appreciate *The Healing Power of Herbs.* This book can help you develop your own self health care program and maximize your potential for a long and vital life.

Terry Lemerond
President, Enzymic Therapy

Foreword to the First Edition

I wish when I first began my journey into the wonders of natural medicine that a book like this had been available. For the intelligent layperson, there has long been a frustrating lack of access to accurate and reliable information about the many aspects of natural medicine. This dearth has been particularly evident in the area of herbal medicine: most of what has been available is an anecdotal rehashing of material written more than 100 years ago.

In the past 50 years, herbal medicines have been the subject of a tremendous amount of research, both in the United States and internationally. This research has resulted in the accumulation of a remarkable body of knowledge that has shown repeatedly, in both clinical and laboratory experimentation, the marvelous healing ability of herbal medicines. Yet little of this information has found its way into lay and professional publications, and few physicians are current in their knowledge of this important area. (Even naturopathic doctors—the only physicians formally trained in the use of botanical medicines—are not as aware of the science of herbal medicine as they should be.) I have often wondered why. I can only conclude, somewhat cynically I must admit, that this is most likely due to several factors: (1) most of today's health care professionals are so enamored with the glitter of high-tech medicine that they lack interest in the less glamorous methods of mother nature; (2) the drug companies can make higher profits only by researching and promoting patentable (chemically modified and synthesized) drugs; (3) doctors of natural medicine are so involved in their practices (traditionally very few teaching and research opportunities have been available) that they have not spent enough time reading the scientific literature; and (4) the publishers of general trade books often require their authors to write to a relatively uneducated audience. This book reaches beyond those constricting factors.

What makes Dr. Murray's work so unique and immensely valuable is his careful blending of concise and understandable clinical recommendations with thorough referencing from the peer-reviewed scientific literature. He has spent thousands of hours combing the international research on herbal medicines. When he makes a recommendation, it is both clinically relevant and scientifically proven.

While I respect and believe in the age-old wisdom of natural medicine and recognize that placebo-controlled scientific studies are not necessary to prove the efficacy of a botanical medicine that has been used for a thousand years, that is no reason to ignore the wealth of information that researchers have gleaned. My belief is that the best information is that which combines and expands the best of clinical experience with applicable scientific research. That is what Dr. Murray has done here.

He has not avoided the challenge of writing to the intelligent reader in a manner that is truly informative. He uses and carefully defines technical terms as appropriate to further understanding while avoiding obscure and excess technicality. On the one hand the book can be used as a simple guide, by using the herbal formulas Dr. Murray has compiled; on the other hand it can serve as a reference manual for the person who is seriously interested in herbal medicine and will pursue the comprehensive references provided at the end of each chapter.

This is a remarkably important and useful work.

Joseph E. Pizzorno, Jr., N.D.
President, John Bastyr College

Preface

Simply stated, practitioners of herbal medicine use plants or plant substances as medicinal agents. But despite our awareness of the medicinal properties of plants, our knowledge of how plants actually affect human physiology remains fragmentary. Whereas many practitioners are content to accept the empirical evidence of a plant's therapeutic indication and effectiveness, others wish to discover whether the plant is truly effective and what its mechanism of action may be. I am largely in the latter category.

What does herbal medicine mean to me? I cannot effectively express my feelings on discovering the remarkable ways in which herbal medicines work. Humility, awe, wonder, joy, and respect often overcome me as I discover the true beauty and harmony that exists in nature.

The more I learn about herbal medicine, the stronger my faith in nature and naturopathic medicine becomes. I want to share not only the information I have discovered, but my faith as well. It is my hope that this book will inspire you.

The bottom line for any practitioner or patient is the result! Herbal medicines must be used successfully if their use is to persist. Challenge yourself to study botanical medicine and you will achieve results.

Live in Good Health with Passion and Joy!

Michael T. Murray, N.D.

Acknowledgments

Dr. Joseph Pizzorno, President of Bastyr University, and Terry Lemerond, President and founder of Enzymatic Therapy, for their integrity and dedication to quality

Joe and Terry, for friendship

Bob and Kathy Bunton, for their love and acceptance

Ben Dominitz and everyone at Prima, for their support

My friends at Enzymatic Therapy, for all of their friendship and support and Karolyn Gazella and everyone at ImpaKt Communications and *Health Counselor Magazine*, for their support

And all the researchers, physicians, and scientists who have striven to increase our understanding of natural medicines. Without their work, this book would not exist.

The Healing Power of Herbs

revised and expanded 2nd edition

SECTION I

Introduction

Herbal medicine: A modern perspective

The term *herb* refers to a plant used for medicinal purposes. Are herbs effective medicinal agents or is their use merely a reflection of folklore, outdated theories, and myth? To the uninformed, herbs are generally thought of as ineffective medicines used prior to the advent of more effective synthetic drugs. To others, herbs are simply sources of compounds to isolate and then market as drugs. But to some, herbs and crude plant extracts are effective medicines to be respected and appreciated.

For many people herbal medicines are the only therapeutic agents available. In 1985, the World Health Organization estimated that perhaps 80 percent of the world population relies on herbs for primary health care needs.[1] This widespread use of herbal medicines is not restricted to developing countries, as it has been estimated that 30 to 40 percent of all medical doctors in France and Germany rely on herbal preparations as their primary medicines.[2]

The rebirth of herbal medicine

Throughout the world, but especially in Europe and Asia, a tremendous renaissance in the use and appreciation of herbal medicine has taken place. In Germany, estimates show that over $4 billion dollars are spent on herbal products each year. In Japan, the figure is thought to be even higher. Herbal products are a major business in the United States as well, with an estimated annual sales figure of $1.3 billion dollars for 1992 and climbing.[3] However, it is interesting to note that while annual sales of ginseng products in the United States in 1992 were roughly $10 million dollars, over 3 million pounds (roughly $100 million dollars) of American ginseng were exported.[4,5]

The rebirth of herbal medicine, especially in developed countries, is largely based on the renewed interest of scientific researchers. During the last 10 to 20 years their efforts have yielded an explosion of scientific information concerning plants, crude plant extracts, and various substances from plants as medicinal agents.

The role of herbs in medicine: American versus European policies

For the past 25 years about 25 percent of all prescription drugs in the United States have contained active constituents obtained from plants. Digoxin, codeine, colchicine, morphine, vincristine, and yohimbine are some popular examples. Many over-the-counter preparations are composed of plant compounds as well. It is estimated that more than $11 billion dollars' worth of plant-based medicines are purchased each year in the United States alone, and $43 billion dollars worldwide.[6]

Because a plant cannot be patented, very little research has been done in this century on whole plants or crude plant extracts as medicinal agents, per se, by the large American pharmaceutical firms. Instead, pharmaceutical firms screen plants for biological activity and then isolate the so-called active constituents (compounds). (Indeed, *pharmacognosy*, the study of natural drugs and their constituents, plays a major role in current drug development.) If the compound is powerful enough, the drug company will begin the formidable process to procure Food and Drug Administration (FDA) approval. I say formidable, because in the United States FDA approval of a plant-based drug typically takes 10 to 18 years at a total cost of roughly $230 million dollars.

In contrast, European policies have made it economically feasible for companies to research and develop herbs as medicines. In Germany, herbal products can be marketed as medicines if they have been proved to be safe and effective.[7] Actually, the legal requirements for herbal medicines are identical to those for all other drugs. Whether the herbal product is available by prescription or over the counter (OTC) is based on its application and safety of use. Herbal products sold in pharmacies are reimbursed by insurance if they are prescribed by a physician.

The proof required by a manufacturer in Germany to illustrate safety and effectiveness for an herbal product is far less than the proof required by the FDA for drugs in the United States. In Germany, a special commission (Commission E) developed a series of 200 monographs on herbal products, similar to the OTC monographs in the United States.[7] An herbal product is viewed as safe and effective if a manufacturer meets the quality requirements of the relevant monograph or produces additional evidence of safety and effectiveness, which can include data from the existing literature, anecdotal information from practicing physicians, as well as limited clinical studies.

The best single illustration of the difference in the regulatory issues on herbal products in the United States compared to Germany concerns *Ginkgo biloba*. In Germany, as well as France, extracts of *Ginkgo biloba* leaves are registered for the treatment of cerebral and peripheral vascular insufficiency.[8] Ginkgo products are available by prescription and OTC purchase. Ginkgo extracts are among the three most widely prescribed drugs in both Germany and France, with a combined annual sales figure of more than $500 million dollars. In contrast, in the United States, extracts, which are identical to those approved in Germany and France, are available as "food supplements."

No medicinal claims are allowed for most herbal products because the FDA requires the same standard of absolute proof as is required for new synthetic drugs. The FDA has rejected the idea of establishing an independent Expert Advisory Panel for the development of monographs similar to Germany's Commission E monographs, as well as other ideas to create a suitable framework for the marketing of herbal products in the United States.

Currently, herbal products continue to be sold as "food supplements," and manufacturers are prohibited from making any therapeutic claims for their products.

The great fallacy

One of the great fallacies promoted by the U.S. medical establishment has been that there is no firm scientific evidence for the use of many natural therapies, including herbal medicine. This assertion is simply not true. In fact, the last 10 to 20 years have produced a tremendous amount of information concerning plants, crude plant extracts, and nutritional substances as medicinal agents.

Compare this to just 30 years ago, at which time it was impossible for the scientific establishment to determine exactly how many herbs promote their healing effects. Take aspirin, for example: you may be surprised to read that the main mechanism of action responsible for aspirin's anti-inflammatory effect was not understood until the early 1970s, and that its mechanism of action for pain relief has yet to be fully understood.

Since in this not-so-distant past the mechanism of therapeutic action of a particular herb could not be fully isolated and understood, many effective plant medicines were erroneously labeled as possessing no pharmacological activity. Today, however, researchers equipped with more sophisticated technology are rediscovering the wonder of plants as medicinal agents. Much of their increased understanding is, ironically, a result of synthetic drug research.

For example, one of the latest classes of so-called "wonder drugs" includes the calcium channel-blocking drugs. These drugs block the entry of calcium into smooth muscle cells, thereby inhibiting contraction and promoting muscular relaxation. Calcium channel-blocking drugs are currently being used in the treatment of high blood pressure, angina, asthma, and other conditions associated with smooth muscle contraction. In many ways, the synthesis and understanding of these drugs symbolizes the level of sophistication of the modern science of pharmacology. After calcium channel-blocking drugs were isolated and their mechanism of action better understood, it was discovered that many herbs contain components that possess calcium channel-blocking activity. In most cases the historical use of these herbs as medicine corresponded to their calcium channel-blocking activity.

In addition to possessing currently understood pharmacological activity, many herbs possess pharmacological actions that are not at all consistent with modern pharmacological understanding. For example, many herbs appear to impact homeostatic control mechanisms to aid normalization of many of the body's processes: when there is a hyperstate the herb exerts a lowering effect and when there is a hypostate it has a heightening effect. This action is baffling to orthodox pharmacologists but not to experienced herbalists, who have used terms such as *alterative, amphiteric, adaptogenic,* or *tonic* to describe this effect.

The advantages of herbal medicines

What advantages do herbal medicines possess over synthetic drugs? As a rule, herbal preparations are less toxic than their synthetic counterparts and offer less risk of side effects (obviously, there are exceptions to this rule). In addition, the mechanism of action of an herb is often to correct the underlying cause of ill health. In contrast, a synthetic drug is often designed to alleviate the symptom or effect without addressing the underlying cause. It has also been demonstrated with many plants that the whole plant or crude extract is much more effective than isolated constituents.

The future of herbal medicine

Herbal medicine will certainly play a major role in future medicine. As modern medicine gains more knowledge and understanding about health and disease it is adopting therapies that are more natural and less toxic. Lifestyle modification, stress reduction, exercise, meditation, dietary changes, and many other traditional naturopathic therapies are becoming much more popular in standard medical circles. This illustrates the paradigm shift that is occurring in medicine. What were once scoffed at are now becoming generally accepted as effective alternatives. In fact, in most instances these natural alternatives offer significant advantages over standard medical practices.

Appreciation is growing for the harmonious healing properties that herbal medicines possess, particularly in Europe and Asia. The United States is becoming more aware of the medicinal value of herbs as well. Without doubt, future medicine will make good use of herbs: the medicine of the past will *be* the medicine of the future.

The difference will be due to the growing sophistication of herbal medicine. With the continuing advancement in science and technology there has been a great improvement in the quality of herbal medicines available. Improvements in cultivation techniques, coupled with improvements in quality control and standardization of potency, will continue to increase the effectiveness of herbal medicines.

References

1. Farnsworth N, *et al.*: Medicinal plants in therapy. *Bull World Health Org* **63**, 965–981, 1985.
2. Interview: An interview with Prof. H. Wagner. *HerbalGram* **17**, 16–17, 1988.
3. Unpublished data from the American Botanical Council. P.O. Box 201660, Austin, Texas 78720.
4. Deveny K: Garlic and ginseng supplements become potent drugstore sellers. *The Wall Street Journal* 10/1/92, pp. B1, B5.
5. Market report. *HerbalGram* **26**, 40, 1992.
6. Principe PP: The economic significance of plants and their constituents as drugs. *Econ Med Plant Res* **3**, 1–17, 1989.
7. Keller K: Legal requirements for the use of phytopharmaceutical drugs in the Federal Republic of Germany. *J Ethnopharamacol* **32**, 225–229, 1991.
8. Kleijnen J and Knipschild P: Drug profiles—*Ginkgo biloba. Lancet* **340**, 1136–1139, 1993.

The history of herbal medicine

The history of the use of plants as medicines is a history full of interesting stories and fascinating facts. The evolution that has occurred in herbal medicine over the centuries is only beginning to be recognized as more natural medicines gain acceptance. Interestingly, this acceptance is largely a result of increased scientific investigation.

What exactly is science?

The term *science* refers to "possession of knowledge as distinguished from ignorance or misunderstanding." Scientific knowledge is based on the scientific method, meaning that the understanding is based on the collection of data through observation and experiment. It must be kept in mind that, while science is evolutionary, the underlying natural laws it tries to explain are constant. In other words, gravity existed long before Sir Isaac Newton was around to explain it.

The scientific method is used to explore the nature of the human body and the environment. Breakthrough developments in many areas of science are occurring at an incredible pace, especially in some areas of medicine. It is interesting to point out that what was once considered scientific medicine is often discarded when a deeper understanding is achieved. For example, in the 1800s scientific medicine involved bloodletting and the administration of toxic substances. Likewise, many current medical treatments involving the use of drugs and surgery will, in all probability, be discarded in the future.

There is a trend toward using substances found in nature, including compounds that are found in the human body (such as interferon, interleukin, insulin, and human growth hormone) as well as foods, food components, herbs, and herbal compounds. More and more researchers are discovering the tremendous healing properties of these natural compounds and their advantages over synthetic medicines and surgery in the treatment of many health conditions. Through these scientific investigations, a trend toward natural medicine is emerging.

To better appreciate this evolutionary trend, let's look at some of the historical aspects of herbal medicine. If you find the history of herbal medicine as interesting as I do, you may want to get Barbara Griggs's *Green Pharmacy: A History of Herbal Medicine*.[1] Much of the information presented in this chapter is derived from this excellent work.

In the beginning

Humans—and animals—have always used plants. The initial use of plants as medicines by humans is thought to have been the result of "instinctive" dowsing. Animals in the wild provide evidence that this phenomenon still occurs: they eat plants that heal them, and avoid plants that do them harm. Presumably humans also possessed this instinct at one time.

As civilizations developed, medicine men and women were responsible for transmitting the information on herbs to their successors. Before the advent of written language, this information was handed down by verbal and experiential means. It was commonly believed that plants had been signed by the "creator" with some sort of clue that would indicate its therapeutic use. This concept was commonly referred to as the "Doctrine of Signatures."

Common examples of this doctrine include ginseng (*Panax ginseng*), whose root bears strong resemblance to a human figure and whose general use is as a tonic; blue cohosh (*Caulophyllum thalictroides*), whose branches are arranged like limbs in spasm, indicating its usefulness in the treatment of muscular spasm; bloodroot (*Sanguinaria canadensis*), whose roots and sap are a beautiful blood color corresponding to its traditional use as a "blood purifier"; lobelia (*Lobelia inflata*), whose flowers are shaped like a stomach, corresponding to its emetic qualities; and goldenseal (*Hydrastis canadensis*), whose yellow-green root signifies its use in jaundice as well as infectious processes. All of these uses have been confirmed by recent research.

Materia medica

With the development of written language, *materia medica* (books providing information on herbs and their prescription) became the vehicle for transmitting information on the medicinal use of herbs to future herbalists. The *materia medica* recorded in ancient China, Babylon, Egypt, India, Greece, and other parts of the world strongly suggest that herbal medicine was highly respected in ancient times.

Galen's influence

No system, rules, or classification was imposed on western materia medicas until the first century A.D., when Galen, a Roman physician, established his system of rules and classification. Galen's classification was based on Hippocratic medicine, that is, on the balance of the four humors—blood, bile, phlegm, and choler.

Galen evaluated each plant and discussed it in terms of its relation to Hippocratic medicine. But despite his apparent reverence for Hippocratic principles, Galen in essence used this system to construct his own elaborate and rigid system of medicine. Galen's work signified the beginning of a clear division between the professional physician and the traditional healer. As only the well educated could understand Galen's system (and even with the best schooling it remained a mystery to many), all challenges were effectively squelched by dogma.

Galen's system effectively paralyzed European medical thinking for 1,500 years. Perhaps if the Roman Empire had continued to flourish someone would have surfaced to rival Galen; instead, Galenic medicine dominated the Middle Ages. The "professional" physician, confident in his superior knowledge, attempted to hasten recovery by bloodletting, purging, and administering exotic medicines. This was in direct contrast to the traditional healer's patient use of traditional herbs and his tremendous faith in the healing power of nature.

The Black Plague and syphilis

Although Galenic medicine dominated the Middle Ages, herbal medicine was still deeply entrenched in European culture. The Black Plague of 1348 A.D. may have marked the beginning of a change in medical thought, as conventional medicine proved itself totally useless in this crisis. As nearly one-third of Europe died as a result of this plague, the public began to lose faith in Galenic medicine.

Nearly 150 years later another blow was dealt to Galenic medicine, when syphilis became a major medical problem. Unlike the Black Death, patients with syphilis tended to survive longer, giving physicians more time to experiment with treatments. At this time perhaps the greatest hoax in the history of medicine began. Mercury became the standard medical treatment for syphilis, despite the fact that even Galen thought mercury too poisonous to use.

Syphilis did, however, open the door for the use of some new herbs from the Americas. A French physician, Nicholas Monardes, published in 1574 a comprehensive account of sarsaparilla and several other "new" drugs in the treatment of syphilis. At that time many Europeans believed that syphilis had come to Europe from the West Indies with Columbus's sailors; since there was a general belief that whatever disease was native to a country might be cured by the medicinal herbs growing in that region, it was only natural for sarsaparilla to become a popular remedy. Because at that time the standard treatment for syphilis involved the use of mercury, which often resulted in greater morbidity than did syphilis, sarsaparilla was a welcome alternative. Despite the initial excitement, Monardes's sarsaparilla cure eventually lost favor, probably owing to other components in the cure—specifically, patients were confined to a warm room for 30 days, and for the following 40 days were to abstain from both wine and sexual intercourse.

Although the public popularity of sarsaparilla waned, it continued to be used in the treatment of syphilis. During military operations in Portugal in 1812, a British Inspector General of Hospitals noted that the Portuguese soldiers suffering from syphilis who used sarsaparilla recovered much faster and more completely than their British counterparts, who were treated with mercury.

Sarsaparilla was also used by the Chinese in the treatment of syphilis. Later clinical observations in China would demonstrate, through the use of blood tests, that sarsaparilla is effective in about 90 percent of cases of acute syphilis and 50 percent of cases of chronic syphilis.

Although sarsaparilla was clearly more beneficial than mercury in the treatment of syphilis, mercury became established as the standard treatment for over four and a half centuries. It has been stated by Leonard Goldwater, author of *Mercury: A History of Quicksilver* that, "the use of mercury in the treatment of syphilis may have been the most colossal hoax ever perpetrated" in the history of medicine. Mercury represented a new kind of medicine, one formulated and prepared in a laboratory using the new techniques of chemistry. It helped prepare the way for future drugs at the expense of herbal medicines.

Challenges to Galenic medicine

The 1500s also saw a strong challenge to Galenic medicine from within traditional circles. Specifically, Paracelsus, an alchemist who believed strongly in the Doctrine of Signatures, was responsible for founding modern pharmaceutical medicine. Paracelsus is probably most remembered for the development of laudanum (tincture of opium). After Paracelsus, Galenic preparations and treatments fell greatly out of favor.

In public circles herbal medicine was regaining some respect as well. In the early 1600s, Nicholas Culpepper, an English pharmacist, published an herbal entitled *The English Physician*. Instead of requiring patients to purchase expensive exotic or imported drugs, Culpepper recommended the herbs his clients and readers had growing in their own back yards. Although Culpepper's herbal is based on astrological rationalizations, it reinforced a strong English tradition of domestic herbal medicine. This came at a time when professional physicians were beginning to become contemptuous of herbal medicine.

Meanwhile, in the Americas during the 1600s and 1700s herbs used traditionally by the native Americans were becoming quite popular, especially in the treatment of malaria and scurvy. Herbal medicine continued to gain even greater respect in the late 1700s, as exemplified by Dr. William Withering's classic description of digitalis. However, mercury, bleeding, and purging were still the "standard" medical treatments, as epitomized by George Washington's death from complications incurred during treatment of a sore throat (i.e., he was bled to death).

The Thomsonian and Eclectic movements

In the early 1800s, standard medicine may have been ready to return to traditional herbal remedies, but for the Thomsonian movement. Samuel Thomson (1769–1843) patented a system of herbal medicine that, in 1839, claimed more than 3 million faithful followers. Although Thomson reinstated the Hippocratic idea of *vis medicatrix naturæ* and gained widespread public support for the use of herbal medicine, the Thomsonian movement was probably detrimental overall to medical reform.

Thomsonianism was founded on ignorance, prejudice, and dogma. Thomsonians insisted that all medical knowledge was complete and could be found in Samuel Thomson's works. These and other claims roused scorn, indignation, rage, and resentment in the average North American doctor. In addition, Thomson's treatments often were as harsh as the standard treatments of the times.

During the 1800s, the Eclectic movement attempted to bridge the gaps between standard medical thought, Thomsonianism, and traditional herbal medicines. Rather than attack the existing medical system, the Eclectic movement sought to bring about reform by educating physicians about the use of herbal medicines. Several Eclectic medical colleges were established and, for a while, it appeared the Eclectic movement was making headway in its attempt to reform the medical system from within.

The movement, however, eventually failed. Several factors were probably responsible for the failure of the Eclectic movement: a split in the ranks that weakened the movement; the discarding of harsh measures such as mercury, calomel, and bloodletting, owing to a decrease in infectious disease as a result of improved sanitation and hygiene; and perhaps most important, the failure to sustain a quality medical school.

The Flexner Report on Medical Education[2] in 1910 spelled doom for the Eclectics: by 1920, seven of the eight Eclectic medical schools that existed prior to the report had closed, with the last closing in 1938. Meanwhile, the standard medical schools flourished, aided by the Rockefeller Foundation, and promoted the growth of the modern pharmaceutical industry and the current near-monopoly of the medical profession.

The growth of the pharmaceutical industry

Because a plant cannot be patented, very little research has been done in this century on plants as medicinal agents, per se, by the large American pharmaceutical firms. Instead, plants have been screened for biological activity and then the so-called active constituents have been isolated. Researchers have been dismayed by the fact that in many instances the isolated constituent was less active biologically than the crude herb. Since the crude herb provided no economic reward to the American pharmaceutical firm, the crude herb or extract never reached the marketplace. In contrast, European policies on herbal medicines made it economically feasible for companies to research and develop crude phytopharmaceuticals.

Another problem for herbal medicine in the United States has been the lack of standardization. The herb that best exemplifies this dilemma is digitalis. One batch of crude digitalis might have an extremely low level of active constituents, making the crude herb ineffective, while the next batch might be unusually high in active constituents, resulting in toxicity or even death, when the standard amount is used. The lack of standardization made it easier for U.S. pharmaceutical firms to rationalize their economic need to isolate, purify, and chemically modify the active constituents of digitalis so that they could market these compounds as drugs. The problem with using the pure active constituent is that the safe dosage range is smaller: digitalis toxicity and death have increased dramatically as a result of purification. Toxicity was less of a factor when using the crude herb because overconsumption of potentially toxic doses resulted in vomiting or diarrhea, thus avoiding the heart disturbance and death that occurs now with pure digitalis cardiac glycoside drugs.

Fortunately, several European and Asian pharmaceutical firms began specializing in phytopharmaceuticals in the early part of the twentieth century. These companies have played a prominent role in researching, developing, and promoting herbal medicines.

Research is demonstrating that crude extracts often have greater therapeutic benefit than the isolated "active" constituent. This has been known for quite some time in other parts of the world, but in the United States isolated plant drugs are still thought of as having the greatest therapeutic effect. This myth is gradually eroding as our knowledge of herbal medicines increases.

If current standardization techniques had been available earlier in this century it is possible that the majority of our current prescription drugs would be crude herbal extracts instead of isolated and modified active constituents.

The future of herbal medicine

As stated earlier, herbs and other plant medicines have been used since antiquity as effective treatments for many common diseases. However, with the advent in this century of synthetic drugs, appreciation of plants as medicinal agents diminished greatly. Currently, a renaissance appears to be occurring in herbal medicine. It is ironic that this renewal comes not from traditional herbalists but rather from renewed scientific investigation into the use of plant medicines. It seems that science and medicine have finally advanced to a level at which they can appreciate nature instead of discounting it. It is worth remembering that although the scientific investigation of plant medicines is taking away some of the mystery and romance of herbalism as a greater understanding of the ways in which herbs work is achieved, herbal medicine is being improved by modern scientific research and technology.

Improvements in plant cultivation techniques and the quality of herbal extracts (quality control and standardization) have led to the development of some very effective plant medicines. It is apparent that many of the "wonder drugs" of the future will be derived from plants or plant cell cultures and from cell cultures producing compounds naturally occurring in the human body (interferon, interleukin 2, various hormones, etc.). Several herbal medicines described here may in fact already fulfill the role of wonder drug, for example, *Ginkgo biloba, Silybum marianum, Panax ginseng,* and *Piper methysticum.*

The future of herbal medicine looks bright. Many of the previous shortcomings of herbal medicine have been overcome (e.g., the lack of scientific support, standardization, and quality control). The future of herbal medicine depends on several factors: (1) continued research into herbal medicine, (2) adoption by manufacturers of recognized standards of quality, (3) continued existence of the naturopathic medical schools, and (4) increased public awareness of the tremendous therapeutic value of herbs. Herbal medicine will undoubtedly play a major role in the medicine of the twenty-first century.

References

1. Griggs B: *Green Pharmacy: A History of Herbal Medicine.* Robert Hale, London, 1981.
2. Flexner A: *Medical Education in the United States and Canada: A report for the Carnegie Foundation for the Advancement of Teaching.* Carnegie Foundation, New York, 1910.

Herbal preparations

Commercial herbal preparations are available in several different forms: bulk herbs, teas, tinctures, fluid extracts, and tablets or capsules. It is important for anyone who routinely uses or recommends herbs to understand the differences between these forms, as well as the methods of expressing strengths of herbal products.

One of the major developments in the herb industry involves improvements in extraction and concentration processes.[1] An *extract* is a concentrated form of the herb, obtained by mixing the crude herb with an appropriate solvent (such as alcohol and/or water).

Understanding herbal extracts

When an herbal tea bag steeps in hot water, it is actually a type of herbal extract known as an *infusion*. The water serves as a solvent in removing some of the medicinal properties from the herb. Teas often are better sources of bioavailable compounds than the powdered herb, but are relatively weak in action compared to tinctures, fluid extracts, and solid extracts. Herbal practitioners often use these forms for medicinal effects.

Tinctures are typically made by using an alcohol and water mixture as the solvent. The herb is soaked in the solvent for a specified amount of time, depending on the herb. This soaking lasts usually from several hours to days; however, some herbs may be soaked for much longer periods of time. The solution is then pressed out, yielding the tincture.

Fluid extracts are more concentrated than tinctures. Although they are most often made from hydroalcoholic mixtures, other solvents may be used (vinegar, glycerin, propylene glycol, etc.). Commercial fluid extracts are usually made by distilling off some of the alcohol, typically by using methods that do not require elevated temperatures, such as vacuum distillation and countercurrent filtration.

A solid extract is produced by further concentration of the extract, using the mechanisms described above for fluid extracts as well as other techniques such as thin-layer evaporation. The solvent is completely removed, leaving a viscous extract (soft solid extract) or a dry solid extract, depending on the plant, plant portion, or solvent used and on whether a drying process was used. The dry solid extract, if not already in powdered form, can be ground into course granules or a fine powder. A solid extract can also be diluted with alcohol and water to form a fluid extract or tincture.

Strengths of extracts

The potencies or strengths of herbal extracts are generally expressed in two ways. If they contain known active principles, their strengths are commonly expressed in terms of the content of these active principles. Otherwise, the strength is expressed in terms of their concentration. For example, tinctures are typically made at a 1:5 concentration. This means one part herb (in grams) is soaked in five parts liquid (in milliliters of volume). This means that there is five times the amount of solvent (alcohol or water) in a tincture as there is herbal material.

A 4:1 concentration means that one part of the extract is equivalent to, or derived from, four parts crude herb. This is the typical concentration of a solid extract. One gram of a 4:1 extract is concentrated from 4 grams of crude herb.

Because a tincture is typically a 1:10 or 1:5 concentration whereas a fluid extract is usually 1:1, a solid extract is typically at least four times as potent when compared to an equal amount of fluid extract and forty times as potent as a tincture if they are produced from the same quality of herb.

Typically, 1 gram of a 4:1 solid extract is equivalent to 4 milliliters of a fluid extract (one-seventh of an ounce) and 40 milliliters of a tincture (almost 1½ ounces). Some solid extracts are concentrated as much as 100:1, meaning it would take nearly 100 grams of crude herb, or 100 milliliters of a fluid extract (approximately 3.5 ounces), or 1,000 milliliters of a tincture (almost 1 quart) to provide an equal amount of herbal material in 1 gram of a 100:1 extract.

Determining quality

In the past, the quality of the extract produced was often difficult to determine, as many of the active principles of the herbs were unknown. However, recent advances in extraction processes, coupled with improved analytical methods, have reduced this problem of quality control.[1-3] Expressing the strength of an extract by the concentration method does not accurately measure potency because there may be great variation among manufacturing techniques and raw materials. By using a high-quality herb (an herb high in active compounds), it is possible to create a more potent dried herb, tincture, or fluid extract compared to the solid extract that was made from a lower quality herb. Standardization is the solution to this problem.[3]

Standardized extracts: the best solution

The term *standardized extract* (or *guaranteed potency extract*) refers to an extract guaranteed to contain a "standardized" level of active compounds. Stating the content of active compounds rather than the concentration ratio allows for more accurate dosages to be made.

The best way to express the quality of an herb is in terms of its active components. Regardless of the form the herb is in, it should be analyzed to ensure that it contains these components at an acceptable standardized level. More accurate dosages can then be given. This form of standardization is generally accepted in Europe and is beginning to be used in the United States as well.

This form of standardization (i.e., stating the content of active constituents versus drug concentration ratio) allows the dosage to be based on active constituents.[3] In Europe *Vaccinium myrtillus*, *Silybum marianum*, and *Centella asiatica* extract dosage levels are based on their active constituent levels rather than drug ratio or total extract weight, for example, 40 milligrams of anthocyanosides for *Vaccinium myrtillus*, 70 milligrams of silymarin for *Silybum marianum*, and 30 milligrams of triterpenic acids for *Centella asiatica*. This type of dosage recommendation provides the greatest degree of consistency and assurance of quality.

Although referred to in terms of active constituents, it must be kept in mind that these are still crude extracts and not isolated constituents. For example, an *Uva ursi* extract standardized for its arbutin content, say

10 percent, still contains all of those synergistic factors that enhance the function of the active ingredient (arbutin).

Techniques used in the production of herbal products

The range of sophistication in the processing of herbs is tremendous—from crude herb to highly concentrated standardized extracts. Nonetheless, there are some common stages. This section describes some of the processes in the production of herbal products and the machines that perform these functions.[4]

Collection/harvesting

When plants are collected from their natural habitat they are said to be "wild-crafted." When they are grown, utilizing commercial farming techniques, they are said to be "cultivated." Collection of plants from cultivated sources ensures that the plant collected is the one that is desired. When an herb is wild-crafted, there is a much greater chance that the wrong herb will be picked, a situation that could lead to serious consequences. The use of analytical methods (discussed following) can be employed to guarantee that the plant collected is the one desired.

Herbs from all over the world are marketed in the United States. The herb collectors vary from uneducated natives and self-proclaimed "herbalists" to skilled botanists. The mode of harvesting varies as well, from hand labor to the use of sophisticated equipment. But the mode of harvesting is not as important as the time: a plant should be harvested when the part of the plant being used contains the highest possible level of active compounds. Again, this is ensured by the use of analytical techniques.

Drying

After harvesting, most herbs have a moisture content of 60 to 80 percent and cannot be stored without drying. Otherwise, important compounds would break down or microorganisms would contaminate the material.

The majority of herbs require relatively mild conditions for drying. Commercially, most plants are dried within a temperature range of 100 to 140 degrees Fahrenheit. During drying the plant material must not be damaged or suffer losses that would prevent it from conforming to accepted standards. With proper drying, the herb's moisture content will be reduced to less than 14 percent.

Garbling

Garbling refers to the separation of the portion of the plant to be used from other parts of the plant, dirt, and other extraneous matter. This step is often done during collection. Although there are machines that perform garbling, garbling is usually performed by hand.

Grinding

Grinding or *mincing* an herb involves mechanically breaking down either leaves, roots, seeds, or other parts of a plant into very small units ranging from larger, coarse fragments to fine powder. Grinding is employed in the production of crude herbal products as well as in the initial phases of extracts.

Often the material must be prechopped or minced before feeding it into a grinder. A number of machines can be used to grind herbs, but the most widely used is the hammer mill. These machines are simple in design. The hammers, arranged radially, follow the rotation of the shaft to which they are attached, breaking up the material that is fed into the machine from above. A grid on the walls of the chamber determines the size of the material that is passed through it. Other types of grinders include knife mills and teeth mills.

Extraction

The process of extraction is used in making tinctures, fluid extracts, and solid extracts. In this context, extraction refers to the separation by physical or chemical means, of the desired material from a plant with the aid of a solvent. The U.S. health food industry often uses alcohol and water mixtures as solvents to extract soluble compounds from herbs. Occasionally liposterolic extractions, involving the use of lipophilic solvents or hypercritical carbon dioxide, are performed.

Most extracts produced by small manufacturers involve the use of maceration procedures. The simplest process consists of soaking the herb in the alcohol/water solution for a period of time, followed by filtering. Typically, this process will yield a lower quality extract at a higher price because the solvent, usually alcohol, cannot be reused. It is, in essence, sold to the customer. Since tinctures are 1:5 concentrates, this means 80 percent of the bottle's content is alcohol and water and only 20 percent herbal material. Tinctures are not as cost effective or as stable as solid extracts.

Larger manufacturers utilize more elaborate techniques to ensure that an herb is fully extracted and that the solvent is reused. For example, countercurrent extraction is often used. In this process, the herb enters into a column of a large percolator composed of several columns. The material to be extracted is pumped at a given temperature and rate of speed through the different columns, where it mixes continuously with solvent. The extract-rich solvent then passes into another column, while fresh solvent once again comes into contact with herbal material as it is passed into a new chamber. In this process, complete extraction of health-promoting compounds can be achieved. The extract-rich solvent is then concentrated by the techniques described below.

Concentration

After extraction of the herb, the resulting solutions can be concentrated into fluid extracts or solid extracts. In large manufacturing operations, the techniques and machines (such as thin-layer evaporators) used ensure that the extracted plant components are not damaged. These machines work by evaporating the solvent, thus isolating the plant compounds. The solvent vapors pass into a condenser, in which they recondense to liquid form and can be used again. The result is separation of the extracted materials from the solvent, so that the final product is a pure extract and the solvent can be used again and again.

Drying of extracts

Although you can still find a number of liquid-form extracts on the market (tinctures, fluid extracts, and soft extracts), a solid form is preferable. The main reason is the greater chemical stability and reduced cost of the solid form (the alcohol in liquid-form extracts is often more expensive than the herb). In addition, tinctures, and fluid and soft extracts, are easily contaminated by bacteria and other microorganisms. Liquid forms of extracts also promote chemical reactions that break down the herbal compounds.

A number of drying techniques are employed, including freeze-drying and spray-drying (atomization). The result is a dried, powdered extract that can then be put into capsules or tablets.

Excipients

An *excipient* is an inert substance added to a prescription to give it a certain form or consistency. The same excipients used in the manufacture of drug preparations as well as vitamin and mineral supplements are often used in the production of tablets and capsules containing herbs or herbal extracts.

Many manufacturers will provide a list of excipients contained in their products.

Analytical methods

Improvements in analytical methods have led to definite improvements in harvesting schedules, cultivation techniques, storage, activity, stability of active compounds, and product purity. All of these gains have resulted in tremendous improvements in the quality of herbal preparations now available.

For example, optimal activity and quality collection should be done at a time when the active ingredient is present in the greatest amount. Improvements in analysis have led to more precise harvesting of many herbs.

Methods currently utilized in evaluating herbs and their extracts include the following:

- Organoleptic
- Microscopic
- Physical
- Chemical/physical
- Biological

Organoleptic means the "impression of the organs." Organoleptic analysis involves the application of sight, odor, taste, touch, and occasionally even sound, to identify the plant. The initial sight of a plant or extract may be so specific that it is sufficient for identification. If this is not enough, perhaps the plant or extract has a characteristic odor or taste. Organoleptic analysis represents the simplest, yet the most human, form of analysis.

Microscopic evaluation is indispensable in the initial identification of herbs, as well as in identifying small fragments of crude or powdered herbs, adulterants (e.g., insects, animal feces, mold, and fungi), and characteristic tissue features of the plant. Every plant possesses a characteristic tissue structure, which can be demonstrated through the study of tissue arrangement, cell walls, and configuration when samples are properly stained and mounted.

In crude plant evaluation, physical methods are often used to determine the solubility, specific gravity, melting point, water content, degree of fiber elasticity, and other physical characteristics.

Various chemical/physical methods are also used to determine the percentage of active principles, alkaloids, flavonoids, enzymes, vitamins, essential oils, fats, carbohydrates, protein, ash, acid-insoluble ash, or crude fiber present.

The final analytical process requires more precise assays to determine quality. Sophisticated techniques, such as high-pressure liquid chromatography and nuclear magnetic resonance, are often used to separate molecules. The readings from these machines provide a chemical "fingerprint" as to the nature of chemicals contained in the plant or extract. These techniques are invaluable in the effort to identify herbs, as well as to standardize extracts.

The plant or extract can then be evaluated by various biological methods, mostly animal tests, to determine pharmacological activity, potency, and toxicity.

Quality control in herbal products

Quality control refers to processes involved in maintaining the quality or validity of a product. Regardless of the form of herbal preparation, some degree of quality control should exist. Currently, no organization or government body certifies the labeling of herbal preparations.

Without quality control, you can't be sure that the herb contained in the bottle is the same as what is stated on the label. The widespread disregard for quality control in the health food industry has tarnished the reputation of many important medicinal herbs. For example, it has been estimated that because of supplier errors in collection, more than 50 percent of the *Echinacea* sold in the United States since 1908 and through 1991 was actually *Parthenium integrifolium*.[5] This highlights the importance of using the Latin name, since both of the above-mentioned herbs are referred to as "Missouri snakeroot," as well as the need for proper plant identification based on organoleptic, microscopic, and chemical analysis.

Recent chemical analysis of commercially available feverfew (*Tanacetum parthenium*) and taheebo (*Tabebuia avellanedae*) for active components (parthenolide and lapachol, respectively) has also shown need for concern. Analysis of over thirty-five different commercial preparations of feverfew indicated a wide variation in the amounts of parthenolide in commercial preparations.[6] The majority of products contained no parthenolide or only traces. Analysis of twelve commercial sources of taheebo could identify lapachol (in trace amounts) in only one product.[7]

Perhaps the best example of problems that can result from a lack of quality control is provided by *Panax ginseng*, as outlined below.

Panax ginseng and quality control

Panax ginseng contains at least thirteen different steroid-like compounds, collectively known as ginsenosides. These compounds are believed to be the most important active constituents of *Panax ginseng*. The usual concentration of ginsenosides in mature ginseng roots is between 1 and 3 percent. Ginsenoside R_{g1} is present in significant concentrations in *Panax ginseng*. In contrast, American ginseng (*Panax quinquefolius*) contains primarily ginsenoside R_{b1} and very little, if any, R_{g1}. This difference is extremely important because R_{b1} and R_{g1} have different effects. In general, R_{b1} possesses a sedative effect whereas R_{g1} possesses a stimulatory effect. Since American ginseng is much higher in R_{b1} than R_{g1}, its action is much different than that of *Panax ginseng*.

Independent research and published studies have clearly documented a tremendous variation in the ginsenoside content of commercial preparations.[8,9] In fact, the majority of products on the market contain only trace amounts of ginsenosides, and many formulations contain no ginseng at all. The lack of quality control has led to several problems, ranging from toxic reactions (discussed below) to absence of medicinal effect. The widespread disregard for quality control in the herbal industry has done much to tarnish the reputation of ginseng, as well as other important herbal medicines.

The problem of quality control is exemplified by a 1979 article, entitled "Ginseng Abuse Syndrome," that appeared in the *Journal of the American Medical Association (JAMA)*.[10] In this article a number of side effects are reported, including hypertension, euphoria, nervousness, insomnia, skin eruptions, and morning diarrhea.

Given the extreme variation in quality of ginseng in the American marketplace and the use both of nonofficial parts of the plant and of adulterants, it is not surprising that side effects were noted. None of the commercial preparations used in the trial had been subjected to controlled analysis. Furthermore, the species of ginseng used included *Panax ginseng, Panax quinquefolius, Eleutherococcus senticosus*, and *Rumex hymenosepalus* in a variety of different forms, that is, roots, capsules, tablets, teas, extracts, cigarettes, chewing gum, and candies.

It is virtually impossible to derive any firm conclusions from the data presented in the *JAMA* article, especially in light of the fact that studies performed on standardized extracts of *Panax ginseng* have demonstrated the absence of side effects, as well as no mutagenic or teratogenic effects.[11,12] These findings further support the superiority of herbal products that were produced using quality control measures.

The "Hairy Baby" Story

To illustrate further the problems that can occur in the absence of proper plant identification and standardization, let's examine the case of the "hairy baby." In another *JAMA* article, it was reported that a 30-year-old woman took "Siberian ginseng" (mistakenly identified in the article as *Panax ginseng*) at a dosage of two 650-milligram tablets twice daily for 9 months of pregnancy and 2 weeks of breast feeding.[13] She had experienced repeated premature uterine contractions during the late stage of pregnancy and had noted increased, thicker hair growth on her head, face, and pubic area. The woman gave birth to a full-term baby boy who was noted to have thick black pubic hair over his entire forehead, along with other signs suggestive of androgenization. The authors of the report went on to warn physicians of the dangers of ginseng.

At first glance, this case report appears to be quite alarming. However, when examined more closely a different picture presents itself. First of all, animal and human studies with *Eleutherococcus senticosus* have shown it to be extremely safe. In fact, in the animal studies *Eleutherococcus* extract actually prevented the teratogenic effects of xenobiotics and in a human study of 1,770 pregnant women it was shown that *Eleutherococcus* improved pregnancy outcome. There were no signs of androgenic effects in either the animal or human studies.[14]

The *JAMA* article caught the attention of Dr. Dennis Awang (at the time Dr. Awang was head of the Natural Products Bureau of Drug Research, Health Protection Branch Health and Welfare Canada). On examining the product the woman had taken, Dr. Awang discovered that the product did not contain Siberian ginseng, but instead consisted of *Periploca sepium*.[15]

Does this mean the woman's reaction was due to *Periploca sepium*? Not necessarily. Studies in animals have determined that *Periploca sepium*, like Siberian ginseng, does not produce an androgenic response.[16] The most likely explanation for the "hairy baby" was that it had nothing to with the herbal product being used.

Addressing the quality control problem

The solution to the quality control problem that exists in the United States is for manufacturers and suppliers of herbal products to adhere to quality control standards and good manufacturing practices. With improvements in the identification of plants by laboratory analysis, consumers should at least be guaranteed that the right plant is being used. Consumers, health food stores, pharmacists, and physicians who use or sell herbal products should ask for information from the suppliers of herbal products on their quality control process. What do they do to guarantee the validity of their product? As more consumers, retailers, and professionals begin asking for quality control from the suppliers, it is possible that more quality control processes will be utilized by manufacturers.

Currently, only a few manufacturers adhere to complete quality control and good manufacturing procedures, including microscopic, physical, chemical/physical, and biological analyses. Companies supplying standardized extracts currently offer the greatest degree of quality control, and hence these products typically offer the highest quality.

Most standardized extracts are currently made in Europe under strict guidelines set forth by individual members of the European Economic Council (EEC) as well as those proposed by the EEC.[1,2,3] Included are guidelines for acceptable levels of impurities such as parasites (bacterial counts), pesticides, residual solvents and heavy metals, and product stability.

The production of standardized extracts serves as a model for quality control processes for all forms of herbal preparations. In general, it is believed that if the active components of a particular herb are known, the herbal product should be analyzed to ensure that it contains these components at an acceptable/standardized level. More accurate dosages can then be prescribed. Products should also be subjected to bacteriological counts.

Currently, in many countries, numerous standardized extracts fulfill the requirements for marketing as drugs. These extracts have typically gone through the quality control steps outlined in Table 1.

Table 1 Quality control steps necessary for the registration of plant-based drug formulation

---

1. Selection of suitable plant material
2. Botanical investigation, using organoleptic and microscopic techniques
3. Chemical analysis, using appropriate laboratory equipment
4. Screening for biological activity
5. Analysis of active fractions of crude extracts
6. Isolation of active principles
7. Determination of chemical structure of active principles
8. Comparison with compounds of similar structure
9. Analytical method developed for formulation
10. Detailed pharmacological evaluation
11. Studies performed to determine activity and toxicity of formulation
12. Studies on absorption, distribution, and elimination of herbal compounds
13. Clinical trials performed to determine activity in humans
14. Registration by National Drug Authorities

Summary

The improvements in extraction and concentration processes represent a major development in herbal medicine. These improvements have led to some very effective herbal products. Your best assurance of quality and results when using herbal products is to use products from those suppliers who employ quality control standards and good manufacturing practices. Standardized extracts that state the level of active compounds provide the greatest benefit, owing primarily to more accurate dosages.

References

1. Bonati A: Formulation of plant extracts into dosage forms. In: *The Medicinal Plant Industry* (Wijeskera ROB, ed.). CRC Press, Boca Raton, FL, 1991, pp. 107–114.
2. Karlsen J: Quality control and instrumental analysis of plant extracts. In: *The Medicinal Plant Industry* (Wijeskera ROB, ed.). CRC Press, Boca Raton, FL, 1991, pp. 99–106.
3. Bonati A: How and why should we standardize phytopharmical drugs for clinical validation? *J Ethnopharmacol* **32**, 195–197, 1991.
4. Bombardelli E: Technologies for the processing of medicinal plants. In: *The Medicinal Plant Industry* (Wijeskera ROB, ed.). CRC Press, Boca Raton, FL, 1991, pp. 85–98.
5. Awang DVC and Kindack DG: Echinacea. *Can Pharmacol J* **124**, 512–516, 1991.
6. Heptinstall S, *et al.*: Parthenolide content and bioactivity of feverfew (*Tanacetum parthenium* (L.) Schultz-Bip.). Estimation of commercial and authenticated feverfew products. *J Pharmaceut Pharmacol* **44**, 391–395, 1992.
7. Awang DVC: Commercial taheebo lacks active ingredient. *Can Pharmacol J* **121**, 323–326, 1988.
8. Liberti LE and Marderosian AD: Evaluation of commercial ginseng products. *J Pharmacol Sci* **67**, 1487–1489, 1978.
9. Soldati F and Sticher O: HPLC separation and quantitative determination of ginsenosides from *Panax ginseng, Panax quinquefolium* and from ginseng drug preparations. *Planta Med* **39**(4), 348–357, 1980.
10. Siegel RK: Ginseng abuse syndrome. *JAMA* **241**, 1614–1615, 1979.
11. Hikino H: Traditional remedies and modern assessment: The case of ginseng. In: *The Medicinal Plant Industry* (Wijeskera ROB, ed.). CRC Press, Boca Raton, FL, 1991, pp. 149–166.
12. Shibata S, *et al.*: Chemistry and pharmacology of *Panax. Econ Med Plant Res* **1**, 217–284, 1985.
13. Koren GS, *et al.*: Maternal ginseng use associated with neonatal androgenization. *JAMA* **264**, 2866, 1990.
14. Farnsworth NR, *et al.*: Siberian ginseng (*Eleutherococcus senticosus*): Current status as an adaptogen. *Econ Med Plant Res* **1**, 156–215, 1985.
15. Awang DVC: Maternal use of ginseng and neonatal androgenization. *JAMA* **265**, 1828, 1991.
16. Waller DP, *et al.*: Lack of androgenicity of Siberian ginseng. *JAMA* **267**, 2329, 1992.

SECTION II

Materia medica

$\mathbf{A}$ *materia medica* refers to a book providing information on the medical prescription of herbs. This section provides detailed information on the history and folk use, pharmacological action, and clinical applications of the herbs most commonly used in the United States. Before using any herb it is important that you follow these important guidelines:

- **Do not self-diagnose**   Proper medical care is critical to good health. If you have symptoms suggestive of an illness discussed in this series, please consult a physician, preferably a naturopath, holistic M.D. or D.O., chiropractor, or other natural health care specialist.
- **Work with your doctor**   If you are currently on a prescription medication, you absolutely must work with your doctor before discontinuing any drug.
- **Use this book**   If you wish to try an herb, discuss it with your physician. Since your physician is most likely unaware of the herb you want to use, you may need to educate him/her. Bring this book along with you to the doctor's office. Most of the herbal preparations recommended here are

based on studies published in medical journals. Key references are provided if your physician wants additional information.

- **Remember** Although many herbs are effective on their own they work even better if they are part of a comprehensive natural treatment plan focusing on diet and lifestyle factors.

The safety of herbs

Most herbs in use are extremely safe. In the 1970s, when herbs began their rise in popularity, numerous articles appearing in medical journals and the lay press questioned the safety of herbal products. Since then, herb usage has increased dramatically, but toxicity reports have not. In a June 1992 article appearing in the *Food and Drug Law Journal*,[1] the results of an extensive review on herbal safety (conducted by the Herbal Research Foundation, a nonprofit organization whose members include experts on pharmacognosy, pharmacology, and toxicology) confirmed the lack of substantial evidence that toxic reactions to herbal products are a major source of concern. The review was based on reports from the American Association of Poison Control Centers and the Centers for Disease Control (Atlanta, GA).

Although numerous herbs growing in the wild can cause significant toxicity, the herbs commonly used in the United States for health purposes are usually safe. Nonetheless, it is important that you be aware of any possible adverse reaction with herbal product use. It is, therefore, essential that you understand the more popular herbal products as detailed in this book.

Reference

1. McCaleb RS: Food ingredient safety evaluation. *Food Drug Law Journal* **47**, 657–665, 1992.

1
Aloe vera

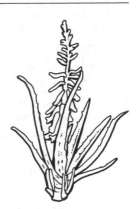

Key uses of *Aloe vera*:

Topical:

- Wound healing
- Sunburn
- Minor skin irritations

Oral:

- Constipation
- Peptic ulcers
- Immune system enhancement
- Diabetes
- Asthma

General description

Of the more than 300 species of aloe, the most popular medicinal variety is currently *Aloe vera*. The nomenclature of *Aloe vera* has been somewhat confused, as the plant has been known by a variety of names, most notably *Aloe barbadensis* and *Aloe vulgari*. Historical records indicate that the medicinal use of aloe may have started in Egypt or the Middle East. Since then aloe has been introduced and naturalized throughout most of the tropics and warmer regions of the world, including the Caribbean, the southern United States, Mexico, Latin America, the Middle East, India, and other parts of Asia.[1]

Aloe vera is a perennial plant with yellow flowers and tough, fleshy, triangular or spearlike leaves arising in a rosette configuration. The leaves are up to 20 inches long and 5 inches across at the base, tapering to a point. There may be as many as 30 leaves per plant. The margins of the leaf are characterized by sawlike teeth. Inside, the meaty leaf is filled with gel that arises from a clear, central, mucilaginous pulp. A mature aloe measures 1½ to 4 feet high, with a base 3 feet or more in diameter.

The leaf is composed of three distinct layers: an outer layer of tough tissue; a corrugated lining just beneath the outer layer; and the major portion of the leaf, the inner layer consisting of parenchymal cells containing large vacuoles of a semisolid, gelatinous transparent gel. The bitter latex of the corrugated layer protects the plants from predators. Should an animal bite the leaf, the sap causes irritation. The dried latex (juice) derived from the corrugated layer is the source of the laxative properties of aloe. The parenchymal tissue, or gel, is the portion of the aloe used in other applications.[2]

Aloe vera terminology

- *Aloe vera* **gel**   Naturally occurring, undiluted gel obtained by stripping away the outer layer of the *Aloe vera* leaf
- *Aloe vera* **concentrate**   *Aloe vera* gel from which the water has been removed
- *Aloe vera* **juice**   An ingestible product containing a minimum of 50 percent *Aloe vera* gel
- *Aloe vera* **latex**   The bitter yellow liquid derived from the pericyclic tubules of the rind of *Aloe vera*, the primary constituent of which is aloin

Chemical composition

Aloe vera contains numerous compounds possessing biological activity. The most important appear to be anthraquinones, polysaccharides (including glycoproteins and mucopolysaccharides), and prostaglandins.

Anthraquinones

In 1851,[1] it was discovered that the cathartic action of aloe was due to aloin, a lemon-yellow powder formed from drying of the bitter latex (Figure 1.1). From this material several compounds known as *anthraquinones* have been isolated, the major anthraquinone being barbaloin. Barbaloin and aloin are often referred to synonymously. Although aloe contains other anthraquinone derivatives including aloe-emodin, barbaloin is considered the most potent cathartic. As a whole, the anthraquinone compounds are water-soluble glycosides easily separated from the water-insoluble resinous material.[1–4]

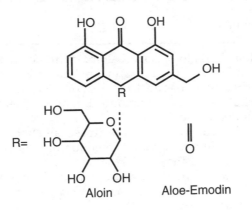

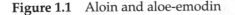

Figure 1.1   Aloin and aloe-emodin

Saccharides

Recent research on *Aloe vera* has focused on the glycoprotein, mucopolysaccharide, and polysaccharide constituents. Aloe contains the polysaccharides galactose, xylose, arabinose, and acetylated mannose. This latter polysaccharide, which is similar to guar and locust bean gums, has received considerable clinical research attention as an antiviral and immunopotentiating agent, especially in the treatment of AIDS (acquired immunodeficiency syndrome). Acemannan, another water-soluble polysaccharide constituent, is discussed below.

Prostaglandins and fatty acids

Recently, several prostaglandin and fatty acid compounds have been discovered in *Aloe vera* extracts.[5] The conversion of essential fatty acids to prostaglandins in a plant such as *Aloe vera* is quite rare. The major unsaturated fatty acid in the plant is gamma-linolenic acid ($C_{18:3}$), which can be converted to prostaglandins of the 1 series. The 1-series prostaglandins are known to exert more favorable effects on inflammation, allergy, platelet aggregation, and wound healing. The presence of gamma-linolenic acid and/or prostaglandins in a stable medium, along with inhibitors of thromboxane synthesis, may be another of the important chemical characteristics of aloe responsible for its wound healing effects.

Other constituents

Other biologically active compounds found in *Aloe vera* include a serine carboxypeptidase, salicylates, minerals, vitamins, sterols, and amino acids.

Table 1.1 Chemical composition of *Aloe vera*[a]

Anthraquinones	Aloin, barbaloin, isobarbaloin, anthranol, aloetic acid, anthracene, ester of cinnamic acid, aloe-emodin, emodin, chrysophanoic acid, ethereal oil, resistannol
Saccharides	Cellulose, glucose, mannose, L-rhamnose, aldopentose
Fatty acids	Gamma-linolenic acid
Enzymes	Oxidase, amylase, catalase, lipase, alkaline phosphatase
Amino acids	Lysine, threonine, valine, methionine, leucine, isoleucine, phenylalanine
Vitamins	Vitamins B_1, B_2, B_6, C, and E, folic acid, choline, beta-carotene
Minerals	Calcium, sodium, manganese, magnesium, zinc, copper, chromium
Miscellaneous	Cholesterol, triglycerides, steroids, uric acid, lignins, beta-sitosterol, gibberellin, salicylic acid

[a]Data from Ref. 4.

Table 1.1 provides a partial listing of the remarkably diverse range of compounds isolated from *Aloe vera*.[2–4]

History and folk use

Aloe vera has a storied history of use. Mesopotamian clay tablets dated 1750 B.C. indicate *Aloe vera* was being used for medicinal purposes. Egyptian records from 550 B.C. also mention aloe for infections of the skin. The ancient Greeks were also aware of aloe's medicinal effects, as both Pliny (23–79 A.D.) and Dioscorides (first century A.D.) wrote of aloe's ability to treat wounds and heal infections of the skin. *Aloe vera* is still widely used in many traditional systems of medicine. In India, for example, in addition to external applications, aloe (whole leaves, the exudate, and the fresh gel) is used as a cathartic, stomachic, and anthelmintic. Many cultures of the world have adopted *Aloe vera* into their materia medicas.[1]

In the United States, the history of aloe can be traced as far back as the United States Pharmacopoeia of 1820, in which a number of aloe preparations were described. Most of these preparations were designed to take advantage of aloe's laxative effects. By the early 1900s more than twenty-seven different aloe preparations were in popular use. In 1920, the cultivation of aloe for pharmaceutical use began.[3]

A major development in the modern use of aloe occurred in 1935 when a group of physicians successfully used the fresh juice to treat a patient suffering from facial burns due to X-rays.[6] The relief offered by aloe in the topical treatment of burns, minor irritations, skin ulcers, and other skin disorders is a major reason why companies supplying dermatological and cosmetic products have incorporated aloe in many of their formulations.

Although more and more of aloe's medicinal effects are being confirmed, aloe is still predominantly administered without direct medical supervision. Therefore, the history and folk use of aloe continues to evolve.

Pharmacology

Aloe vera has demonstrated a wide range of pharmacological activity. Some of these activities are discussed in this section; others are discussed in Clinical Applications (below).

Antibacterial and antifungal activity

Aloe has demonstrated activity against many common bacteria and fungi in several studies.[7-10] The antimicrobial effects of *Aloe vera* compare quite favorably to those of silver sulfadiazine, a potent antiseptic used in the treatment of extensive burns.[7] A 60 percent *Aloe vera* extract was found to be bactericidal against *Pseudomonas aeruginosa, Klebsiella pneumoniae, Serratia marcescens, Citrobacter* species, *Enterobacter cloacae, Streptococcus pyogenes,* and *Streptococcus agalactiae.* Seventy-percent concentrations of aloe were bactericidal for *Staphylococcus aureus,* 80 percent for *Escherichia coli,* and 90 percent for *Streptococcus faecalis* and *Candida albicans.* Organisms inhibited in other studies include *Mycobacterium tuberculosis, Trichophyton* species, and *Bacillus subtilis.*[2-4]

As evident in Table 1.2, the antimicrobial activity against common skin pathogens of *Aloe vera* gel in a cream base was shown to be slightly better than silver sulfadiazine.[7]

Antiviral effects

Acemannan (acetylated mannose) in injectable form has been approved for veterinary use in fibrosarcomas and feline leukemia. Its action in feline leukemia is quite impressive. Feline leukemia, like AIDS, is caused by a retrovirus (feline leukemia virus, or FeLV). The virus is so lethal that once cats develop clinical symptoms they are usually euthanized. Typically more than 70 percent of cats die within 8 weeks of the onset of clinical signs. In a study of 44 cats with clinically confirmed feline leukemia, acemannan was injected (2 milligrams per kilogram) weekly for 6 weeks and reexamined 6 weeks

Table 1.2 Antimicrobial effects of *Aloe vera* extract in cream base compared to silver sulfadiazine (AgSD) in agar well (6-millimeter) diffusion

	Inhibition zone (mm)[a]	
Organism	Aloe vera	AgSD
Gram negative		
E. coli	16	12
Ent. cloacae	14	12
K. pneumoniae	14	6
P. aeruginosa	17	12
Gram positive		
S. aureus	18	12
Strep. pyogenes	16	12
Strep. agalactiae	16	12
Strep. faecalis	6	11
B. subtilis	19	14

[a]Inhibition zones measured in millimeters.

after termination of treatment.[11] At the end of the 12-week study, 71 percent of the cats were alive and in good health.

Acemannan has demonstrated significant antiviral activity against several viruses, including human immunodeficiency virus type 1 (HIV-1), influenza virus, and measles virus.[12–14] Although acemannan has demonstrated some direct antiviral activity against HIV-1 by inhibiting glycosylation of viral glycoproteins, its main promise in treating AIDS and HIV may be to enhance the action of azidothymidine (AZT), the antiviral drug used to combat AIDS. *In vitro* studies have shown that acemannan, combined with suboptimal noncytotoxic concentrations of AZT or acyclovir, acts synergistically to inhibit the replication of HIV and herpes simplex type 1 (HSV-1).[14] On the basis of these studies, as well as preliminary human studies, researchers believe that the use of acemannan may reduce the amount of AZT required by as much as 90 percent.[15] This is quite significant. In addition to AZT being extremely expensive, AZT's use is often associated with severe side effects, including anemia and depression of white blood cell production.

Preliminary clinical studies suggest acemannan and *Aloe vera* may be beneficial when administered orally in HIV-positive individuals.[16,17]

Immune enhancement

Acemannan is a potent immune system stimulant.[11,18–20] Prominent among the effects noted are the enhancement of macrophage activity as well as the release of immune system potentiators. Acemannan also enhances the function of T cells and interferon production, although these actions may also be due to enhanced macrophage function. Clinical animal research has shown promising results in sarcomas and spontaneous tumors.[20,21]

Antiallergy and antiinflammatory aspects

Aloe vera exerts a number of antiinflammatory actions (including blocking of the generation of inflammatory mediators such as thromboxanes and bradykinin), thereby reducing swelling.[2–4,7,22–25] Several compounds in aloe are responsible for these actions. The most important are glycoproteins, which inhibit and actually break down bradykinin, a major mediator of pain and inflammation; various anthraquinones; and salicylates. These antiinflammatory substances may be of significance in both topical (discussed in the next section) and oral applications.

Wound healing

Aloe vera contains a number of compounds necessary for wound healing, including vitamin C, vitamin E, and zinc. Unlike many other antiinflammatory substances, *Aloe vera* has been shown to stimulate fibroblast and connective tissue formation, thereby promoting wound repair. In addition, aloe appears to stimulate the epidermal growth and repair process, presumably due to its polysaccharides.[1–4,26–28]

Diabetes

The results of experimental studies in rats and mice suggest that *Aloe vera* may be effective, both topically and internally, in the treatment of diabetic leg ulcers. In addition to exerting positive effects on wound healing,[29] *Aloe vera* also exhibits a blood sugar-lowering effect in both normal and chemical-induced diabetic mice.[30]

Clinical applications

Aloe vera has many uses in clincal medicine. *Aloe vera* products can be ingested or applied to the skin to take advantage of its wound healing and antiinflammatory properties. Oral preparations are also useful in constipation, peptic ulcers, immune system enhancement, diabetes, and asthma.

Constipation

Although physicians have prescribed the whole aloe leaf as a cathartic for more than 2,000 years, it was not until 1851 that the active principle, aloin, was discovered.[1] In small doses, aloin acts as a tonic to the digestive system, giving tone to the intestinal muscle. At higher dosages, it becomes a strong purgative. Its most obvious actions are on the large intestine, where it increases colonic secretions and peristaltic contractions. In combination with strychnine and belladonna, aloin became (in the 1800s) one of the most popular laxatives for chronic constipation for many years. Because aloin often causes painful contraction, other anthraquinone laxatives such as cascara and senna are now much more popular.[31,32]

Peptic ulcer

The use of *Aloe vera* gel internally to treat peptic ulcers was studied in 1963.[33] Twelve patients with X-ray-confirmed duodenal ulcers were given a tablespoon of an emulsion of *Aloe vera* gel in mineral oil once daily. At the end of 1 year, all patients demonstrated complete recovery and no recurrence. On the basis of experimental evidence, the following factors were thought to be responsible for the effectiveness:

1. *Aloe vera* gel inactivates pepsin in a reversible fashion. When the stomach is empty, pepsin is inhibited by *Aloe vera* gel; however, in the presence of food, pepsin is released and allowed to digest the food.
2. The gel inhibits the release of hydrochloric acid by interfering with the binding of histamine to the parietal cells.
3. *Aloe vera* gel is an extremely good demulcent; demulcents heal and prevent aggravating irritants from reaching sensitive ulcers.

Gastrointestinal tonic

Aloe vera juice may exert benficial tonic effects on the gastrointestinal system. In 1985, Jeffrey Bland, Ph.D., reported the effect of orally consumed *Aloe vera* juice on urinary indican, gastrointestinal pH, stool culture, and stool specific gravity in a study of ten (five men and five women) healthy human subjects.[34] Urinary indican indicates the degree to which dietary protein is malabsorbed, or the degree to which intestinal bacteria are engaged in putrefactive processes. After 1 full week of drinking 6 ounces of *Aloe vera* juice three times daily, urinary indican levels decreased one full unit. This result suggests that regular *Aloe vera* juice consumption can lead to improved protein digestion and assimilation and/or reduced bacterial putrefaction.

With gastric analysis, *Aloe vera* juice was shown to increase gastric pH by an average of 1.88 units. This result supports the findings of other researchers, that *Aloe vera* gel can inhibit the secretion of hydrochloric acid. The gastric analysis also demonstrated that *Aloe vera* juice can slow down gastric emptying, possibly leading to improved digestion.

Six of the ten subjects showed marked alterations in stool cultures after the week-long study. This implies that *Aloe vera* juice may exert some anti-bacterial or anti-*Candida* activity. In the four subjects with positive cultures for *Candida albicans*, there was a reduction in the number of yeast colonies.

Stool specific gravity was reduced after the week of *Aloe vera* juice consumption. This result implies improved water retention, yet none of the subjects complained of diarrhea or loose stools while taking the *Aloe vera* juice.

The use of *Aloe vera* juice for health-promoting effects is a popular practice, yet very little scientific evidence supports for this practice. Additional research is required before such widespread use can be justified.

AIDS and other viral infections

Acemannan shows some promise when administered in the early stages of AIDS. In one study, fourteen HIV patients prescribed oral acemannan (800 milligrams per day) demonstrated significant increases in circulating monocytes/macrophages. In particular, the number of large circulating monocytes increased significantly, indicating improvement in phagocytizing, processing, and presenting cells in the blood.[15] In another study of fifteen AIDS patients receiving an oral dose of acemannan (800 milligrams per day), the average Modified Walter Reed (MWR) Clinical (a scoring system commonly used in AIDS research), absolute T-4, absolute T-8, and p24 core antigen level scores all improved in surviving patients (Table 1.3) at the end of 900 days. (Two patients died of AIDS; another committed suicide.[16])

In another study, *Aloe vera* juice (20 ounces per day) was used in conjunction with essential fatty acids and a multiple vitamin, mineral, and amino acid supplement to treat twenty-nine patients.[35] The fifteen AIDS, twelve AIDS-related complex (ARC), and two HIV-seropositive patients continued with regular medication, including AZT. After 180 days, all patients showed clinical improvement, 25 percent of those positive for the p24 core antigen converted to nonreactive, anemia induced by AZT showed improvement in all patients, and the patients gained an average of 7 percent in body weight.

Although acemannan may be helpful in the beginning stages of AIDS, a recent study[36] indicates that it may be of little value in patients with advanced HIV disease, that is, AIDS. In one study, sixty-two male patients with advanced HIV disease (they had CD4 counts of 50 to 300 per cubic millimeter

Table 1.3 Acemannan in the treatment of AIDS[a]

Test	Score	
	Pretreatment	*After 900 days*
Modified Walter Reed (MWR) clinical score	65	2.0
Absolute T-4	322/mm^3	324/mm^3
Absolute T-8	469/mm^3	660/mm^3
p24 core antigen	5 of 15	4 of 12

[a]Data from Ref. 38.

within 1 month of entry, and had received antiretrovirals [e.g., AZT or ddI] for 6 months or more at a stable dose for the month prior to entry) received either acemannan (400 milligrams four times daily) or a placebo.[36] Helper T cell counts were done every 4 weeks for 48 weeks. p24 antigen was measured at entry and every 12 weeks thereafter. Quantitative viral cultures were similarly done in a subset of patients. AZT pharmacokinetics were assessed at baseline, and at 4 and 24 weeks. Helper T cells numbered 165 and 144 per cubic millimeter in the placebo and acemannan groups, respectively; 90 percent were on AZT at entry (30 percent were later switched to dideoxyinosine [ddI]). Ten patients in each group discontinued the study therapy prematurely, none due to serious adverse reactions. Seven patients in the acemannan group and five in the placebo group developed AIDS-defining illnesses. There was no difference between groups in terms of helper T cell count at 48 weeks. Among AZT-treated patients, the median rate of change in helper T cell count in the initial 16 weeks was –121 and –120 cells per year in the acemannan and placebo groups, respectively; the change in helper T cell count from week 16 to 48 was 0 and –65 cells per year in the acemannan and placebo groups, respectively. There was no statistical difference between groups with regard to adverse events, p24 antigen, quantitative virology, or pharmacokinetics. At the dose tested, acemannan was well tolerated and had no pharmacokinetic interaction with AZT. Although the rate of decline in the helper T cell count from 16 to 48 weeks favored the acemannan group, there was no difference between groups in helper T cell count at 48 weeks. In summary, acemannan showed no significant benefit.

From this study, as well as others, it has been suggested that the prognostic criteria on which to determine whether an AIDS patient will benefit from acemannan are an absolute T-4 count greater than 150 per cubic millimeter and a p24 level less than 300.

Asthma

The oral administration of an extract of *Aloe vera* for 6 months produced good results in the treatment of asthma.[26] The exception to this was the fact that the *Aloe vera* extract was not effective at all in patients dependent on corticosteroids. The mechanism of action is thought to be via restoration of protective mechanisms, followed by improvements in the immune system.

The extract used in the study was produced from the supernatant of fresh leaves stored in the dark at 4°C for 7 days. The dosage was 5 milliliters, twice daily for 24 weeks, of a 20 percent solution of the aloe extract in saline. Eleven of twenty-seven patients (40 percent) without corticosteroid dependence reported significant improvement at the study's conclusion.

Studies indicate that subjecting the leaves to conditions of cold and darkness results in an increase in the polysaccharide fraction. One gram of the crude extract obtained from leaves stored under cold/dark conditions produced 400 milligrams of neutral polysaccharide, compared to only 30 milligrams produced from leaves not subjected to cold or dark.

Topical applications

The topical effects of *Aloe vera* appear to be due to a combination of enhancement of wound healing along with antiinflammatory, moisturizing, emollient, and antimicrobial actions.[7,28,29,37–39]

Research into the topical applications of *Aloe vera* gel began in the 1930s with the treatment of radiation burns. During the 1930s, X-rays were used therapeutically for cancer, eczema, and other skin complaints, and as a depilatory agent. A paper by Collins and Collins in 1935[6] reported the success of *Aloe vera* gel in a single case, a woman with a patch of severe X-ray dermatitis on her forehead. The woman had tried various medical treatments for 8 months, only to see her condition worsen. The authors were going to perform a skin graft, but as a temporary measure applied a preparation of fresh, whole *Aloe vera* leaves to reduce the itching. The result was as follows: "Twenty-four hours later she reported that the sensation of itching and burning had entirely subsided," and by 5 weeks "there was complete regeneration of the skin of the forehead and scalp, new hair growth, complete restoration of sensation, and absence of scar" (Collins and Collins).[6] Five months after the start of treatment healing was complete. Subsequent case reports clearly indicated that, although not as positive as this initial study, *Aloe vera* was effective in some cases.

Up until the 1940s most of the studies on aloe consisted of reported case histories.[3] To substantiate these case studies, animal studies began to appear in the literature. Rowe and co-workers[3,37,38] performed several studies in rats with radiation-induced ulcers and determined that fresh aloe pulp was effective whereas dried aloe powder was not effective.

In 1953, Lushbaugh and Hale,[39] working for the U.S. Atomic Energy Commission, produced one of the most convincing studies of the efficacy of *Aloe vera* gel. Twenty albino rats were exposed to beta radiation and different treatments were used on quadrants of the affected area of each animal. The treatments used were fresh *Aloe vera* leaf, a commercial *Aloe vera* ointment, application of a dry gauze bandage, and an untreated control. Both fresh *Aloe vera* and the *Aloe vera* ointment produced clear improvements. At the end of 2 months the *Aloe vera*-treated areas were completely healed; the other two areas had still not healed at the end of 4 months.

Despite growing consumer awareness of *Aloe vera*'s soothing effects on burns and wound healing, few human studies have been carried out. Most of the studies on *Aloe vera* have utilized different animals in various models of inflammation and wound healing. Virtually all of the studies support the topical use of *Aloe vera* gel, especially in minor burns or skin inflammation.

Although limited, the human research on wound healing has been promising. For example, in one study *Aloe vera* gel was used quite successfully in three patients with chronic leg ulcers (5, 7, and 15 years in duration).[40] The gel was applied to the ulcers on gauze bandages. Rapid reduction in ulcer size was noted in all three subjects and complete resolution occurred in two. Encouraging results were also reported for acne and seborrhea.

Dosage

Aloe vera gel can be applied liberally for topical applications. A wide range of products is available; however, simple, pure *Aloe vera* gel is sufficient.

Aloe vera juice can be consumed orally as a beverage or tonic. Detailed information on the optimal dose for these types of products is currently lacking; it is recommended that no more than 1 quart be consumed in any one day.

The dose of acemannan being used in HIV/AIDS patients is 800–1,600 milligrams per day. This would correspond to a dose of approximately ½ to 1 liter per day for most *Aloe vera* juice products. However, it appears that there may be great variation in the amount of acemannan in various products.

Toxicity

Although rare, allergic reactions manifesting as generalized nummular, eczematous, and papular dermatitis as a result of topically applied *Aloe vera* preparations have been reported.

It should be noted that *Aloe vera* gel has been shown to delay wound healing in cases of surgical wounds such as those produced during laparotomy or cesarean delivery.[41] Topical aloe preparations are therefore not useful in the treatment of deep, vertical wounds.

References

1. Haller JS: A drug for all seasons, medical and pharmacological history of aloe. *Bull NY Acad Sci* **66**, 647–657, 1990.
2. Klein AD and Penneys NS: *Aloe vera. J Am Acad Dermatol* **18**, 714–719, 1988.
3. Grindlay D and Reynolds T: The *Aloe vera* leaf phenomena: A review of the properties and modern use of the leaf parenchyma gel. *J Ethnopharmacol* **16**, 117–151, 1986.
4. Shelton RW: *Aloe vera*, its chemical and therapeutic properties. *Int J Dermatol* **30**, 679–683, 1991.
5. Afzal M, *et al.*: Identification of some prostanoids in *Aloe vera* extracts. *Planta Medica* **57**, 38–40, 1991.
6. Collins CE and Collins C: Roentgen dermatitis treated with fresh whole leaf *Aloe vera. Am J Roentgenol* **33**, 396–397, 1935.
7. Robson MC, Heggers JP, and Hagstron WJ: Myth, magic, witchcraft, or fact? *Aloe vera* revisited. *J Burn Care Rehab* **3**, 157–162, 1982.
8. Fly LB and Keim I: Tests of *Aloe vera* for antibiotic activity. *Econ Bot* **17**, 46–48, 1963.
9. Lorenzetti LJ, *et al.*: Bacteriostatic property of *Aloe vera. J Pharmacol Sci* **53**, 1287, 1964.
10. Heggers JP, Pineless GR, and Robson MC: Dermaide *Aloe/Aloe vera* gel: Comparison of the antimicrobial effects. *J Am Med Technol* **41**, 293–294, 1979.
11. Sheets MA, *et al.*: Studies of the effect of acemannan on retrovirus infections: Clinical stabilization of feline leukemia virus-infected cats. *Mol Biother* **3**, 41–45, 1991.
12. Kemp MC, *et al.*: In-vitro evaluation of the antiviral effects of acemannan on the replication and pathogenesis of HIV-1 and other enveloped viruses: Modification of the processing of glycoprotein precursors. *Antiviral Res Suppl* **1**, 83, 1990.
13. Kahlon JB, *et al.*: Inhibition of AIDS virus replication by acemannan in vitro. *Mol Biother* **3**, 127–135, 1991.
14. Kahlon JB, *et al.*: *In vitro* evaluation of the synergistic antiviral effects of acemannan in combination with azidothymidine and acyclovir. *Mol Biother* **3**, 214–223, 1991.
15. Anonymous: *Aloe vera* may boost AZT. *Med Tribune*, August 22, 1991, p. 4.
16. McDaniel HR, *et al.*: An increase in circulating monocyte/macrophages (MM) is induced by oral acemannan (ACE-M) in HIV-1 patients. *Am J Clin Pathol* **94**, 516–517, 1990.
17. McDaniel HR, *et al.*: Extended survival and prognostic criteria for acemannan (ACE-M) treated HIV-1 patients. *Antiviral Res Suppl* **1**, 117, 1990.
18. Hart LA, *et al.*: Effects of low molecular weight constituents from *Aloe vera* gel on oxidative metabolism and cytotoxic and bactericidal activities of human neutrophils. *Int J Immunol Pharmacol* **12**, 427–434, 1990
19. Womble D and Helderman JH: Enhancement of alloresponsiveness of human lymphocytes by acemannan (Carrisyn™). *Int J Immunopharmacol* **10**, 967–974, 1988.
20. Peng SY, *et al.*: Decreased mortality of Norman murine sarcoma in mice treated with the immunomodulator, acemannan. *Mol Biother* **3**, 79–87, 1991.
21. Harris C, *et al.*: Efficacy of acemannan in treatment of canine and feline spontaneous neoplasms. *Mol Biother* **3**, 207–213, 1991.

22. Davis RH, Shapiro E, and Agnew PS: Topical effect of aloe with ribonucleic acid and vitamin C on adjuvant arthritis. *J Am Pod Med Assoc* **75**, 229–237, 1985.
23. Yagi A, *et al.*: Antibradykinin active material in *Aloe saponaria. J Pharmaceut Sci* **71**, 1172–1174, 1982.
24. Davis RH, *et al.*: Isolation of a stimulatory system in an *Aloe* extract. *J Am Pod Med Assoc* **81**, 473–478, 1991.
25. Davis RH, *et al.*: Anti-inflammatory activity of *Aloe vera* against a spectrum of irritants. *J Am Pod Med Assoc* **79**, 263–266, 1989.
26. Shida T, *et al.*: Effect of *Aloe* extract on peripheral phagocytosis in adult bronchial asthma. *Planta Medica* **51**, 273–275, 1985.
27. Henry R: An updated review of *Aloe vera. Cosmet Toilet* **94**, 42–50, 1979.
28. Davis RH, Kabbani JM, and Maro NP: *Aloe vera* and wound healing. *J Am Pod Med Assoc* **77**, 165–169, 1987.
29. Davis RH, Leitner MG, and Russo JM: *Aloe vera*, a natural approach for treating wounds, edema, and pain in diabetes. *J Am Pod Med Assoc* **78**, 60–68, 1988.
30. Ajabnoor MA: Effect of aloes on blood glucose levels in normal and alloxan diabetic mice. *J Ethnopharmacol* **28**, 215–220, 1990.
31. Godding EW: Therapeutics of laxative agents with special reference to anthraquinones. *Pharmacology* **14**(Suppl 1), 78–101, 1976.
32. Anton R and Haag-Berrurier MH: Therapeutic use of natural anthraquinones for other than laxative actions. *Pharmacology* **14**(Suppl 1), 104–112, 1976.
33. Blitz JJ, Smith JW, and Gerard JR: *Aloe vera* gel in peptic ulcer therapy: Preliminary report. *J Am Osteopathol Soc* **62**, 731–735, 1963.
34. Bland J: Effect of orally-consumed *Aloe vera* juice on human gastrointestinal function. *Natural Foods Network Newslett*, August, 1985.
35. Pulse TL and Uhlig E: A significant improvement in a clinical pilot study utilizing nutritional supplements, essential fatty acids and stabilized *Aloe vera* juice in 29 seropositive, ARC and AIDS patients. *J Adv Med* **3**, 209–230, 1990.
36. Singer J: A randomized placebo-controlled trial of oral acemannan as an adjunctive to anti-retroviral therapy in advanced HIV disease. *Int Conf AIDS* **9**(1), 494, 1993. [Abstract No. PO-B28-2153]
37. Rowe TD, Lovell BK, and Parks LM: Further observations on the use of *Aloe vera* leaf in the treatment of third-degree X-ray reactions. *J Am Pharm Assoc* **30**, 266–269, 1941.
38. Rowe TD: Effect of fresh *Aloe vera* gel in the treatment of third-degree Roentgen reactions on white rats. *J Am Pharmacol Assoc* **29**, 348–350, 1940.
39. Lushbaugh CC and Hale DB: Experimental acute radiodermatitis following beta radiation. V. Histopathological study of the mode of action of therapy with *Aloe vera. Cancer* **6**, 690–698, 1953.
40. El Zawahry M, Hegazy MR, and Helal M: Use of aloe in treating leg ulcers and dermatoses. *Int J Dermatol* **12**, 68–73, 1973.
41. Schmidt JM and Greenspoon JS: *Aloe vera* dermal wound gel is associated with a delay in wound healing. *Obstet Gynecol* **78**, 115–117, 1991.

2

Angelica species

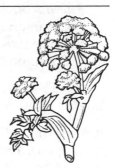

Key uses of *angelica* species:

- Menopausal symptoms
- Premenstrual syndrome
- Allergies
- Smooth muscle spasm

General description

Angelica species are biennial or perennial plants with hollow fluted stems that rise to a height of 3 to 7 feet. The umbels of greenish-white flowers bloom from May to August. The plants are found in damp mountain ravines and meadows, on river banks, and in coastal areas; *angelica* is also a widely cultivated species. In Asia, it is grown primarily for its medicinal action, whereas in the United States and Europe angelica is cultivated for use as a flavoring agent in most major categories of food products, including alcoholic (e.g., bitters, liqueurs, and vermouths) and nonalcoholic beverages, ice cream, candy, gelatins, and puddings. With all species, the roots and rhizomes are the most extensively used portions of the plant.

Latin and common names of *angelica* species

Angelica sinensis or *polymorpha* (family Umbelliferae or Apiaceae)
  Common names: Chinese angelica, dong quai
Angelica acutiloba (family Umbelliferae or Apiaceae)
  Common name: Japanese angelica

Angelica archangelica (family Umbelliferae or Apiaceae)
  Common name: European angelica
Angelica atropurpurea (family Umbelliferae or Apiaceae)
  Common name: American angelica
Angelica sylvestris (family Umbelliferae or Apiaceae)
  Common name: Wild angelica

Angelica sinensis and Angelica acutiloba

In Asia, the authentic and original medicinal angelica is *Angelica sinensis* (dong quai), a native to China. While at least nine other *angelica* species are used in China, dong quai is by far the most highly regarded. For several thousand years, dong quai has been cultivated for medicinal use in the treatment of a wide variety of disorders, in particular "female" disorders. It is often referred to as the "female ginseng."[1]

Several hundred years ago, when the supply of Chinese angelica was scarce, the Japanese began to cultivate *Angelica acutiloba*, an *angelica* species indigenous to Japan, as a substitute.[1] The two species appear to have very similar therapeutic effects, although it is interesting to note that in China, the Japanese angelica is thought to have no therapeutic value while in Japan, Chinese angelica is thought of as being without effect. Experimentally, both species exhibit very similar therapeutic effects, and each country's claim to produce a superior dong quai is based more on emotion than scientific investigation.

Angelica archangelica and Angelica atropurpurea

Historical usage suggests that European angelica (*Angelica archangelica*) and American angelica (*Angelica atropurpurea*) have properties different from those of the Asian species. These differences have not, however, been evaluated by chemical analysis.

Chemical composition

Angelica sinensis and Angelica acutiloba

Chinese and Japanese angelica are similarly composed of various coumarins, essential oils, and flavonoids, which are responsible for their medicinal actions. The essential oil of oriental angelica contains *n*-butylphthalide, cadinene, carvacrol, *n*-dodecanal, isosafrole, linoleic acid, palmitic acid, safrole, sesquiterpene, and *n*-tetradecanol.[2,3]

Angelica archangelica

Also very rich in coumarins, *Angelica archangelica* is particularly phototoxic (causes severe sunburn). Coumarins, including osthole, angelicin, osthenol, umbelliferone, archangelicine, bergapten, and ostruthol, are found in significant concentrations, with osthole composing nearly 0.2 percent of the root. The root is also a good source of flavonoids, including archangelenone and caffeic acids. The root contains 0.3 to 1.0 percent volatile oil (which is composed mainly of beta-phyllamdrene), alpha-pinene, borneol, limonene, and four macrocylic lactones.[2,4]

History and folk use

Angelica sinensis and Angelica acutiloba

In Asia, angelica's reputation is perhaps second only to that of ginseng. Predominantly regarded as a "female" remedy, angelica has been used to treat such conditions as dysmenorrhea (painful menstruation), amenorrhea (absence of menstruation), metrorrhagia (abnormal menstruation), menopausal symptoms (especially hot flashes), and to assure a healthy pregnancy and easy delivery. Angelica is also used in the treatment of abdominal pain, anemia, injuries, arthritis, migraine headache, and many other conditions.[2,3,5]

Angelica archangelica

One of the most highly praised herbs in old herbal texts, archangelica was used in all northern European countries for protection against contagion, for purifying the blood, and for curing every conceivable malady; it was considered a sovereign remedy for poisons, agues, and all infectious maladies.

According to one legend, archangelica was revealed in a dream as a cure for the plague. One explanation for the name is related to its blooming near May 8, the feast day of Michael the Archangel. It was therefore seen as a "protector against evil spirits and witchcraft."[6]

Archangelica has been used for a wide variety of conditions, including flatulent dyspepsia, pleurisy, respiratory catarrh, and bronchitis. The plant was believed to possess carminative, spasmolytic, diaphoretic, expectorant, and diuretic activity.[6]

Angelica atropurpurea

The therapeutic use of American angelica mirrors that of European angelica. Its most common use is for heartburn and flatulent colic.[7]

Pharmacology

The pharmacology of *Angelica* species relates to their high coumarin content. However, unlike other scientific investigations of herbal medicines, much of the research done on *Angelica* species has been done on plant extracts, rather than isolated constituents. The overwhelming majority of the studies have been done on the Asian species. Some of the pharmacological activities demonstrated include phytoestrogen activity, analgesic activity, cardiovascular effects, smooth muscle relaxing effects, antiallergy and immunomodulating activity, and antibacterial activity.

Phytoestrogen effects

Plant estrogenic substances, or *phytoestrogens*, are components of many medicinal herbs historically used to treat conditions now treated with synthetic estrogens. Chinese and Japanese angelicas contain highly active phytoestrogens, although these compounds are much lower in activity than animal estrogens (1:400 as active). This helps to explain why angelica is used ito treat conditions characterized by both high and low estrogen levels. Phytoestrogens demonstrate an alterative effect by competing with estrogen for binding sites on cells. When estrogen levels are low, phytoestrogens exert some estrogenic activity; when estrogen levels are high, phytoestrogens reduce overall estrogenic activity by occupying estrogen receptor sites. This alterative action of angelica phytoestrogens is probably the basis of much of the plant's use in amenorrhea and menopause.

Japanese angelica has demonstrated uterine tonic activity, causing an initial increase in uterine contraction followed by relaxation.[8,9] In addition, administration of Japanese angelica to mice resulted in increased uterine weight, increased DNA content of the uterus and liver, and increased glucose utilization by the liver and uterus.[1,8] Because of these and other effects, angelica has been referred to as a uterine tonic.

Cardiovascular effects

Although not used historically for these purposes, angelica does possess significant blood pressure-lowering action.[1,3,8] This effect is largely due to its ability to dilate blood vessels. Dihydropyranocoumarins and dihydrofuranocoumarins from umbelliferous plants such as the *Angelica* species have been shown to possess significant ability to dilate coronary vessels and relieve vasospasms.[10] The mechanism of action appears to be largely a result of calcium channel antagonism. Agents that interact with calcium channels (calcium channel blockers) are quickly coming into prominence in the treatment of a wide variety of conditions, including hypertension and angina. Angelica and other umbelliferous plants may offer similar effects. Other cardiovascular effects noted for angelica include antiarrhythmic actions; inhibition of platelet aggregation; lowering of blood pressure; and increase in blood flow to the heart, brain, and extremities.[1-3]

Smooth muscle relaxing activity

Calcium channel-blocking compounds are also capable of relaxing the smooth muscles of visceral organs. Angelica (essential oil) relaxes the smooth muscles of the intestines and uterus, whereas the water extract produces an initial contraction and then prolonged relaxation.[1,8,9] This confirms its historical use in the treatment of intestinal spasm and uterine cramps. Its action on other smooth muscles could explain its hypotensive action (vascular smooth muscle) and historical use in asthma (bronchial smooth muscle).

Analgesic activity

Both Chinese and Japanese angelica have demonstrated pain-relieving and mild tranquilizing effects in experimental studies in animals.[1,8,11,12] Angelica's pain-relieving action was 1.7 times that of aspirin in one study.[12] Its analgesic activity, combined with its smooth muscle-relaxing activity, supports its historical use in such conditions as uterine cramps, trauma, headaches, and arthritis.

Antiallergy and immunomodulating activity

Chinese and Japanese herbalists have long used angelica in the prevention and treatment of allergic symptoms in individuals who are sensitive to a variety of substances (pollen, dust, animal dander, food, etc.).[1,13] Its action is related to its ability to inhibit selectively the production of allergy-related antibodies (IgE). Because IgE levels in patients with allergic conditions are typically three to ten times greater than is considered normal, angelica may offer some benefit by reducing these elevated antibody levels.

Coumarin compounds have demonstrated immune-enhancing activity in both healthy and cancer patients.[14,15] Coumarins have been shown to stimulate white blood cells and increase their ability to destroy foreign particles and cancer cells.[14] Such activity is thought to offer significant protection against the growth and spread of tumor cells. On coumarin administration, specific white blood cells known as macrophages are said to be "activated" and thus capable of entering the tumor, where they can destroy tumor cells.[14,15]

Coumarin compounds of angelica and the polysaccharides of the water extract of Japanese angelica have immune-modulating activity: they enhance the activity of white blood cells, increase interferon production, increase antitumor activity, and stimulate nonspecific host defense mechanisms.[16–19] These effects on the immune system by coumarins, polysaccharides, and extracts of *Angelica* species would seem to support their historical anticancer effects and their use as support agents in modern cancer therapy.

Antibacterial activity

Extracts of Chinese angelica have been shown to possess antibacterial activity against both gram-negative and gram-positive bacteria, whereas extracts of Japanese angelica exhibited no antibacterial action.[8] The inconsistency could be due to different essential oil concentrations of the extracts used in the studies. The oil of *Angelica archangelica* exhibits significant antifungal properties but virtually no antibacterial activity.[3,5] Because other herbs have much greater antimicrobial activity, *Angelica* species should be considered a less than optimum agent if this effect is desired.

Clinical applications

Angelica species have been used throughout the world in the treatment of a wide variety of conditions. At this time it appears that *Angelica archangelica* and *Angelica atropurpurea* are most indicated as expectorants, antispasmodics, and carminatives in the treatment of such conditions as respiratory ailments, gas, and abdominal spasm. Chinese angelica (*Angelica sinensis* or *polymorpha*) and Japanese angelica (*Angelica acutiloba*) appear most useful in the treatment of disorders of menstruation, menopause (especially hot flashes), atopic conditions, smooth muscle spasm (e.g., uterine cramps, migraines, and abdominal spasm), and possibly as an immunostimulatory adjunct in cancer therapy. Further human research is needed to document the degree of clinical efficacy of *Angelica* species.

Dosage

Take three times per day:

Powdered root or as tea: 1 to 2 grams

Tincture (1:5): 4 milliliters (1 teaspoon)
Fluid extract: 1 milliliter ($\frac{1}{4}$ teaspoon)

Toxicity

Angelica is generally considered to be of extremely low toxicity. However, it does contain many substances that can react with sunlight to cause a rash or severe sunburn. This possible side effect should be kept in mind when using any umbelliferous plant. This side effect can be used therapeutically in the treatment of vitiligo and psoriasis.

References

1. Hikino H: Recent research on Oriental medicinal plants. *Econ Med Plant Res* **1**, 53–85, 1985.
2. Duke JA: *Handbook of Medicinal Herbs*. CRC Press, Boca Raton, FL, 1985. pp. 43–44.
3. Zhu DPQ: Dong quai. *Am J Chin Med* **15**, 117–125, 1987.
4. Duke JA and Ayensu ES: *Medicinal Plants of China*. Reference Publications, Algonac, MI, 1985, pp. 74–77.
5. Opdyke DLJ: Angelica root oil. *Food Cosmet Toxicol* **13**(Suppl.), 713–714, 1975.
6. Grieve M: *A Modern Herbal*. Dover Publications, New York, 1971. pp. 35–40.
7. Lust J: *The Herb Book*. Bantam Books, New York, 1974. pp. 97–99.
8. Yoshiro K: The physiological actions of tang-kuei and cnidium. *Bull Orient Healing Arts Inst USA* **10**, 269–278, 1985.
9. Harada M, Suzuki M, and Ozaki Y: Effect of Japanese angelica root and peony root on uterine contraction in the rabbit in situ. *J Pharmacol Dynam* **7**, 304–311, 1984.
10. Thastrup O, Fjalland B, and Lemmich J: Coronary vasodilatory, spasmolytic and cAMP-phosphodiesterase inhibitory properties of dihydropyranocoumarins and dihydrofuranocoumarins. *Acta Pharmacol Toxicol* **52**, 246–253, 1983.
11. Tanaka S, *et al.*: Anti-nociceptive substances from the roots of *Angelica acutiloba*. *Arzneim Forsch* **27**, 2039–2045, 1977.
12. Tanaka S, *et al.*: Effects of "Toki" (*Angelica acutiloba* Kitawaga) extracts on writhing and capillary permeability in mice (analgesic and anti-inflammatory effects). *Yakugaku Zassh* **91**, 1098–1104, 1971.
13. Sung CP, *et al.*: Effects of *Angelica polymorpha* on reaginic antibody production. *J Natural Prod* **45**, 398–406, 1982.
14. Casley-Smith JR: The actions of benzopyrenes on the blood-tissue-lymph system. *Folia Angiol* **24**, 7–22, 1976.
15. Berkarda B, Bouffard-Eyuboglu H, and Derman U: The effect of coumarin derivatives on the immunological system of man. *Agents Actions* **13**, 50–52, 1983.
16. Ohno N, Matsumoto SI, Suzuki I, *et al.*: Biochemical characterization of a mitogen obtained from an oriental crude drug, tohki (*Angelica acutiloba* Kitawaga). *J Pharmacol Dynam* **6**, 903–912, 1983.
17. Yamada H, Kiyohara H, Cyong JC, *et al.*: Studies on polysaccharides from *Angelica acutiloba*. *Planta Medica* **48**, 163–167, 1984.
18. Yamada H, Kiyohara H, Cyong JC, *et al.*: Studies on polysaccharides from *Angelica acutiloba*. IV. Characterization of an anti-complementary arabinogalactan from the roots of *Angelica acutiloba* Kitagawa. *Mol Immunol* **22**, 295–304, 1985.
19. Kumazawa Y, Mizunoe K, and Otsuka Y: Immunostimulating polysaccharide separated from hot water extract of *Angelica acutiloba* Kitagawa (Yamato Tohki). *Immunology* **47**, 75–83, 1982.

3
Bilberry

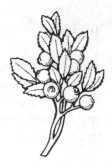

Key uses of bilberry:

- Diabetic retinopathy
- Macular degeneration
- Cataract
- Glaucoma
- Varicose veins

General description

Bilberry or European blueberry (*Vaccinium myrtillus*) is a member of the genus *Vaccinium*, which comprises nearly 200 species of berries including cranberry, cowberry, and American blueberry. Bilberry is a shrubby perennial plant that grows in the woods and forest meadows of Europe. The angular, green, branched stem grows from a creeping rootstock to a height of 1 to 1.5 feet. The 0.5 to 1.0-inch long leaves are oval, slightly dentate, and bright green, while the flowers are reddish- or greenish-pink and bell-shaped. The flowering season is April to June. The fruit is a blue-black or purple berry.[1] Bilberry differs from the American blueberry in that the meat of the fruit is also purple, while the American variety has a cream- or white-colored interior.

Chemical composition

The pharmacologically active constituents of bilberries include flavonoid compounds known as *anthocyanosides*. An anthocyanoside consists of a backbone molecule known as anthocyanidin bound to one of three sugars (arabinose, glucose, or galactose). More than fifteen different anthocyanosides originate from the five different anthocyanidins found in bilberry.[2]

Other members of the genus *Vaccinium*, as well as *Ribes nigum* (black currant) and *Vitis vinifera* (grape), contain similar anthocyanosides.[3] Extracts of these fruit are also used for medicinal purposes in Europe.

The concentration of anthocyanosides in the fresh fruit is approximately 0.1 to 0.25 percent, whereas concentrated extracts of bilberry yield an anthocyanidin content of 25 percent.[2] An extract with an anthocyanidin content of 25 percent actually contains about 38 percent anthocyanosides owing to the conjugation of the anthocyanidin with a sugar. For analytical purposes, the anthocyanoside content should always be expressed in terms of anthocyanidin. Only very small amounts of free anthocyanidins exist in nature and in bilberry extracts.

History and folk use

Bilberries have, of course, been used as food and for their high nutritive value. Medicinally, they have been utilized in the treatment of scurvy and urinary complaints (including infection and stones).[1]

The dried berries have been used primarily for their astringent qualities in the treatment of diarrhea and dysentery. Decoctions of the leaves have been used in the treatment of diabetes.[1]

Renewed interest in the medicinal use of bilberry was first aroused when it was observed during World War II that British Royal Air Force pilots reported improved nighttime visual acuity on bombing raids after consuming bilberries. Subsequent studies showed that administration of bilberry extracts to healthy subjects resulted in improved nighttime visual acuity, quicker adjustment to darkness, and faster restoration of visual acuity after exposure to glare.

In Europe, bilberry extracts are now part of the conventional medical treatment of many eye disorders including cataracts and macular degeneration, as well as retinitis pigmentosa, diabetic retinopathy, and night blindness. This use is supported by positive results in controlled clinical trials.

Pharmacology

The pharmacology of bilberry is discussed almost entirely in relationship to its anthocyanoside content, as research has focused primarily on the anthocyanosides.

Collagen-stabilizing action

Anthocyanosides, like procyanidolic oligomers (see Chapter 16), possess significant collagen-stabilizing action.[4-15] Collagen, the most abundant protein of the body, is responsible for maintaining the integrity of "ground substance" as well as tendons, ligaments, and cartilage. Collagen is destroyed during the inflammatory processes that occur in rheumatoid arthritis, periodontal disease, and other inflammatory conditions involving bones, joints, cartilage, and other connective tissue.

The anthocyanidins in bilberry extracts affect collagen metabolism in several ways:

1. Anthocyanosides have the ability to actually cross-link collagen fibers, resulting in reinforcement of the natural cross-linking of collagen that forms the collagen matrix of connective tissue (ground substance, cartilage, tendon, etc.).[4-7,14]
2. Anthocyanosides prevent free radical damage with their potent antioxidant and free radical-scavenging action.[4-8]
3. Anthocyanosides inhibit enzymatic cleavage of collagen by enzymes secreted by leukocytes during inflammation.[4-6,8,13,14]
4. Anthocyanosides and other flavonoid components of bilberry prevent the release and synthesis of compounds that promote inflammation, such as histamine, serine proteases, prostaglandins, and leukotrienes.[4-6,11,12,15]
5. Anthocyanosides promote mucopolysaccharide and collagen biosynthesis and stimulate reticulation of collagen fibrils.[9,10,16]

Normalization of capillary permeability

Anthocyanosides have strong "vitamin P" activity.[4] Their effects include an ability to increase intracellular vitamin C levels and decrease capillary permeability and fragility.[4-6] Their effect in reducing capillary fragility and permeability is roughly twice that of rutin, both in intensity and duration of action.[17]

One interesting effect of the normalization of collagen structures and capillaries is the demonstration that anthocyanosides from bilberry decrease the permeability of the blood–brain barrier.[14,18] Increased blood–brain permeability has been linked to autoimmune diseases of the central nervous system, schizophrenia, "cerebral allergies," and a variety of other psychiatric disorders. Presumably, the anthocyanosides inhibit both enzymatic and nonenzymatic degradation of the basement membrane collagen of brain capillaries, thus helping maintain or restore the brain's protection from drugs, pollutants, naturally occurring degradation products, and other cerebral toxins.

Antiaggregation effect on platelets

Anthocyanosides, like many other flavonoids, have been shown to exert significant antiaggregation effects on platelets.[19–21] Excessive platelet aggregation is linked to atherosclerosis and blood clot formation.

Blood sugar-lowering effect

A decoction of blueberry leaves has a long history of folk use in the treatment of diabetes. This use is supported by research, which has shown that oral administration reduces hyperglycemia in normal and depancreatized dogs, even when glucose is concurrently injected intravenously.[22,23]

The anthocyanoside myrtillin is apparently the most active hypoglycemic component of bilberry. On injection, myrtillin is somewhat weaker than insulin, but it is also less toxic, even at 50 times the therapeutic dose of 1 gram per day. It is of interest to note that a single dose can produce beneficial effects lasting for several weeks.[22]

Smooth muscle-relaxing activity

Anthocyanoside extracts have demonstrated significant vascular smooth muscle-relaxing effects in a variety of experimental models.[24–26] The clinical application of this research may be in the treatment of dysmenorrhea, for which a preliminary study has demonstrated positive effects.[27]

Antiulcer effects

Oral administration of bilberry anthocyanosides to rats exerted a significant preventive and curative antiulcer activity in various experimental models of gastric ulcer, without affecting gastric secretion.[28] This activity can be attributed, at least partly, to an increase in gastric mucus.

Clinical applications

Bilberry extracts have been widely used in Europe in the treatment of various eye conditions as well as for vascular disorders, peptic ulcers, and dysmenorrhea.

Eye disorders

Perhaps the most significant clinical applications of bilberry extracts are in the field of ophthalmology. Although many aspects of vision remain a mystery, certain requirements must be met for normal vision to occur: light must interact with the specialized nerve cells of the eye—rods and cones—to create a nerve impulse, and the nerve impulse must then be transmitted to the visual areas of the brain. Many nutritional compounds are important in vision, both in terms of protecting the eye from damage as well as in the actual process of vision.

The health of the eye is largely dependent on a rich supply of nutrients and oxygen. Relatively speaking, the amount of blood flow through the eye is the greatest in the body. This high blood flow emphasizes the importance of nutrition and the circulatory system for optimal eye health and function.

When normal mechanisms designed to deliver oxygen and other nutrients to the eye fail, or if protective mechanisms intended to protect the eye from damage begin to fail, a variety of disorders develop including cataracts and macular degeneration. These disorders are almost always associated with aging.

Bilberry extracts appear to offer significant benefit to the eyes, presumably via an ability to improve the delivery of oxygen and blood to the eye. The extracts also exert other important pharmacological effects, including acting as an antioxidant.

The origin of many eye diseases including cataract formation and macular degeneration is ultimately related to damage caused by free radicals. In a nutshell, a free radical is a highly reactive molecule that can bind to and destroy body components. Free radical or "oxidative" damage is what makes us age. In addition to their role in causing cataracts and macular degeneration, free radicals have also been shown to be responsible for the initiation of many diseases, including the two biggest killers of Americans—heart disease and cancer.

Bilberry extracts may also play a significant role in the prevention and treatment of glaucoma via its effect on collagen structures in the eye. In the eye, collagen provides tensile strength and integrity to the tissues.

Bilberry extract improves vision   Some of the first scientific studies on bilberry extract confirmed the effects noticed by Royal Air Force pilots during World War II. The administration of bilberry extract to healthy subjects resulted in improved nighttime visual acuity, quicker adjustment to darkness, and faster restoration of visual acuity after exposure to glare.[29,30]

Further studies confirmed these results.[31–34] Results were most impressive in individuals with retinitis pigmentosa and hemeralopia. Hemeralopia refers to "day blindness," or an inability to see as distinctly in bright light as in dim light.

It appears that the purple bilberry anthocyanosides have an affinity for the pigmented epithelium or visual purple area of the retina. This portion of the retina is responsible for vision and controls the adaptation from dark to light and vice versa.[35] This affinity for visual purple is consistent with several of the clinical effects observed. The outcome is that anthocyanoside extracts of bilberry appear to be of great value in the treatment of both poor night vision and poor day vision.

Cataracts   Cataracts are the leading cause of impaired vision and blindness in the United States. Approximately 4 million people have some degree of vision-impairing cataract, and at least 40,000 people in the United States are blind due to cataracts. Cataracts are a source of a tremendous financial burden on our society; cataract surgery is the most common major surgical procedure done in the United States each year (600,000 per annum) for persons on Medicare, at a cost of over $4 billion.

Bilberry anthocyanosides may offer significant protection against the development of cataracts. The occurrence of cataracts in rats can be retarded by changing their diet from a commercial lab chow to a "well-defined diet."[36] Preliminary research suggests that flavonoid components in the well-defined diets may be responsible for the protective effects.[37]

In one human study, bilberry extract plus vitamin E stopped progression of cataract formation in 97 percent of fifty patients with senile cortical cataracts.[38]

Macular degeneration   The macula is the portion of the eye responsible for fine vision. Degeneration of the macula is the leading cause of severe visual loss in the United States and Europe in persons aged 55 years or older. The risk factors for macular degeneration include aging, atherosclerosis, and high blood pressure. There is no current medical treatment for the most common form of macular degeneration. Laser surgery is used for those individuals who develop a less common type of macular degeneration (exudative macular degeneration).

Bilberry anthocyanosides may offer significant protection against the development of macular degeneration. The rate of retinal degeneration can be retarded by changing their diet from a commercial lab chow to a "well-defined diet."[39] Preliminary research suggests that flavonoid components in the well-defined diets may be responsible for the protective effects.[37]

In one study, thirty-one patients with various types of retinopathy (twenty with diabetic retinopathy, five with retinitis pigmentosa, four with macular degeneration, and two with hemorrhagic retinopathy due to anti-coagulant therapy) were treated with bilberry extract.[40] A tendency toward reduced permeability and a tendency to hemorrhage were observed in all patients, especially those with diabetic retinopathy.

Diabetes mellitus

Although bilberry may lower blood glucose levels, the most important benefits of the use of anthocyanosides in the treatment of diabetes relate to their ability to improve diabetic retinopathy, collagen integrity, and capillary permeability.

Bilberry anthocyanoside extracts are widely used in Europe in the prevention and treatment of diabetic retinopathy.[44-46]

Bilberry anthocyanosides also exert a protective effect on capillary fragility in diabetics and reduce serum cholesterol and triglyceride levels in primary dyslipidemia.[41]

Although studies in rabbits have not confirmed a cholesterol-lowering effect, anthocyanosides did decrease significantly the development of atherosclerotic plaque. Presumably, this is a result of increasing collagen cross-linking, thus diminishing the permeability in small, as well as large, blood vessels.[42]

Vascular disorders

Clinical studies have demonstrated the positive effect of bilberry extract in the treatment of capillary fragility, blood purpuras, various circulation disturbances of the brain (similar to *Ginkgo biloba*), venous insufficiency, varicose veins, and microscopic blood loss in the urine caused by kidney capillary fragility.[15,43-53]

Capillary fragility   The ability of bilberry extract to reduce capillary fragility is discussed in Pharmacology (above). In one human study, following oral administration of anthocyanosides, patients with varicose veins and ulcerative dermatitis experienced a substantial drop in capillary leakage.[43] Anthocyanosides were found to protect altered capillary walls by increasing the endothelium barrier effect through stabilization of membrane phospholipids, and through restoration of the altered sheath of connective tissue surrounding the blood vessels.

Bilberry's reduction of microscopic blood loss in the urine caused by kidney capillary fragility may reflect its tissue distribution. Absorption and distribution studies in rats have demonstrated the affinity of bilberry anthocyanosides for the kidneys.[54] Anthocyanosides reflect the high concentration of collagen and mucopolysaccharides in the kidneys along with the fact that these flavonoid compounds are excreted via the kidneys.

Varicose veins   Bilberry's efficacy in the treatment of a variety of venous disorders relates to the ability of anthocyanosides to protect altered veins (post-phlebitic veins as well as varicose veins) via two mechanisms: (1) increasing the endothelium barrier effect through stabilization of the membrane phospholipids, and (2) increasing the biosynthesis of the connective ground substance, thus restoring the connective tissue sheath that surrounds the vein.[15] This latter effect leads to a marked increase in newly formed capillaries and collagen fibrils.

In one study, forty-seven patients with varicose veins were treated with bilberry extract (480 milligrams per day).[44] Significant improvements were found in abnormal capillary permeability, edema, feelings of heaviness, paresthesia, pain, and skin dystrophy and dyschromia. Bilberry anthocyanosides improve vein function by reducing capillary flow, converting richly branched vascular units into terminal units, and eliminating blood stasis.

Dosage

The standard dose for bilberry should be based on its anthocyanoside content, as calculated by its anthocyanidin percentage. Widely used pharmaceutical preparations in Europe are standardized for anthocyanidin content (typically 25 percent). The following doses should be taken three times daily:

Anthocyanosides (calculated as anthocyanidin): 20–40 milligrams
Bilberry extract (25 percent anthocyanidin content): 80–160 milligrams

Toxicity

Extensive toxicological investigation confirms that bilberry anthocyanoside extracts are devoid of toxic effects. Rats administered doses as high as 400 milligrams per kilogram showed no apparent side effects, and excess levels were quickly excreted through the urine and bile.[17,54]

References

1. Grieve M: *A Modern Herbal*, Vol. 1. Dover Publications, New York, 1971, pp. 385–386.
2. Baj A, *et al*.: Qualitative and quantitative evaluation of *Vaccinium myrtillus* anthocyanins by high-resolution gas chromatography and high-performance liquid chromatography. *J Chromatogr* **279**, 365–372, 1983.

3. Andersen OM: Anthocyanins in fruits of *Vaccinium uliginosum* L. (bog whortleberry). *J Food Sci* **52**, 665–666, 680, 1987.

4. Kuhnau J: The flavonoids, a class of semi-essential food components: Their role in human nutrition. *World Rev Nutr Diet* **24**, 117–191, 1976.

5. Gabor M: Pharmacologic effects of flavonoids on blood vessels. *Angiologica* **9**, 355–374, 1972.

6. Havsteen B: Flavonoids, a class of natural products of high pharmacological potency. *Biochem Pharmacol* **32**, 1141–1148, 1983.

7. Monboisse JC, *et al*.: Non-enzymatic degradation of acid-soluble calf skin collagen by superoxide ion: Protective effect of flavonoids. *Biochem Pharmacol* **32**, 53–58, 1983.

8. Monboisse JC, Braquet P, and Borel JP: Oxygen-free radicals as mediators of collagen breakage. *Agents Actions* **15**, 49–50, 1984.

9. Rao CN, Rao VH, and Steinman B: Influence of bioflavonoids on the collagen metabolism in rats with adjuvant induced arthritis. *Ital J Biochem* **30**, 54–62, 1981.

10. Ronziere MC, *et al*.: Influence of some flavonoids on reticulation of collagen fibrils in vitro. *Biochem Pharmacol* **30**, 1771–1776, 1981.

11. Middleton E: The flavonoids. *Trends Pharm Sci* **5**, 335–338, 1984.

12. Amella M, *et al*.: Inhibition of mast cell histamine release by flavonoids and biflavonoids. *Planta Medica* **51**, 16–20, 1985.

13. Jonadet M, *et al*.: Anthocyanosides extracted from *Vitis vinifera*, *Vaccinium myrtillus* and *Pinus maritimus*. I. Elastase-inhibiting activities in vitro. II. Compared angioprotective activities in vivo. *J Pharm Belg* **38**, 41–46, 1983.

14. Detre A, *et al*.: Studies on vascular permeability in hypertension: Action of anthocyanosides. *Clin Physiol Biochem* **4**, 143–149, 1986.

15. Blau LW: Cherry diet control for gout and arthritis. *Tex Rep Biol Med* **8**, 309–311, 1950.

16. Mian E, *et al*.: Anthocyanosides and the walls of the microvessels: Further aspects of the mechanism of action of their protective effect in syndromes due to abnormal capillary fragility. *Minerva Med* **68**, 3565–3581, 1977.

17. Lietti A and Forni G: Studies on *Vaccinium myrtillus* anthocyanosides. I. Vasoprotective and anti-inflammatory activity. *ArzneimiHel-Forsch* **26**, 829–832, 1976.

18. Robert AM, *et al*.: Action of the anthocyanosides of *Vaccinium myrtillus* on the permeability of the blood brain barrier. *J Med* **8**, 321–332, 1977.

19. Zaragoza F, Iglesias I, and Benedi J: Comparison of thrombocyte antiaggregant effects of anthocyanosides with those of other agents. *Arch Pharmacol Toxicol* **11**, 183–188, 1985.

20. Morazzoni P and Magistretti MJ: Effects of *Vaccinium myrtillus* anthocyanosides on prostacyclin like activity in rat arterial tissue. *Fitoterapia* **57**, 11–14, 1986.

21. Bottecchia D, *et al*.: Preliminary report on the inhibitory effect of *Vaccinium myrtillus* anthocyanosides on platelet aggregation and clot retraction. *Fitoterapia* **48**, 3–8, 1987.

22. Bever B and Zahnd G: Plants with oral hypoglycemic action. *Q J Crude Drug Res* **17**, 139–196, 1979.

23. Allen FM: Blueberry leaf extract: Physiologic and clinical properties in relation to carbohydrate metabolism. *JAMA* **89**, 1577–1581, 1927.

24. Bettini V, *et al*.: Effects of *Vaccinium myrtillus* anthocyanosides on vascular smooth muscle. *Fitoterapia* **55**, 265–272, 1984.

25. Bettini V, *et al*.: Inhibition by *Vaccinium myrtillus* anthocyanosides of barium-induced contractions in segments of internal thoracic vein. *Fitoterapia* **55**, 323–327, 1984.

26. Bettini V, *et al*.: Mechanical responses of isolated coronary arteries to barium in the presence of *Vaccinium myrtillus* anthocyanosides. *Fitoterapia* **56**, 3–10, 1985.

27. Colombo D and Vescovini R: Controlled clinical trial of anthocyanosides from *Vaccinium myrtillus* in primary dysmenorrhea. *G Ital Obstet Ginecol* **7**, 1033–1038, 1985.

28. Criston A and Magistretti MJ: Antiulcer and healing activity of *Vaccinium myrtillus* anthocyanosides. *Il Farmaco* **42**(2), 29–43, 1986.

29. Jayle GE and Aubert L: Action des glucosides d'anthocyanes sur la vision scotopique et mesopique du sujet normal. *Therapie* **19**, 171–185,1964.

30. Terrasse J and Moinade S: Premiers resultats obtenus avec un nouveau facteur vitamininique P "les anthocyanosides" extraits du *Vaccinium myrtillus*. *Presse Med* **72**, 397–400, 1964.

31. Sala D, Rolando M, Rossi PL, and Pissarello L: Effect of anthocyanosides on visual performances at low illumination. *Minerva Oftalmol* **21**, 283–285, 1979.

32. Gloria E and Peria A: Effect of anthocyanosides on the absolute visual threshold. *Ann Ottalmol Clin Ocul* **92**, 595–607, 1966.

33. Junemann G: On the effect of anthocyanosides on hemeralopia following quinine poisoning. *Klin Monatsbl Augenheilkd* **151**, 891–896, 1967.

34. Caselli L: Clinical and electroretinographic study on activity of anthocyanosides. *Arch Med Int* **37**, 29–35, 1985.
35. Wegmann R, Maeda K, Tronche P, and Bastide P: Effects of anthocyanosides on photoreceptors. Cyto-enzymatic aspects. *Ann Histochim* **14**, 237–256, 1969.
36. Hess H, Knapka JJ, Newsome DA, *et al.*: Dietary prevention of cataracts in the pink-eyed RCS rat. *Lab Anim Sci* **35**, 47–53, 1985.
37. Pautler EL, Maga JA, and Tengerdy C: A pharmacologically potent natural product in the bovine retina. *Exp Eye Res* **42**, 285–288, 1986.
38. Bravetti G: Preventive medical treatment of senile cataract with vitamin E and anthocyanosides: Clinical evaluation. *Ann Ottalmol Clin Ocul* **115**, 109, 1989.
39. Pautler EL and Ennis SR: The effect of diet on inherited retinal dystrophy in the rat. *Curr Eye Res* **3**, 1221–1224, 1984.
40. Scharrer A and Ober M: Anthocyanosides in the treatment of retinopathies. *Klin Monatsbl Augenheilkd* **178**, 386–389, 1981.
41. Passariello N, Bisesti V, and Sgambato S: Influence of anthocyanosides on the microcirculation and lipid picture in diabetic and dyslipidic subjects. *Gaz Med Ital* **138**, 563–566, 1979.
42. Kadar A, *et al.*: Influence of anthocyanoside treatment on the cholesterol-induced atherosclerosis in the rabbit. *Paroi Arterielle* **5**, 187–206, 1979.
43. Mian E, *et al.*: Anthocyanosides and the walls of microvessels: Further aspects of the mechanism of action of their protective effect in syndromes due to abnormal capillary fragility. *Minerva Med* **68**, 3565–3581, 1977.
44. Ghiringhelli C, Gregoratti F, and Marastoni F: Capillarotropic activity of anthocyanosides in high doses in phlebopathic stasis. *Min Cardioangiol* **26**, 255–276, 1978.
45. Treviso A: Therapeutic value of the association of anthocyanin glucosides with glutamine and phos-phorylserine in the treatment of learning disturbances at different ages. *Gaz Med Ital* **138**, 217–232, 1979.
46. Grismond GL: Treatment of pregnancy-induced phlebopathies. *Minerva Ginecol* **33**, 221–230, 1981.
47. Piovella F, *et al.*: Results with anthocyanidins in the treatment of haemorrhagic diathesis due to defec-tive primary haemastasis. *Gaz Med Ital* **140**, 445–449, 1981.
48. Pennarola R, *et al.*: The therapeutic action of the anthocyanosides in microcirculatory changes due to adhesive-induced polyneuritis. *Gaz Med Ital* **139**, 485–491, 1980.
49. Amouretti M: Therapeutic value of *Vaccinium myrtillus* anthocyanosides in an internal medicine department. *Therapeutique* **48**, 579–581, 1972.
50. Coget J and Merlen JF: Clinical study of a new chemical agent for vascular protection. Difrarel 20, com-posed of anthocyanosides extracted from *Vaccinium myrtillus*. *Phlebologie* **21**, 221–228, 1968.
51. Spinella G: Natural anthocyanosides in treatment of peripheral venous insufficiency. *Arch Med Int* **37**, 21–29, 1985.
52. Coget JM and Merlen JF: Anthocyanosides and microcirculation. *J Mal Vasc* **5**, 43–46, 1980.
53. Neumann L: Long-term therapy of vascular permeability disorders using anthocyanosides. *Munch Med Wochenschr* **115**, 952–954, 1973.
54. Lietti A and Forni G: Studies on *Vaccinium myrtillus* anthocyanosides. II. Aspects of anthocyanin pharmacokinetics in the rat. *ArzneimiHel-Forsch* **26**, 832–835, 1976.

4

Bromelain

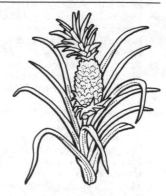

Key uses of bromelain:

- Inflammation
- Sports injuries
- Respiratory tract infections
- Painful menstruation
- Adjunct in cancer therapy

General description

Bromelain refers to a group of sulfur-containing enzymes that digest protein (proteolytic enzymes or proteases) obtained from the pineapple plant (*Ananas comusus*). Commercial bromelain is usually derived from the stem, which differs from the bromelain derived from the fruit. Commercial bromelain contains a mixture of several proteases and small amounts of several other enzymes, and organically bound calcium. Japan, Taiwan, and Hawaii are the major suppliers of commercial bromelain.[1]

History and folk use

Bromelain was introduced as a therapeutic agent in 1957, and since that time more than 200 scientific papers on its therapeutic applications have appeared in the medical literature.[2,3] Many of the early studies were performed using Ananase (Rorer), an enteric-coated bromelain tablet. Later studies implied that bromelain failed in some of these early studies because of the enteric coating as well as inadequate dosages.[3]

Pharmacology

Commercial bromelain has been reported to exert a wide variety of pharmacological effects: digestion assistance, antiinflammatory activity, burn debridement, prevention of swelling (edema), smooth muscle relaxation, inhibition of blood platelet aggregation, enhancement of antibiotic absorption, cancer treatment, ulcer prevention, sinusitis relief, appetite inhibition, shortening of labor, and enhancement of wound healing.[1-3] Most of these effects are discussed below.

Activating and deactivating factors

Being sulfhydryl proteases, like papain and ficin, both stem and fruit bromelains are inhibited by oxidizing agents, such as hydrogen peroxide, methyl bromide, and iodoacetate, and by certain metallic ions, such as lead, mercury, cadmium, copper, and iron. Human serum also inhibits bromelain protein-digesting activity. Magnesium and cysteine are activators of commercial bromelain.[1]

Strength

The activity of bromelain is expressed in a variety of enzyme units. The Food Chemistry Codex (FCC) officially recognizes the use of milk clotting units (mcu). The gelatin digesting unit (gdu) is another enzyme unit that is acceptable and equal in numerical value to the milk clotting unit. Different grades of bromelain are available on the basis of the milk clotting unit. For most indications the recommended milk clotting unit range is 1,200 to 1,800.

Absorption

Bromelain is absorbed via a number of routes, and has been effectively administered orally, parenterally, and through intravenous infusion.[4-6] Experiments with dogs have shown oral administration to result in peak levels at 10 hours, while detectable levels are still apparent at 48 hours. Intravenous infusion peaks in 50 minutes and remains detectable for 5 hours.[5] There is definite evidence that, in both animals and humans, up to 40 percent of the absorbed orally administered bromelain can be absorbed intact.[4-6]

Digestive activity

Bromelain is quite effective as a substitute for trypsin or pepsin in cases of pancreatic insufficiency.[2,3] Because of bromelain's ability to remain active over a wide pH range, it can act on substrates in the stomach (a low-pH environment) as well as in the small intestine (a high-pH environment). The combination of bromelain with pancreatin and ox bile has been demonstrated via double-blind studies to be highly effective in the treatment of patients with pancreatic insufficiency.[7]

Antiinflammatory activity

Several mechanisms may account for bromelain's antiinflammatory effects: (1) activation of proteolytic activity at sites of inflammation (although bromelain's proteolytic actions are inhibited by serum factors), (2) fibrinolysis activity via the plasminogen–plasmin system, (3) depletion of kininogen, and (4) inhibition of biosynthesis of proinflammatory prostaglandins and induction of prostaglandin E_1 accumulation (which tends to inhibit inflammation).[8–10]

The first hypothesis has not been substantiated, while the latter three may be part of the same mechanism of action. After tissue injury the kinin, complement, fibrinolytic, and clotting systems are activated (Figure 4.1). These systems are closely interrelated via activation of the Hageman factor (XII) and feedback mechanisms.

What fibrin does to promote the inflammatory response is to form a matrix that walls off the area of inflammation, resulting in blockage of blood vessels and inadequate tissue drainage and edema; in the meantime the kinin system cascade causes the production of kinins (e.g., bradykinin and kallidin). These compounds increase vascular permeability, causing edema (swelling) as well as evoking pain.

Bromelain reduces inflammation at first by breaking down fibrin, a process known as *fibrinolysis*. Bromelain does this by stimulating the production of plasmin, which breaks down the fibrin, thereby preventing fibrin from producing localized swelling.[8,9,11,12] Plasmin also blocks the formation of proinflammatory compounds.

Bromelain has also been shown to reduce plasma kininogen levels. The net result of this action is inhibition of the production of kinins.[13] As kinins cause much inflammation, swelling, and pain, inhibiting their production is warranted in the treatment of traumatic injuries such as sports injuries.

These actions—the activation of plasmin and the reduction of kinin levels—are probably the main pharmacological effects of bromelain. Brome-

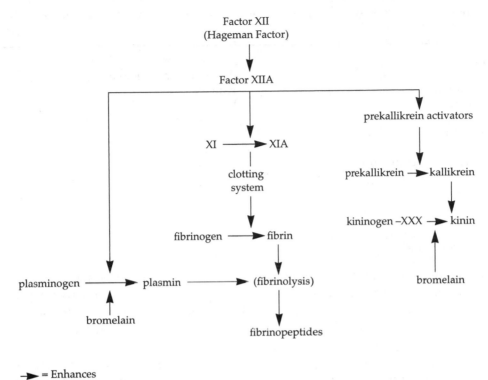

Figure 4.1 Bromelain's Effects on the Fibrin and Kinin Pathways

lain's ability to reduce inflammation has been documented in a variety of experimental models and clinical studies.

Antibiotic activity

Bromelain has been shown in clinical studies to increase serum levels of a variety of antibiotics (e.g., amoxycillin, tetracycline, and penicillin) in many different tissues and body fluids (e.g., cerebrospinal fluid, sputum, mucus, blood, urine, uterus, salpinx, ovary, gallbladder, appendix, and epithelial tissue).[14-16] In these studies the researchers concluded that bromelain itself possesses significant effects. Bromelain was as effective as antibiotics in treating a variety of infectious processes, that is, pneumonia, perirectal abscess, cutaneous staphylococcus infection, pyelonephritis, and bronchitis.[14]

Table 4.1 Conditions for which documented clinical evidence supports the use of bromelain

Angina	Maldigestion
Arthritis	Pancreatic insufficiency
Athletic injury	Pancreatitis
Bronchitis	Pneumonia
Burn debridement	Scleroderma
Cellulitis	Sinusitis
Dysmenorrhea	Staph infection
Ecchymosis (bruising)	Surgical trauma
Edema (swelling)	Thrombophlebitis

Anticancer activities

Bromelain exerts a number of unique anticancer effects. When added to the diet of mice with cancer, bromelain (0.3 percent of the diet by weight) decreased lung metastases by 90 percent.[17] This antimetastatic potential was demonstrated by both the active and inactive forms of bromelain, with or without proteolytic or anticoagulant activity.

In a study conducted at the Cancer Research Center of Hawaii (University of Hawaii, Honolulu, HI) bromelain significantly inhibited the growth of tumor cells in cell cultures.[18] (It should be noted that this study found another enzyme, known as *peroxidase*, to be the major antitumor component.)

Other animal and *in vitro* studies have shown that bromelain exerts substantial anticancer properties.[3,19] These studies indicate that the anticancer effects go beyond the proteolytic and fibrinolytic effect of bromelain.

Clinical applications

Bromelain is one of the most popular natural agents in use. Because of its ability to impact many aspects of inflammation, it is used predominantly in cases of injury, sprains, strains, arthritis, and other inflammatory conditions. However, it is also used as a digestive aid and in respiratory tract infections, thrombophlebitis, varicose veins, dysmenorrhea, and as an adjunct in cancer therapy (see Table 4.1).

Arthritis

Bromelain can be useful in both rheumatoid arthritis and osteoarthritis. It is especially effective alone or in combination with curcumin in reducing the need for corticosteroids (such as prednisone) in rheumatoid arthritis. In one study, twenty-five patients with severe rheumatoid arthritis, along with one patient with both rheumatoid arthritis and osteoarthritis, two patients with osteoarthritis alone, and one patient with gout who had residual joint swelling and impairment in mobility following long-term corticosteroid therapy, were given bromelain.[20] Their corticosteroid doses were tapered to small maintenance doses and they received enteric-coated bromelain (20 to 40 milligrams three to four times daily). Most patients experienced a significant reduction in residual joint swelling, and joint mobility was increased soon after supplementation was started. After 3 weeks to 13 months of observation, eight of twenty-nine (28 percent) had excellent results, thirteen of twenty-nine (45 percent) had good results, four of twenty-nine (14 percent) had fair results, and four of twenty-nine (14 percent) had poor results. The patient with gout had poor results. One of the osteoarthritis patients reported good results; the other described fair results. Smaller amounts of steroids were needed when bromelain was given concurrently. Even better results may have been obtained by using a non-enteric-coated product.

Surgical procedures

The effect of orally administered bromelain on the reduction of swelling, bruising, healing time, and pain following various surgical procedures has been demonstrated in several clinical studies.[21-24] Studies of patients undergoing oral surgery concluded that, while giving bromelain after surgery is effective, a regimen of giving bromelain before and after surgery is recommended.[21,22]

In one double-blind study of patients undergoing oral surgery, bromelain was found to be significantly superior to the placebo: swelling decreased in 3.8 days with bromelain, compared with 7 days for the placebo; and the duration of pain was reduced to 5.1 days in the bromelain group, compared with 8.1 days in the placebo group.[22] Similar observations were made in studies of episiotomy cases. Bromelain reduced edema, inflammation, and pain, and preoperative administration potentiated the effects.[23,24]

Athletic injuries

Bromelain has been used in a variety of sports-related injuries. Perhaps the most interesting was a 1960 study involving boxers.[25] Fifty-eight of seventy-four boxers receiving bromelain reported that all signs of bruising had cleared completely within 4 days. Of the remaining sixteen, complete clearance took 8 to 10 days. Of the seventy-two controls, only ten showed bruises completely cleared at the end of 4 days, the remainder taking 7 to 14 days.

It is important to recognize that, while bromelain has been shown to reduce pain effectively, this is probably the result of a reduction in tissue inflammation and edema, rather than a direct analgesic effect.

Respiratory tract diseases

Bromelain exerts an antitussive effect (suppression of cough) when used to treat chronic bronchitis, and reduces the viscosity of sputum (mucolytic activity). Patients examined with a specialized apparatus for determining respiratory function (a spirometer) before and after bromelain treatment showed increased lung capacity and function. These favorable effects were believed to be the results of enhanced resolution of respiratory congestion, owing to bromelain's ability to fluidify and decrease bronchial secretions. It appears that bromelain's mucolytic activity is responsible for its particular effectiveness in respiratory tract diseases.[26]

Acute sinusitis also responds to bromelain therapy. Good to excellent results were obtained in 87 percent of bromelain-treated patients, compared with 68 percent of the placebo group.[27]

Thrombophlebitis

Numerous investigators have demonstrated that orally administered bromelain has a very favorable effect on acute thrombophlebitis (inflammation of a vein), deep vein thrombosis, cellulitis, bruises, and edema.[28-31] In a double-blind study involving seventy-three patients with acute thrombophlebitis, bromelain, as an adjunct to analgesics, was shown to reduce all the symptoms of inflammation: pain, edema, redness, tenderness, elevated skin temperature, and disability.[29] In this study and others, the common daily dose of bromelain was 60 to 160 milligrams of 1,200-mcu bromelain. According to some researchers, doses of 400 to 800 milligrams are needed to achieve consistent results in patients with thrombophlebitis; this probably holds true for most other conditions as well.[28]

Varicose veins

Individuals with varicose veins have a decreased ability to break down fibrin. Vein walls are an important source of plasminogen activator, which promotes the breakdown of fibrin. Veins that have become varicosed have decreased levels of plasminogen activator, leading to the deposition of fibrin in the tissue near the varicose veins and causing the surrounding skin to become hard and "lumpy." Decreased fibrinolytic activity increases the risk of thrombus formation, which may result in thrombophlebitis, myocardial infarction, pulmonary embolism, or stroke. Bromelain acts in a manner similar to plasminogen activator to cause fibrin breakdown.[8]

Bromelain should be used before and after going through any surgical preparation for stripping or ligating varicose veins.[32] In one study concerning a series of 180 consecutive operations for varicose veins, bromelain was given to alternate patients at a dose of 40 milligrams four times daily from the first to the third postoperative day and 20 milligrams four times daily from the fourth to the seventh day, as a prophylactic (i.e., preventative) treatment of hematomas and excessive bruising. The number of hematomas and bruises was significantly lower in the treated group. After 2 weeks, sixty-five of the ninety treated patients had no hematomas whereas only thirty-two of the ninety untreated patients had no hematomas.

Dysmenorrhea

Bromelain and papain have been used successfully in the treatment of dysmenorrhea (painful menstruation).[33] Bromelain is believed to be a smooth muscle relaxant, since it decreases the spasms of the contracted cervix in these patients. Note, however, that the active agent in this treatment may not be the main protease—when used alone, bromelain protease (purified by adsorption) failed to produce the desired effect.

Cancer

Bromelain may augment standard chemotherapy treatment. In one study conducted in Germany, administration of oral bromelain, sometimes given with subtoxic doses of chemotherapeutic drugs such as 5-fluorouracil and vincristine, resulted in significant tumor regression.[34] Doses less than 100 milligrams daily of active bromelain were inadequate. It appears that up to 2.4 grams per day may be necessary for optimal effects. Furthermore, not all bromelain preparations were equally beneficial. The most effective preparations were nonenteric coated, with a milk clotting unit activity between 1,200 and 1,800. Nieper[34] believes the therapeutic effect may be due to bromelain's ability to "deshield" the tumor cell's fibrin coat, providing the immune system with more ready access to them.

In another study, this one in France, twelve patients with different tumors were treated with 600 milligrams of bromelain daily for 6 months to several years.[35] Cancerous masses of ovarian carcinoma resolved, and most breast cancers and metastases decreased markedly compared to standard therapy alone.

These results are quite promising and suggest that bromelain, in addition to enhancing the effectiveness of standard chemotherapy, may exert effects on its own.

Dosage

Unless bromelain is being used as a digestive aid, administration should be made on an empty stomach (between meals). The dosage depends largely on the potency of the bromelain preparation. Most currently available bromelain is in the 1,200- to 1,800-mcu range, with the typical dosage being 250 to 500 milligrams three times per day between meals.

Toxicity

Very large doses of bromelain (nearly 2.0 grams) have been given with no side effects.[36] It is virtually nontoxic, as no LD_{50} (50 percent lethal dose) exists up to 10 grams per kilogram. Chronic use appears to be well tolerated. Although no significant side effects have been noted, allergic reactions may occur (as with most therapeutic agents) in sensitive individuals or with prolonged occupational exposure.[37,38] Other possible, but unconfirmed, reactions include nausea, vomiting, diarrhea, metrorrhagia, and menorrhagia.[39]

References

1. Leung A: *Encyclopedia of Common Natural Ingredients Used in Foods, Drugs, and Cosmetics.* John Wiley & Sons, New York, 1980, pp. 74–76.
2. Taussig S, *et al.*: Bromelain, a proteolytic enzyme and its clinical application. A review. *Hiroshima J Med Sci* **24**, 185–193, 1975.
3. Taussig S and Batkin S: Bromelain, the enzyme complex of pineapple (*Ananas comosus*) and its clinical application. An update. *J Ethnopharmacol* **22**, 191–203, 1988.
4. Miller J and Opher A: The increased proteolytic activity of human blood serum after oral administration of bromelain. *Exp Med Surg* **22**, 277–280, 1964.
5. Izaka K, Yamada M, Kawano T, and Suyama T: Gastrointestinal absorption and anti-inflammatory effect of bromelain. *Jpn J Pharmacol* **22**, 519–534, 1972.
6. Seifert J, Ganser R, and Brendel W: Absorption of a proteolytic enzyme of plant origin from the gastrointestinal tract into the blood and lymph of adult rats. *Z Gastroenterol* **17**, 1–18, 1979.
7. Balakrishnan V, Hareendran A, and Nair C: Double-blind cross-over trial of an enzyme preparation in pancreatic steatorrhoea. *J Assoc Phys Ind* **29**, 207–209, 1981.
8. Ako H, Cheung A, and Matsura P: Isolation of a fibrinolysis enzyme activator from commercial bromelain. *Arch Int Pharmacodyn* **254**, 157–167, 1981.
9. Taussig S: The mechanism of the physiological action of bromelain. *Med Hypothesis* **6**, 99–104, 1980.
10. Felton G: Does kinin released by pineapple stem bromelain stimulate production of prostaglandin E_1-like compounds? *Hawaii Med J* **36**, 39–47, 1977.

11. Pirotta F and de Giuli-Morghen C: Bromelain—a deeper pharmacological study. Note I. Anti-inflammatory and serum fibrinolytic activity after oral administration in the rat. *Drugs Exp Clin Res* **4**, 1–20, 1978.

12. de Giuli-Morghen C and Pirotta F: Bromelain—a deeper pharmacological study. Note II. Interaction with some protease inhibitors and rabbit specific antiserum. *Drugs Exp Clin Res* **4**, 21–37, 1978.

13. Katori M, *et al.*: A possible role of prostaglandins and bradykinin as a trigger of exudation in carrageenan-induced rat pleurisy. *Agents Actions* **8**, 108–112, 1978.

14. Neubauer R: A plant protease for the potentiation of and possible replacement of antibiotics. *Exp Med Surg* **19**, 143–160, 1961.

15. Luerti M and Vignali M: Influence of bromelain on penetration of antibiotics in uterus, salpinx and ovary. *Drugs Exp Clin Res* **4**, 45–48, 1978.

16. Tinozzi S and Venegoni A: Effect of bromelain on serum and tissue levels of amoxycillin. *Drugs Exp Clin Res* **4**, 39–44, 1978.

17. Batkin S, *et al.*: Antimetastatic effect of bromelain with or without its proteolytic and anticoagulant activity. *J Cancer Res Clin Oncol* **114**, 507–508, 1988.

18. Taussig SJ, Szekerczes J, and Batkin S: Inhibition of tumour growth in vitro by bromelain, an extract of the pineapple plant (*Ananas comosus*). *Planta Med* **52**, 538–539, 1985.

19. Maurer HR, *et al.*: Bromelain induces the differentiation of leukemic cells in vitro: An explanation for its cytostatic effects? *Planta Medica* **54**, 377–381, 1988.

20. Cohen A and Goldman J: Bromelain therapy in rheumatoid arthritis. *Pennsyl Med J* **67**, 27–30, June 1964.

21. Tassman G, Zafran J, and Zayon G: Evaluation of a plant proteolytic enzyme for the control of inflammation and pain. *J Dent Med* **19**, 73–77, 1964.

22. Tassman G, Zafran J, and Zayon G: A double-blind crossover study of a plant proteolytic enzyme in oral surgery. *J Dent Med* **20**, 51–54, 1965.

23. Howat R and Lewis G: The effect of bromelain therapy on episiotomy wounds—a double blind controlled clinical trial. *J Obstet Gynecol Br Common* **79**, 951–953, 1972.

24. Zatuchni G and Colombi D: Bromelain therapy for the prevention of episiotomy pain. *Obstet Gynecol* **29**, 275–278, 1967.

25. Blonstein J: Control of swelling in boxing injuries. *Practitioner* **203**, 206, 1960.

26. Rimoldi R, Ginesu F, and Giura R: The use of bromelain in pneumological therapy. *Drugs Exp Clin Res* **4**, 55–66, 1978

27. Ryan R: A double-blind clinical evaluation of bromelains in the treatment of acute sinusitis. *Headache* **7**, 13–17, 1967.

28. Taussig S and Nieper H: Bromelain: Its use in prevention and treatment of cardiovascular disease: Present status. *J Int Assoc Prev Med* **6**, 139–151, 1979.

29. Seligman B: Oral bromelains as adjuncts in the treatment of acute thrombophlebitis. *Angiology* **20**, 22–26, 1969.

30. Seligman B: Bromelain: An anti-inflammatory agent. *Angiology* **13**, 508–510, 1962.

31. Felton G: Fibrinolytic and antithrombotic action of bromelain may eliminate thrombosis in heart patients. *Med Hypothesis* **6**, 1123–1133, 1980.

32. Durant JH and Waibel PP: Prevention of hematoma in surgery of varices. *Praxis* **61**, 950–951, 1972.

33. Hunter RG, Henry GW, and Henicke RM: The action of papain and bromelain on the uterus. *Am J Obstet Gynecol* **73**, 867–880, 1957.

34. Nieper HA: Bromelain in der kontrolle malignen Washstums. *Krebsgeschehen* **1**, 9–15, 1976.

35. Gérard G: Therapeutique anti-cancreuse et bromelaines. *Agressologie* **3**, 261–274, 1972.

36. Gutfreund A, Taussig S, and Morris A: Effect of oral bromelain on blood pressure and heart rate of hypertensive patients. *Hawaii Med J* **37**, 143–146, 1978.

37. Baur X: Studies on the specificity of human IgE-antibodies to the plant proteases papain and bromelain. *Clin Allergy* **9**, 451–457, 1979.

38. Baur X and Fruhman G: Allergic reactions, including asthma, to the pineapple protease bromelain following occupational exposure. *Clin Allergy* **9**, 443–450, 1979.

39. Ananase (Rorer). In: *Physicians Desk Reference*. Medical Economics Company, Oradell, NJ, 1982, p. 1645.

5
Cayenne pepper

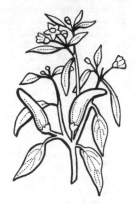

Key uses of cayenne pepper:

Oral:

- Antioxidant support
- Atherosclerosis

For asthma:

- Pain disorders
- Diabetic neuropathy
- Cluster headaches
- Arthritis
- Psoriasis

General description

Cayenne pepper (also known as chili or red hot pepper) is the fruit of *Capsicum annuum*, a shrubby, tropical plant that can grow to a height of up to 3 feet. The fruit is technically a berry. Paprika is a milder and sweeter-tasting fruit produced from a different variety of capsicum. Although cayenne pepper is native to tropical America, it is now cultivated in tropical locations throughout the world and has found its way into the cuisine of many parts of the world, particularly Southeast Asia, China, southern Italy, and Mexico.

Chemical composition

Capsaicin is the active component of cayenne pepper.[1] It is also the component responsible for the pungent and irritating effects of cayenne pepper—

in other words, it's what makes red pepper hot. Typically, cayenne pepper contains about 1.5 percent capsaicin and related principles.

Other active constituents present include carotenoids, vitamins A and C, and volatile oils.

History and folk use

The folk use of cayenne pepper is quite extensive; it was used for asthma, fevers, sore throats, and other respiratory tract infections, digestive disturbances, poultices, and cancers.

Pharmacology

The pharmacology of cayenne pepper centers on its capsaicin content.

Antioxidant activity

The carotene molecules of cayenne pepper and paprika exert powerful antioxidant effects.

Cardiovascular effects

Cayenne pepper exerts a number of benefical effects on the cardiovascular system. In addition to possessing excellent antioxidant compounds, studies have shown that cayenne pepper reduces the likelihood of developing atherosclerosis by reducing blood cholesterol and triglyceride levels; in addition, it reduces platelet aggregation and increases fibrinolytic activity.[2–4] (For the significance of these effects, see Chapter 11—Garlic.) Cultures consuming large amounts of cayenne pepper have a much lower rate of cardiovascular disease.

Topical effects

When topically applied to the skin or mucous membranes, capsaicin is known to stimulate and then block small-diameter pain fibers by depleting them of a neurotransmitter called substance P. Substance P is thought to be the principal chemomediator of pain impulses from the periphery. In addition, substance P has been shown to activate inflammatory mediators in joint tissues in osteoarthritis and rheumatoid arthritis.[1]

Clinical applications

Cayenne pepper should be recommended as a food for its beneficial antioxidant and cardiovascular effects. Although people with active peptic ulcers may be bothered by "spicy" foods containing cayenne pepper, spicy foods do not cause ulcers in normal individuals. In fact, cayenne pepper exerts several beneficial effects on gastrointestinal function.[5]

Interestingly enough, capsaicin, although hot to the taste, actually lowers body temperature by stimulating the cooling center of the hypothalamus in the brain.[6] The ingestion of cayenne peppers by cultures native to the tropics appears to help these people deal with high temperatures.

Modern clinical use of cayenne pepper has focused on the use of topical capsaicin-containing preparations. Commercial ointments containing 0.025 or 0.075 percent capsaicin are available over the counter. These preparations may offer significant benefit in a number of conditions, including pain disorders (e.g., postamputation pain, postmastectomy pain, post-herpetic neuralgia), diabetic neuropathy, cluster headaches, osteoarthritis, and rheumatoid arthritis. In addition, topically applied capsaicin may be useful in the treatment of psoriasis.

Post-herpetic neuralgia

Initial studies examined the use of topically applied capsaicin in relieving the pain associated with shingles (herpes zoster), a clinical condition known as post-herpetic neuralgia. Numerous studies now document this Food and Drug Administration (FDA)-approved application.

For example, in one study[7] thirty-nine patients with chronic post-herpetic neuralgia (average duration, 24 months) were treated with 0.025 percent capsaicin cream for 8 weeks. During therapy the patients rated their pain. Nineteen patients (48.7 percent) substantially improved after the 8-week trial; five (12.8 percent) discontinued therapy owing to side effects such as intolerable capsaicin-induced burning sensations (four patients) or mastitis (one patient); fifteen (38.5 percent) reported no benefit. The decrease in pain ratings was significant after 2 weeks of continuous application. Of the responders, 72.2 percent were still improved 10 to 12 months after the study, with most continuing to apply the cream regularly.

In general, the results of this study are consistent with other studies, that is, about 50 percent of people with post-herpetic neuralgia respond to topically applied capsaicin (0.025 percent).[8-11] Although this may not be a great response, it is better than the 10 percent response noted in the placebo group. A higher concentration (0.075 percent versus 0.025 percent) may produce better results (as high as 75 percent response).[12]

Trigeminal neuralgia

Topically applied capsaicin may be effective in reducing the pain of trigeminal neuralgia (also known as *tic douloureux*)—a painful disorder of the main nerve of the face characterized by severe, stabbing pain affecting the cheek, lips, gums, or chin on one side of the face. In one study,[13] twelve patients were followed up for 1 year after a topical application of capsaicin (three times a day for several days) over the painful area. Six patients experienced complete relief and four patients had partial relief from pain; the remaining two patients felt no relief from pain. Of the ten patients who did respond to therapy, four relapsed in 95–149 days. None relapsed, following a second round of therapy, for the remainder of the year. These results are quite promising for a condition that usually does not respond to any therapy short of surgery.

Postmastectomy pain

Topically applied capsaicin may help relieve the pain following breast reconstruction or mastectomy. In one double-blind study, twenty-three patients with postmastectomy pain syndrome (PMPS) applied either capsaicin (0.075 percent) or vehicle-only cream four times daily for 4–6 weeks.[14] There was a significant difference in jabbing pain, in category pain severity scales, and in overall pain relief scales in favor of capsaicin. Five of thirteen patients on capsaicin were categorized as good-to-excellent responses, with eight (62 percent) having 50 percent or greater improvement. Only one of ten patients reported a good response to vehicle, with three rated as 50 percent or better.

In another study, fourteen patients with postmastectomy pain experienced significant pain relief following application of 0.025 percent capsaicin cream four times daily for 4–6 weeks.[15] Unpleasant or painful sensations in response to light touch or pressure in the painful area (hyperesthesia, allodynia) were also improved.

Mouth pain due to chemotherapy or radiation

In a study conducted at the Yale Pain Management Center (New Haven, CT), capsaicin was shown to reduce dramatically the pain of mouth sores resulting from chemotherapy or radiation treatment.[16] The interesting feature in this study was the vehicle used to deliver the capsaicin—taffy. The researchers chose taffy because it could be held in the mouth long enough to desensitize the neurons, its sugar decreased the initial burning sensation, and its soft edges would not aggravate sore mouths as did hard candy. All eleven patients in the Yale study said their pain decreased—in two cases stopping entirely—after eating the capsaicin-laced candy.

Diabetic neuropathy

Diabetic neuropathy is a painful nerve disorder caused by long-term diabetes. Topically applied capsaicin has been shown in numerous double-blind studies[17–22] to be of considerable benefit in relieving the pain of diabetic neuropathy.

For example, in one large, double-blind, 8-week study investigators at twelve sites enrolled 277 men and women with painful diabetic neuropathy of the hands and feet; 69.5 percent of the group applied capsaicin cream (0.075 percent) showed improvement compared to 53.4 percent who applied a vehicle (i.e., inert substance) cream.

In another study, forty patients applied either 0.075 percent capsaicin cream or placebo to their affected extremities daily. After 4 weeks, 76 percent of treated patients had some pain relief, compared to 50 percent of placebo patients. In addition, those responding to capsaicin said their pain was cut in half, while those on placebo averaged between 15 and 20 percent relief.

Cluster headaches

Cluster headaches are migraine-like headache characterized by severe pain, usually localized around one eye. They are called cluster headaches because they tend to occur in clusters of one to three headaches a day for a few days, recurring every few months. Unlike migraines, there are no warning symptoms. Double-blind studies indicate that intranasal application of a special capsaicin ointment by a physician may relieve cluster headaches.

In one double-blind study, patients with acute cluster headaches were randomized to receive either capsaicin or placebo in the nostril for 7 days.[23] Patients recorded the severity of each headache for 15 days. Headaches on days 8–15 of the study were significantly less severe in the capsaicin group versus the placebo group. There was also a significant decrease in headache severity in the capsaicin group on days 8–15 compared to days 1–7, but not in the placebo group. Episodic patients appeared to benefit more than chronic patients.

Arthritis

Topically applied capsaicin may be effective in relieving the pain of either osteoarthritis or rheumatoid arthritis. While one study showed it to be more effective in osteoarthritis, another study showed just the opposite.

In the double-blind study showing more effect in osteoarthritis,[24] seven patients with rheumatoid arthritis and fourteen patients with osteoarthritis, all of whom had painful involvement of the hands, applied either capsaicin 0.075 percent or vehicle-only cream to the hands four times daily. Capsaicin reduced tenderness and pain associated with osteoarthritis, but not rheumatoid arthritis.

In the study showing greater benefit for rheumatoid arthritis,[25] seventy patients with osteoarthritis and thirty-one with rheumatoid arthritis received capsaicin or placebo for 4 weeks. The patients were instructed to apply 0.025 percent capsaicin cream or its vehicle (placebo) to painful knees four times daily. Significantly more relief of pain was reported by the capsaicin-treated patients than by the placebo patients throughout the study; after 4 weeks of capsaicin treatment, rheumatoid and osteoarthritis patients demonstrated mean reductions in pain of 57 and 33 percent, respectively. These reductions in pain were statistically significant compared with those reported for the placebo group. According to overall evaluations, 80 percent of the capsaicin-treated patients experienced a reduction in pain after 2 weeks of treatment.

Psoriasis

Excessive substance P levels in the skin have been linked to psoriasis. This finding prompted researchers to study the effects of topically applied capsaicin. In one double-blind study, forty-four patients with symmetrically distributed psoriasis lesions applied topical capsaicin to one side of their body and a placebo to the other side.[26] After 3–6 weeks, significantly greater reductions in scaling and redness were observed on the capsaicin-treated side. Burning, stinging, itching, and skin redness were noted by nearly half of the patients initially, but these diminished or vanished on continued application.

In a more recent study, 197 patients applied capsaicin 0.025 percent cream or placebo cream four times a day for 6 weeks.[27] Efficacy was based on a physician's evaluation and a combined psoriasis severity score including scaling, thickness, erythema, and itchiness (pruritus). Capsaicin-treated patients demonstrated significantly greater improvement in physician's evaluation and in pruritus relief, as well as a significantly greater reduction in combined psoriasis severity.

Dosage

Cayenne pepper can be used liberally in the diet. Creams containing 0.025 or 0.075 percent capsaicin may be applied to affected areas up to four times daily.

Toxicity

Cayenne pepper is generally recognized as safe (GRAS) in the United States. Topically applied capsaicin may produce a local burning sensation; however, this effect fades away with time and is rarely severe enough to prevent use of the cream.

References

1. Cordell GA and Araujo OE: Capsaicin: Identification, nomenclature, and pharmacotherapy. *Ann Pharmacother* **27**, 330–336, 1993.
2. Kawada T, *et al.*: Effects of capsaicin on lipid metabolism in rats fed a high fat diet. *J Nutr* **116**, 1272–1278, 1986.
3. Wang JP, *et al.*: Antiplatelet effect of capsaicin. *Thrombosis Res* **36**, 497–507, 1984.
4. Visudhiphan S, *et al.*: The relationship between high fibrinolytic activity and daily capsicum ingestion in Thais. *Am J Clin Nutr* **35**, 1452–1458, 1982.
5. Horowitz M, *et al.*: The effect of chilli on gastrointestinal transit. *J Gastroenterol Hepatol* **7**, 52–56, 1992.
6. Dib B: Effects of intrathecal capsaicin on autonomic and behavioral heat loss responses in the rat. *Pharmacol Biochem Behav* **28**, 65–70, 1987.
7. Peikert A, *et al.*: Topical 0.025% capsaicin in chronic post-herpetic neuralgia: Efficacy, predictors of response and long-term course. *J Neurol* **238**, 452–456, 1991.
8. Bjerring P, *et al.*: Argon laser induced cutaneous sensory and pain thresholds in post-herpetic neuralgia. Quantitative modulation by topical capsaicin. *Acta Derm Venereol (Stockh)* **70**, 121–125, 1990.
9. Bernstein JE, *et al.*: Topical capsaicin treatment of chronic post-herpetic neuralgia. *J Am Acad Dermatol* **21**, 265–270, 1989.
10. Watson CP, *et al.*: Post-herpetic neuralgia and topical capsaicin. *Pain* **33**, 333–340, 1988.
11. Watson CPN, *et al.*: Post-herpetic neuralgia: 208 cases. *Pain* **35**, 289–297, 1988.
12. Bernstein JE, *et al.*: Treatment of chronic post-herpetic neuralgia with topical capsaicin. A preliminary study. *J Am Acad Dermatol* **17**, 93–96, 1987.
13. Fusco BM and Alessandri M: Analgesic effect of capsaicin in idiopathic trigeminal neuralgia. *Anesth Analg* **74**, 375–377, 1992.
14. Watson CP and Evans RJ: The postmastectomy pain syndrome and topical capsaicin: A randomized trial. *Pain* **51**, 375–379, 1992.
15. Watson CPN, *et al.*: The post-mastectomy pain syndrome and the effect of topical capsaicin. *Pain* **38**, 177–186, 1989.
16. Nelson C: Heal the burn: Pepper and lasers in cancer pain therapy. *J Natl Cancer Inst* **86**, 1381, 1994.
17. The Capsaicin Study Group: Effect of treatment with capsaicin on daily activities of patients with painful diabetic neuropathy. *Diabetes Care* **15**, 159–165, 1992.
18. Chad, D: *Med World News*, February 27, 1989.
19. Tandan R, *et al.*: Topical capsaicin in painful diabetic neuropathy. Controlled study with long-term follow-up. *Diabetes Care* **15**, 8–14, 1992.
20. Tandan R, *et al.*: Topical capsaicin in painful diabetic neuropathy. Effect on sensory function. *Diabetes Care* **15**, 15–18, 1992.
21. Basha KM and Whitehouse FW: Capsaicin: A therapeutic option for painful diabetic neuropathy. *Henry Ford Hosp Med J* **39**, 138–140, 1991.
22. Pfeifer MA, *et al.*: A highly successful and novel model for treatment of chronic painful diabetic peripheral neuropathy. *Diabetes Care* **16**, 1103–1115, 1993.
23. Marks DR, *et al.*: A double-blind placebo-controlled trial of intranasal capsaicin for cluster headache. *Cephalalgia* **13**, 114–116, 1993.
24. McCarthy GM and McCarty DJ: Effect of topical capsaicin in the therapy of painful osteoarthritis of the hands. *J Rheumatol* **19**, 604–607, 1992.
25. Deal CL, *et al.*: Treatment of arthritis with topical capsaicin: A double-blind trial. *Clin Ther* **13**, 383–395, 1991.
26. Bernstein JE, *et al.*: Effects of topically applied capsaicin on moderate and severe psoriasis vulgaris. *J Am Acad Dermatol* **15**, 504–507, 1986.
27. Ellis CN, *et al.*: A double-blind evaluation of topical capsaicin in pruritic psoriasis. *J Am Acad Dermatol* **29**(3), 438–442, 1993.

6

Coleus forskohlii

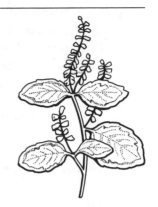

Key uses of *Coleus forskohlii*:

- Eczema
- Asthma
- Psoriasis
- Angina
- High blood pressure

General description

Coleus forskohlii is a small, perennial member of the mint family (Labiatae). It grows on the sun-exposed, dry slopes of the mountains of India, Nepal, Sri Lanka, and Thailand, at an altitude of 1,000 to 6,000 feet. Its Latin name comes from the word *coleos*, which means sheath and refers to the fused filaments that form a sheath around the stylus of the flower. The epithet *forskohlii* was given to commemorate the Finnish botanist Forskal, who traveled extensively in Egypt and Arabia in the eighteenth century.

The radially spread rootstock is the portion of the plant used for medicinal purposes. The rootstock is also the source of a compound of unique biological importance—forskolin. No other species of coleus contains forskolin.

Chemical composition

The primary chemical of interest contained in *C. forskohlii* is forskolin. Forskolin was discovered during a large-scale screening of medicinal plants by the Indian Central Drug Research Institute in 1974.[1] The screening revealed the presence of a hypotensive and spasmolytic component of

C. forskohlii, which was named coleanol.[1] Additional investigation determined the exact chemical structure and the name was changed to forskolin. Between 1981 and 1994 forskolin has been used in more than 5,000 *in vitro* research studies designed to better understand cellular processes governed by cyclic adenosine monophosphate (cAMP; discussed below). While most of these studies have used isolated forskolin, there is evidence that other components within the plant extract enhance the absorption and biological activity of forskolin. However, no detailed analysis of the chemical composition of *C. forskohlii* could be found.

History and folk use

Coleus forskohlii has a long history of use in Ayurvedic, Siddha, and Unani systems of medicine. The pharmacological activity of forskolin substantiates the traditional uses of *C. forskohlii*, which includes the treatment of cardiovascular disease, eczema, abdominal colic, respiratory disorders, painful urination, insomnia, and convulsions.[1]

Pharmacology

The basic mechanism of action of forskolin is the activation of an enzyme, adenylate cyclase, which increases the amount of cyclic adenosine monophosphate (cAMP) in cells.[2] Cyclic AMP is perhaps the most important cell-regulating compound. Once formed it activates many other enzymes involved in diverse cellular functions.

Under normal conditions cAMP forms when a stimulatory hormone (e.g., epinephrine) binds to a receptor site on the cell membrane and stimulates the activation of adenylate cyclase. This enzyme is incorporated into all cellular membranes, and only the specificity of the receptor determines which hormone will activate it in a particular cell. Forskolin appears to bypass this need for direct hormonal activation of adenylate cyclase via transmembrane activation. As a result of this activation of adenylate cyclase, intracellular cAMP levels rise.

The physiological and biochemical effects of a raised intracellular cAMP level include the following: inhibition of platelet activation and degranulation, inhibition of mast cell degranulation and histamine release, increased force of contraction of heart muscle, relaxation of the arteries and other smooth muscles, increased insulin secretion, increased thyroid function, and increased lipolysis.

Recent studies have found forskolin to possess additional mechanisms of action independent of its ability to stimulate adenylate cyclase and cAMP-dependent responses directly.[3] Specifically, forskolin inhibits a number of membrane transport proteins and channel proteins through a mechanism that does not involve the production of cAMP. The result, once again, is a transmembrane signal that results in activation of other cellular enzymes. Research is under way in an attempt to determine the exact receptors to which forskolin binds.

Forskolin also antagonizes the action of platelet-activating factor (PAF) by interfering with the binding of PAF to receptor sites on cells.[4] Platelet-activating factor plays a central role in many inflammatory and allergic processes, including neutrophil activation, increasing vascular permeability, smooth muscle contraction (including bronchoconstriction), and reduction in coronary blood flow. After treatment of platelets with forskolin prior to PAF binding, a 30–40 percent decrease in PAF binding was observed. The decrease in PAF binding caused by forskolin was concomitant with a decrease in the physiological responses of platelets induced by PAF. However, this forskolin-induced decrease in PAF binding was not a consequence of cAMP formation, as the addition of a cAMP analog could not mimic the action of forskolin. In addition, the inactive analog of forskolin, dideoxyforskolin, which does not activate adenylate cyclase, also reduced PAF binding to its receptor. Researchers speculate that the action of forskolin on PAF binding is due to a direct effect of this molecule and its analog on the PAF receptor itself or to components of the postreceptor signaling for PAF.

Clinical applications

The therapeutic ramifications of *C. forskohlii*, based on the pharmacology of forskolin, are immense. There are many conditions in which a decreased intracellular cAMP level is thought to be a major factor in the development of the disease process. At present *C. forskolii* appears to be extremely well indicated in these types of conditions, which include eczema (atopic dermatitis), asthma, psoriasis, angina, and hypertension. Although *C. forskohlii* can be used alone, it may prove to be most useful when combined with other botanicals and/or other measures in the treatment of these disorders.

Asthma and other allergic conditions

Allergic conditions such as asthma and eczema are characterized by a relative decrease in cAMP in the bronchial smooth muscle and skin, respectively. As a result of this derangement, mast cells degranulate and smooth muscle cells contract. In addition, these allergic conditions are also characterized by excessive levels of PAF.

Current drug therapy for allergic conditions such as asthma and eczema is largely designed to increase cAMP levels by using substances that bind to receptors to stimulate adenylate cyclase (e.g., corticosteroids) or inhibit the enzyme phosphodiesterase, which breaks down cAMP once it is formed (e.g., methylxanthines). These actions are not like that of forskolin, which increases the initial production of cAMP via a transmembrane activation of adenylate cyclase. The cAMP-elevating action of forskolin supports the use of *C. forskohlii* extracts alone or in combination with standard drug therapy in the treatment of virtually all allergic conditions.

Coleus forskohlii extracts may be particularly useful in the treatment of asthma, as increasing cellular levels of cAMP result in relaxation of bronchial muscles and relief of asthma symptoms. Forskolin has been shown to have remarkable effects in relaxing constricted bronchial muscles in asthmatics.[5–7] The bronchials are composed of what is known as smooth muscle. This type of muscle is also found in the gastrointestinal tract, uterus, bladder, and arteries. Forskolin exerts a tremendous antispasmodic action on these various smooth muscles.[1] This antispasmodic action of forskolin supports the long history of use of *C. forskholii* in the treatment not only of asthma, but also intestinal colic, uterine cramps (menstrual cramps), painful urination, angina, and hypertension.

Forskolin's ability to relax smooth muscle in bronchial asthma is most probably due to an increase in cAMP, although forskolin has other antiallergic activities, such as inhibiting the release of histamine and the synthesis of allergic compounds.[8]

One double-blind clinical study sought to determine the antiasthmatic effects of forskolin compared to the drug fenoterol.[7] Sixteen patients with asthma were given single inhalative doses of fenoterol dry powder capsules (0.4 milligrams), metered doses of fenoterol (0.4 milligrams), and forskolin dry powder capsules (10.0 milligrams). All substances caused a significant improvement in respiratory function and bronchodilation. However, while the fenoterol preparations caused tremors and a decrease in blood potassium levels, no such negative effects were seen with forskolin.

In another study, the bronchodilating effect (after 5 minutes) of forskolin was as good as that produced by fenoterol in twelve healthy volunteers (nonsmokers) as determined by whole-body plethysmography.[9] Both substances were administered by metered dose inhalers. At the beginning (after 3 and 5 minutes) the protective effect of forskolin against inhaled acetylcholine was as good as that produced by fenoterol, whereas later on (after 15 and 30 minutes) fenoterol performed better.

Whether orally administered forskolin in the form of *C. forskohlii* extract would produce similar bronchodilatory effects has yet to be determined. However, on the basis of the plant's historical use and additional mechanisms of action it is extremely likely.

Psoriasis

Psoriasis is an extremely common skin disorder that seems to be caused by a decrease in cAMP in relation to another cell-regulating compound, cyclic guanine monophosphate (cGMP). The result is a tremendous increase in cell division. In fact, psoriatic cells divide at a rate 1,000 times greater than do normal cells. Preliminary studies have indicated that forskolin may be of great benefit to individuals with psoriasis, because of its ability to normalize the balance that exists between cAMP and cGMP.[1]

Cardiovascular effects

Perhaps the most useful clinical applications of *C. forskohlii* extracts will turn out to be in the treatment of cardiovascular diseases such as hypertension, congestive heart failure, and angina. The cardiovascular effects of *C. forskohlii* and its components have been studied in great detail.[1,10,11] Forskolin's basic cardiovascular actions involve the lowering of blood pressure along with improved contractility of the heart. Again, this is related to increasing cAMP levels throughout the cardiovascular system, which results in relaxation of the arteries and increased force of contraction. The net effect is tremendous improvement in cardiovascular function.

Several clinical and animal studies have suggested that forskolin may lower blood pressure significantly as well as improve heart function in patients.[10–13] In one human study involving seven patients with dilated cardiomyopathy, forskolin was shown to improve left ventricular function primarily via reduction of preload and without rising metabolic costs.[12] This study confirmed earlier animal studies showing that forskolin increases the contractile force of heart muscle.[11]

Another human study evaluated the hemodynamic effects of intravenous forskolin given to patients with dilated cardiomyopathy (dosage, 3 micrograms per kilograms per minute).[13] Although systemic vascular resistance and diastolic pressure fell, forskolin had no effect on cardiac index, ejection fraction, or myocardial oxygen consumption at this very low dosage.

However, when a small dosage of dobutamine was given along with the forskolin, an increase in all four parameters was observed. At a higher dosage (4 micrograms per kilogram per minute) forskolin improved heart function by 19 percent and produced a 16 percent rise in heart rate. However, these changes were associated with symptomatic flush syndromes. These results indicate that forskolin may best be used in congestive heart failure in combination with other botanicals such as *Crataegus* species.

Forskolin has also been shown to be a direct cerebral vasodilator, indicating that it may prove to be useful in cerebral vascular insufficiency and poststroke recovery.[14]

An additional mechanism of action particularly beneficial in a wide range of cardiovascular conditions is the inhibition of platelet aggregation. In this case solid evidence indicates that a standardized *C. forskohlii* extract is superior to pure forskolin.[15] In this study, an animal model evaluating *in vivo* inhibition of platelet aggregation, rats were divided into four groups. Group 1 received *C. forskohlii* extract (480 milligrams per kilogram, supplying 20 milligrams per kilogram of forskolin); group 2 received forskolin (20 milligrams per kilogram); group 3 received dipyridamole; and group 4 served as the control. All treatments were given orally once daily. ADP-induced platelet aggregation was measured on days 1 through 15. All three treatments produced significant inhibition of platelet aggregation. On day 15, the percentages of inhibition were approximately 42 percent for group 1, 37 percent for group 2, and 52 percent for group 3. Hence, the extract of *C. forskohlii* produced greater inhibition than did pure forskolin.

Glaucoma

In clinical studies, forskolin reduces intraocular pressure when it is applied directly to the eyes.[16-19] This effect indicates that topical forskolin preparations may be of great benefit in the treatment of glaucoma. Unlike current drug therapy, forskolin actually increases intraocular blood flow, has no side effects, and does not cause the pupils to constrict. Because topical preparations containing forskolin are not yet available commercially, oral preparations may be tried instead.

Other possible clinical applications

Coleus forskohlii extracts concentrated and standardized for forskolin content may prove to be useful in a number of other clinical applications, including weight loss programs, hypothyroidism, malabsorption and digestive disorders, depression, prevention of cancer metastasis, and immune system enhancement. Here's why:

- **Weight loss programs**   Lipolysis, the breakdown of stored fat, is regulated by cAMP. Forskolin has been shown to stimulate lipolysis as well as inhibit the synthesis of fat in adipocytes.[20-23] Forskolin also counteracts the decreased response of fat cells to lipolytic hormones, such as epinephrine, associated with aging.[24]

- **Hypothyroidism**   Forskolin increases thyroid hormone production, and stimulates thyroid hormone release.[25-27]

- **Malabsorption and digestive disorders**   Forskolin stimulates digestive secretions including the release of hydrochloric acid, pepsin, amylase, and pancreatic enzymes.[1,2] Forskolin has been shown to promote nutrient absorption in the small intestine.[28] *Coleus forskohlii* extracts may prove useful in treating dry mouth, as forskolin increases salivation.[29]

- **Depression**   Forskolin has been shown to exert antidepressant activity in animal studies.[30]

- **Cancer metastases**   Forskolin is a potent inhibitor of cancer metastasis in mice injected with malignant cells.[31] As little as 82 micrograms administered to mice inhibited metastasis by over 70 percent.

- **Immune system enhancement**   Forskolin exhibits potent immune system enhancement (primarily through activation of macrophages and lymphocytes) in several models.[32-34]

Dosage

The forskolin content of coleus root is typically 0.2–0.3 percent; therefore the forskolin content of crude coleus products may not be sufficient to produce a pharmacological effect. Use standardized extracts with a concentrated forskolin content. The recommended dosage should be based on the level of forskolin. The current recommendation for a *Coleus forskohlii* extract standardized to contain 18 percent forskolin is 50 milligrams (9 milligrams of forskolin) two to three times daily.

Toxicity

Animal studies on forskolin indicate an extremely low order of toxicity for forskolin. On the basis of its pharmacology, you might be wise to restrict the use of *C. forskohlii* preparations in cases of low blood pressure and peptic ulcers. Furthermore, *C. forskohlii* preparations should be used with caution by patients on prescription medications, especially antiasthmatics and antihypertensives, because forskolin could possibly potentiate the effects of these drugs.

References:

1. Ammon HPT and Muller AB: Forskolin: From Ayurvedic remedy to a modern agent. *Planta Medica* **51**, 473–477, 1985.
2. Seamon KB and Daly JW: Forskolin: A unique diterpene activator of cAMP-generating systems. *J Cyclic Nucleotide Res* **7**, 201–224, 1981.
3. Laurenza A, Sutkowski EM, and Seamon KB: Forskolin: A specific stimulator of adenylyl cyclase or a diterpene with multiple sites of action? *Trends Pharmacol Sci* **10**, 442–447, 1989.
4. Wong S, *et al.*: Forskolin inhibits platelet-activating factor binding to platelet receptors independently of adenylyl cyclase activation. *Eur J Pharmacol* **245**, 55–61, 1993.
5. Kreutner W, *et al.*: Bronchodilatory and antiallergy activity of forskolin. *Eur J Pharmacol* **111**, 1–8, 1985.
6. Lichey J, *et al.*: Effect of forskolin on methacholine-induced bronchoconstriction in extrinsic asthmatics. *Lancet* **ii**, 167, 1984.
7. Bauer K, *et al.*: Pharmacodynamic effects of inhaled dry powder formulations of fenoterol and colforsin in asthma. *Clin Pharmacol Ther* **53**, 76–83, 1993.
8. Marone G, *et al.*: Forskolin inhibits the release of histamine from human basophils and mast cells. *Agents Actions* **18**, 96–99, 1986.
9. Kaik G and Witte PU: Protective effect of forskolin in acetylcholine provocation in healthy probands. Comparison of 2 doses with fenoterol and placebo. *Wien Med Wochenschr* **136**, 637–641, 1986.
10. Dubey MP, *et al.*: Pharmacological studies on coleonol, a hypotensive diterpene from *Coleus forskohlii*. *J Ethnopharmacol* **3**, 1–13, 1981.
11. Lindner E, Dohadwalla AN, and Bhattacharya BK: Positive inotropic and blood pressure lowering activity of a diterpene derivative isolated from *Coleus forskohlii*: Forskolin. *Arzneimittel-Forsch* **28**, 284–289, 1978.
12. Kramer W, *et al.*: Effects of forskolin on left ventricular function in dilated cardiomyopathy. *Arzneimittel-Forsch* **37**, 364–367, 1987.
13. Schlepper M, Thormann J, and Mitrovic V: Cardiovascular effects of forskolin and phosphodiesterase-III inhibitors. *Basic Res Cardiol* **84**(Suppl 1), 197–212, 1989.
14. Wysham DG, Brotherton AF, and Heistad DD: Effects of forskolin on cerebral blood flow: Implications for a role of adenylate cyclase. *Stroke* **17**, 1299–1303, 1986.
15. De Souza NJ: Industrial development of traditional drugs: The forskolin example. A mini-review. *J Ethnopharmacol* **38**, 177–180, 1993.
16. Potter DE, Burke JA, and Temple JR: Forskolin suppresses sympathetic neuron function and causes ocular hypotension. *Cur Eye Res* **4**, 87–96, 1985.
17. Caprioli J and Sears M: Forskolin lowers intraocular pressure in rabbits, monkeys, and man. *Lancet* **i**, 958–960, 1983.
18. Meyer BH, *et al.*: The effects of forskolin eye drops on intraocular pressure. *S Afr Med J* **71**(9), 570–571, 1987.
19. Seto C, *et al.*: Acute effects of topical forskolin on aqueous humor dynamics in man. *Jpn J Ophthalmol* **30**, 238–244, 1986.
20. Allen DO and Quesenberry JT: Quantitative differences in the cyclic AMP-lipolysis relationships for isoproterenol and forskolin. *J Pharmacol Exp Ther* **244**, 852–858, 1988.
21. Allen DO, Ahmed B, and Naseer K: Relationships between cyclic AMP levels and lipolysis in fat cells after isoproterenol and forskolin stimulation. *J Pharmacol Exp Ther* **238**, 659–664, 1986.
22. Okuda H, Morimoto C, and Tsujita T: Relationship between cyclic AMP production and lipolysis induced by forskolin in rat fat cells. *J Lipid Res* **33**, 225–231, 1992.
23. Bianco AC, Kieffer JD, and Silva JE: Adenosine 3',5'-monophosphate and thyroid hormone control of uncoupling protein messenger ribonucleic acid in freshly dispersed brown adipocytes. *Endocrinology* **130**, 2625–2633, 1992.

24. Hoffman BB, Chang H, and Reaven GM: Stimulation and inhibition of lipolysis in isolated rat adipocytes: Evidence for age-related changes in responses to forskolin and PGE$_1$. *Horm Metab Res* **19**, 358–360, 1987.

25. Saunier B, *et al.*: Cyclic AMP regulation of Gs protein. Thyrotropin and forskolin increase the quantity of stimulatory guanine nucleotide-binding proteins in cultured thyroid follicles. *J Biol Chem* **265**, 19942–19946, 1990.

26. Roger PP, Servais P, and Dumont JE: Regulation of dog thyroid epithelial cell cycle by forskolin, an adenylate cyclase activator. *Exp Cell Res* **172**, 282–292, 1990.

27. Haye B, *et al.*: Chronic and acute effects of forskolin on isolated thyroid cell metabolism. *Mol Cell Endocrinol* **43**, 41–50, 1990.

28. Reymann A, Braun W, and Woermann C: Proabsorptive properties of forskolin: Disposition of glycine, leucine and lysine in rat jejunum. *Arch Pharmacol* **334**, 110–115, 1986.

29. Larsson O, Detsch T, and Fredholm BB: VIP and forskolin enhance carbachol-induced K$^+$ efflux from rat salivary gland fragments by a Ca^{2+}-sensitive mechanism. *Am J Physiol* **259**, C904–910, 1990.

30. Wachtel H and Loschmann PA: Effects of forskolin and cyclic nucleotides in animal models predictive of antidepressant activity: Interactions with rolipram. *Psychopharmacol* **90**, 430–435, 1986.

31. Agarwal KC and Parks RE: Forskolin: A potential antimetastatic agent. *Int J Cancer* **32**, 801–804, 1983.

32. Schorlemmer HU, *et al.*: Forskolin for immune stimulation. *Chem Abstr* **102**, 1009, 1985.

33. Krall JF, *et al.*: Human aging: Effect on the activation of lymphocyte cyclic AMP-dependent protein kinase by forskolin. *Proc Soc Exp Biol Med* **184**, 396–402, 1987.

34. Chang J, *et al.*: Effect of forskolin on prostaglandin synthesis by mouse resident peritoneal macrophages. *Eur J Pharmacol* **103**, 303–312, 1984.

7
Dandelion

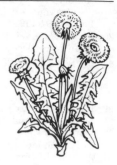

Key uses of dandelion:

Root:

- Liver tonic

Leaves:

- Diuretic
- Weight loss aid

General description

Dandelion (*Taraxacum officinale*) is a member of the Compositae family and is closely related to chicory.[1] Several origins have been attributed to the name *Taraxacum*—the most likely is a combination of the Greek words *taraxo* (disorder, disturbance), *akos* (remedy), and *akeomai* (I heal); another possibility is *tharakhcharkon* (edible), a derivative of a Persian–Arabic word and the name by which the plant is referred to in a thirteenth-century Arabian botanical work.

Taraxacum is known around the world by a variety of names. In English-speaking countries, dandelion (from the French *dent-de-lion*, referring to the plant's lion's tooth leaves) is its most common name. It is also known as wet-a-bed (after its diuretic action), lion's tooth, fairy clock, priest's crown, swine's snout, blowball, milk gowan, wild endive, white endive,[2] canker-wort,[3] puffball, and Irish daisy.[1]

The appearance of dandelion is well known. Technically speaking, it is a variable perennial, growing to a height of 12 inches. Its spatula-like leaves are deeply toothed, shiny, hairless, and arranged in a ground-level rosette. The yellow flowers bloom for most of the year, and are sensitive to light—weather-opening at daybreak and closing at nightfall, and opening in fine weather and closing in wet weather (a closed dandelion flower signals rain).

When the flower matures, it closes up, the petals wither, and it forms a puff-ball containing seeds that are dispersed by the breeze.

The rosette formation of grooved leaves channels rain water into its center and down to a taproot that is thick and dark brown (almost black) on the outside. The root is cylindrical, tapering, and somewhat branched. It has a slight odor and a sweetish taste. The inside of a dried dandelion root is yellowish, very porous, and without pith.

It is believed that the plant originated in central Asia and spread throughout most of the world, preferring the cooler climates.[1] Although *Taraxacum* is very adaptable, it prefers moist, nitrogen-rich soils at altitudes less than 6,000 feet. Most species occur in the temperate zones of the northern hemisphere, with the greatest concentration in northwest Europe.

The portion of the plant that is most commonly used is the root; however, the leaves and whole plant can also be used. In addition to its medicinal use, dandelion is also consumed as a nutritious food and beverage. Tender leaves are used raw in salads and sandwiches, or lightly cooked as a vegetable. Tea is made from the leaves, coffee substitute from the roots, and wine and schnapps from the flowers.

Chemical composition

The primary therapeutic actions of dandelion are believed to be due to the bitter principle taraxacin, various terpenoids, inulin, and its excellent nutritional profile. The seasonal changes in the levels of these components in different parts of the plant have interested researchers for more than 160 years. Other constituents of dandelion that may contribute to its pharmacology include resin, pectin, taraxanthin (a carotenoid pigment in the flowers), fatty acids, and flavonoids.

Many studies show that dandelion is a rich source of vitamins and minerals.[1] The leaves have the highest vitamin A content of all greens (14,000 international units [IU] per 100 grams raw greens) as well as ample amounts of vitamins D, B complex, and C, and minerals such as iron, silicon, magnesium, sodium, potassium, zinc, manganese, copper, and phosphorus.[1,4] Dandelion also contains relatively high amounts of choline—an important nutrient for the liver.[5]

History and folk use

While many individuals may consider the common dandelion an unwanted weed, herbalists revere this valuable herb. Generally regarded as a liver remedy, dandelion has a long history of folk use. In Europe, dandelion was used in the treatment of fevers, boils, eye problems, diarrhea, fluid retention, liver congestion, heartburn, and various skin problems. In China, dandelion has been used to treat breast problems (cancer, inflammation, lack of milk flow, etc.), liver diseases, appendicitis, and digestive ailments. Dandelion's use in India, Russia, and most other parts of the world revolved primarily around its action on the liver.

Pharmacology

The primary pharmacological activities relate to digestion, liver function, and diuresis.

Digestive effects

The use of bitter herbs, such as dandelion, to aid digestion is based on the belief that bitter principles stimulate the initial phase of digestion, including the secretion of salivary and gastric juices. Dandelion exceeds this initial stimulation by stimulating the release of bile by the liver and gallbladder.

Liver effects

Studies in humans and laboratory animals show that dandelion root enhances the flow of bile, improving such conditions as liver congestion, bile duct inflammation, hepatitis, gallstones, and jaundice.[2,3,6] Dandelion's action in increasing bile flow is twofold: (1) it affects the liver directly by causing an increase in bile production and flow to the gallbladder (choleretic effect); and (2) it exerts a direct effect on the gallbladder, causing contraction and release of stored bile (cholagogue effect). The high choline content of the root may be a major factor in dandelion's ability to act as a "tonic" to the liver. Historically, dandelion's positive effect on such a wide variety of conditions is probably closely related to its ability to improve liver function.

Diuretic and weight loss effects

Dandelion leaves have confirmed diuretic activity. In one study in mice, dandelion exerted a diuretic activity comparable to that of furosemide (Lasix).[7] Because dandelion replaces potassium lost through diuresis, it does not have the potential side effects of furosemide, such as hepatic coma and circulatory collapse. The dose given was 8 milliliters of the aqueous fluid extract of the leaf per kilogram body weight. This dose produced a 30 percent loss of body weight in mice and rats in a 30-day period. Much of the weight loss was attributed to the significant diuretic effects.

Cancer

A Japanese study performed in 1979 found that dandelion alcoholic extract administered to mice for 10 days markedly inhibited the growth of inoculated Ehrlich ascites cancer cells within a week after treatment.[8] A freeze-dried warm water extract of the root for use as an antitumor agent was patented by the Japanese in 1979 and TOf-CFr, a glucose polymer isolated by Japanese researchers in 1981, was found to have antitumor properties in laboratory mice.[1] These findings lend support to the Chinese use of dandelion for breast cancer. Similarly, in a U.S. study performed in 1987, antibodies to the active polypeptides in tumor-induced mouse ascites fluid were produced from dandelion.[9]

Diabetes

Dandelion and inulin have demonstrated experimental hypoglycemic activity in animals.[10] Because inulin is composed of fructose chains it may act to buffer blood glucose levels, thus preventing sudden and severe fluctuations.

Clinical applications

Although dandelion's specific action is on the liver, as an alterative or tonic it benefits the body as a whole. It is often used as a diuretic, laxative, cholagogue, general stimulant for the urinary system, choleretic, depurative (purifier), hypoglycemic, and antitumor agent.

Liver conditions

Two studies in humans have demonstrated the liver-healing properties of dandelion. In a 1938 study in Italy, twelve patients with severe liver imbalances, many exhibiting classic symptoms of loss of appetite, low energy, and jaundice, were treated with dandelion extract (one 5-milliliter injection per day for 20 days).[1] Eleven of the twelve patients showed a considerable drop in blood cholesterol. In the other study dandelion extract was used to successfully treat hepatitis, swelling of the liver, jaundice, and dyspepsia with deficient bile secretion.[2]

Dandelion's gentle effects on the liver, particularly its lipotropic effects, may be put to good use in the treatment of premenstrual syndrome. Decreased clearance of estrogen and other hormones by the liver is believed to be responsible for these symptoms in some women. If dandelion can improve the liver's ability to detoxify these hormones, symptoms may be likewise improved.

Dosage

As a general tonic and mild liver remedy, the root can be used at the following dosages three times daily:

- Dried root: 2–8 grams by infusion or decoction
- Fluid extract (1:1): 4–8 milliliters (1–2 teaspoons)
- Tincture: alcohol-based tinctures of dandelion are not recommended because of the extremely high dosage required
- Juice of fresh root: 4–8 milliliters (1–2 teaspoons)
- Powdered solid extract (4:1): 250–500 milligrams

Preparations of the leaves can be used as a mild diuretic and weight loss agent at the following dosages three times daily:

- Dried leaf: 4–10 grams by infusion
- Fluid extract (1:1): 4–10 milliliters

Toxicity

Dandelion is extremely safe. Its toxicity has been found by researchers to be extremely low, and it is considered safe to use, even in large amounts.[1] No toxic or adverse effects have ever been reported, either for external or internal use.

References

1. Hobbs C: *Taraxacum officinale*: A monograph and literature review. In: *Eclectic Dispensatory*. Eclectic Medical Publications, Portland, OR, 1989.
2. Faber K: The dandelion *Taraxacum officinale*. *Pharmazie* **13**, 423–436, 1958.
3. Susnik F: Present state of knowledge of the medicinal plant *Taraxacum officinale* Weber. *Med Razgledi* **21**, 323–328, 1982.
4. Leung AY: *Encyclopedia of Common Natural Ingredients Used in Food, Drugs and Cosmetics*. John Wiley & Sons, New York, 1980.
5. Broda B and Andrzejewska E: Choline content in some medicinal plants. *Farm Polska* **22**, 181–184, 1966.

6. Bohm K: Choleretic action of some medicinal plants. *Arzneimittel-Forsch* **9**, 376–378, 1959.
7. Racz-Kotilla E, Racz G, and Solomon A: The action of *Taraxacum officinale* extracts on the body weight and diuresis of laboratory animals. *Planta Medica* **26**, 212–217, 1974.
8. Kotobuki Seiyaku KK: *Taraxacum* extracts as antitumour agents. *Chem Abstr* **94**, 14530m, 1979.
9. Salvucci ME, *et al.*: Purification and species distribution of rubisco activase. *Plant Physiol* **84**, 930–936, 1987.
10. Yamashita K, Kawai K, and Itakura M: Effects of fructooligosaccharides on blood glucose and serum lipids in diabetic subjects. *Nutr Res* **4**, 491–496, 1984.

8
Echinacea

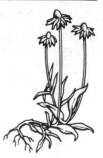

Key uses of *Echinacea*:

- Common cold
- Infections
- Low immune status
- Cancer

General description

Echinacea (purple coneflower) species are perennial herbs native to midwestern North America, from Saskatchewan to Texas. The genus derives its name from the Greek *echinos* (from the word for sea urchin). This refers to the prickly scales of the dried seed head portion of the flower.

Of the nine *Echinacea* species, *E. angustifolia*, *E. purpurea*, and *E. pallida* are the most commonly used.[1] *Echinacea angustifolia*, with a typical height of up to 2 feet, is shorter than *E. purpurea* (1.5 to 5 feet) and *E. pallida* (1 to 3 feet). Another key to species identification is that *E. angustifolia* and *E. purpurea* have yellow pollen whereas *E. pallida* is noticeably paler and has white pollen. The portions of the plant used for medicinal purposes include the aerial portion, the whole plant including the root, and the root itself. The tap root of *E. angustifolia* can reach a length of 3 to 4 feet.[2,3]

Echinacea angustifolia has thick, hairy leaves 3 to 8 centimeters long, found at the base of a purple seed head shaped like a cone. The only exception in this family of "purple" coneflowers is *E. paradoxa*, which has a yellow flower.

Chemical composition

Analysis of *Echinacea* species has yielded an assortment of chemical constituents with pharmacological activities. The broad chemical composition of this medicinal plant suggests possible synergistic effects among its constituents. For example, in some experimental models, echinacea's water-soluble polysaccharides stimulate the cellular immune system more so than the fat-soluble components, which enhance macrophage phagocytosis.[3]

The important constituents, from a pharmacological perspective, of echinacea can be divided into seven categories: (1) polysaccharides, (2) flavonoids, (3) caffeic acid derivatives, (4) essential oils, (5) polyacetylenes, (6) alkylamides, and (7) miscellaneous chemicals. These are discussed below.

Polysaccharides

A number of immunostimulatory and mild antiinflammatory polysaccharides have been isolated from *Echinacea* species.[2–8] Most notable are inulin, found in high concentration (5.9 percent) in *E. angustifolia* root, and the high molecular weight (25,000–50,000) polysaccharides found in the aerial part of *E. purpurea*. These components possess significant immune-enhancing properties. The most potent immune-enhancing polysaccharides are the water-soluble, acidic, branched-chain heteroglycans, which are composed of many types of sugar rather than one type of sugar. (Inulin, on the other hand, consists of fructose units.)

Flavonoids

The leaves and stems of *E. angustifolia* and *E. purpurea* contain numerous flavonoids, with rutoside being the most abundant.[3,8] The total flavonoid content (calculated as quercetin) for *E. angustifolia* and *E. purpurea* is 0.48 and 0.38 percent, respectively.[2,3,8,9]

Caffeic acid derivatives

Caffeic acid (Figure 8.1) serves as the backbone for a number of important medicinal plant compounds in other plants as well as in echinacea. The first compound believed to be unique to echinacea was echinacoside,[10] a compound eventually shown to be composed of caffeic acid, a caffeic acid derivative (similar to catechol), glucose, and rhamnose, all attached to a central glucose molecule (Figure 8.2). Echinacoside accumulates in the roots, but is

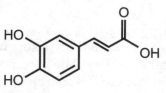

Figure 8.1 Caffeic acid

also found in smaller concentrations in the flowers. According to recent investigations, the roots of *E. angustifolia* contain 0.3–1.3 percent while the roots of *E. pallida* contain a similar concentration of 0.4–1.7 percent.[11] It is assumed that *E. purpurea* has similar echinacoside levels as well.

Other caffeic acid derivatives important in the pharmacology of echinacea include: cichoric acid, chlorogenic acid, and cynarin.[3] Cichoric acid was originally isolated from *E. purpurea* and is found in much higher concentrations in this species compared to *E. angustifolia* and *E. pallida*.[2,3,8] However, *E. angustifolia* and *E. pallida* have greater amounts of other types of caffeic acid derivatives.[2,3,12] These differences are not thought to have much clinical significance; rather, they may prove to be valuable in quick chemical differentiation of species.

Essential oils

The essential oil content varies among the three common species: *E. angustifolia* root and leaves have a content of less than 0.1 percent; *E. purpurea* root

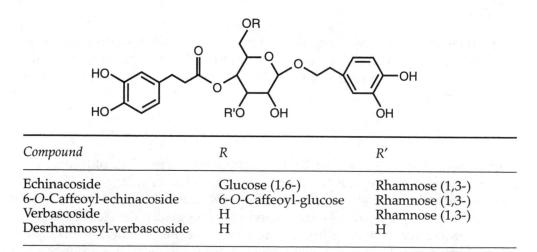

Compound	R	R'
Echinacoside	Glucose (1,6-)	Rhamnose (1,3-)
6-O-Caffeoyl-echinacoside	6-O-Caffeoyl-glucose	Rhamnose (1,3-)
Verbascoside	H	Rhamnose (1,3-)
Desrhamnosyl-verbascoside	H	H

Figure 8.2 Echinacoside and other caffeic acid derivatives

has 0.2 percent, and flowers and leaves 0.6 percent; and *E. pallida* root has up to 2 percent, while its leaves have less than 1 percent.[13] Interestingly, in one study the essential oil content of *E. pallida* root was found to rise to 3.5–4 percent in April and May, only to fall to 1–1.5 percent for the rest of the year.[14] The major essential oil components are sesquiterpene derivatives, borneol, alphapinine, and related aromatic compounds.[2,3]

Polyacetylenes

A number of polyacetylenes have been identified in the roots of all three commercial species.[15] The difference in the type of polyacetylene and susceptibility to breakdown may help differentiate between species.[16]

Alkylamides

Alkylamides typically cause a tingling sensation on the tongue. This feature is representative of their mild anesthetic effect. These compounds are found in highest concentrations in the roots. The roots of *E. angustifolia* contain higher concentrations (0.009 percent) than *E. purpurea* (0.004 percent) and *E. pallida* (0.001 percent).[8,17]

Miscellaneous chemicals

Other constituents undoubtedly contribute to the pharmacology of echinacea. The occurrence of a "colorless alkaloid" was first reported by the great John Uri Lloyd in 1897[2] and substantiated recently by the isolation of the alkaloids tussilagine and isotussilagine.[18] Other compounds isolated from *Echinacea* species include resins, glycoproteins, sterols, minerals, and fatty acids.[2,3]

History and folk use

Native Americans used echinacea extensively. In fact, American Indians used echinacea more than any other plant in the treatment of illness and injury. The root was used externally for the healing of wounds, burns, abscesses, and insect bites; internally for infections, toothache, and joint pains; and as an antidote for snake (rattlesnake) bites.[19]

A commercial product containing echinacea was introduced to Americans around 1870 by H. C. F. Meyer, a German lay healer, who recommended it as a wonder cure called "Meyer's blood purifier."[2,3] Meyer recommended it for almost every conceivable malady and there were numerous case reports of successful treatments for snake bites, typhus, diphtheria, and other infections.

Echinacea angustifolia became a favorite with Eclectic physicians, as it was thought to be greater in activity than other *Echinacea* species. Eclectics used it externally as a local antiseptic, stimulant, deodorant, and anesthetic; and internally for "bad blood," that is, to correct "fluid depravation with tendency to sepsis and malignancy."[20]

Although many physicians began to investigate and use echinacea as a serious medicine, in 1909 the Council on Pharmacy and Chemistry of the American Medical Association refused to recognize echinacea as an active drug, stating, "in view of the lack of any scientific scrutiny of the claims made for it, *Echinacea* is deemed unworthy of further consideration until more reliable evidence is presented in its favor."[2] Despite this opposition, echinacea was included in the National Formulary of the United States and remained there until 1950.[2,3]

With the demise of the Eclectic movement, the popularity of echinacea in the United States waned except among naturopathic physicians. Around 1980 echinacea was "rediscovered," owing to increased consumer interest in immune system disorders such as candidiasis, chronic fatigue syndrome, acquired immunodeficiency syndrome (AIDS), and cancer. Although interest in echinacea had decreased in America between the 1930s and 1980s, European physicians continued research. Much of this research was initiated by a 1932 study by Gerhard Madaus. Madaus demonstrated the immune-enhancing effects of a preparation made from the fresh juice of the aerial portion of *E. purpurea*. This was followed by the development of a commercial product and a great deal of scientific study. Thus, *E. purpurea* began to be as respected as *E. angustifolia* among herbal practitioners in Europe.[2,3]

Pharmacology

The chemistry, pharmacology, and clinical applications of echinacea have been the subject of over 350 scientific studies.[2,3] The overwhelming majority of the clinical studies have utilized an extract of the juice of the aerial (above-ground) portion of *E. purpurea* along with 22 percent ethanol (for preservation).

The following subsections summarize some of the vast pharmacological information on echinacea, with particular attention given to the species used, part of the plant used, solvent used for extraction, and other relevant features. When no species delineation is made, the activity described is similar in all species.

Tissue regeneration and antiinflammatory properties

The fresh-pressed juice of *E. purpurea*, as well as the polysaccharide components of all *Echinacea* species, promote tissue regeneration and reduce inflammation in experimental studies.[7,21-24] This is apparently largely due to inhibition of the enzyme hyaluronidase. Hyaluronidase is referred to as the "spreading factor." It is secreted by microorganisms and is found in snake venom; its purpose is to break down hyaluronic acid, a major component of the ground substance (intracellular cement) that holds body cells together. Echinacea maintains the structure and integrity of the connective tissue and ground substance.

In addition to increased hyaluronic acid stabilization, echinacea also stimulates cells (fibroblasts) that manufacture ground substance.[24]

Echinacea exerts a mild, direct, cortisone-like effect and enhances the secretion of adrenal cortex hormones.[2,3,22] Echinacea's polysaccharide portion appears to be responsible for the direct antiinflammatory effects, although the alkylamide fraction has also demonstrated some activity.[25]

Immunostimulatory properties

Echinacea contains a diverse range of active components affecting different aspects of immune function.[2,3] To fully appreciate echinacea's effect, you must understand some aspects of the immune system.

The immune system is perhaps one of the most complex and fascinating systems of the human body. The immune system's prime function is to protect the body against infection and the development of cancer. The immune system is composed of the lymphatic vessels and organs (thymus, spleen, tonsils, and lymph nodes), white blood cells (lymphocytes, neutrophils, basophils, eosinophils, monocytes, etc.), specialized cells residing in various tissue (macrophages, mast cells, etc.), and specialized chemical factors such as complement, interferon, and interleukin.

Effect of echinacea on the alternate complement pathway

Echinacea exerts many "nonspecific" effects on the immune system. For example, inulin, the major component in the root of echinacea, activates a part of the immune system known as the alternate complement pathway. As a result, the movement of white blood cells into areas of infection is enhanced; immune complexes solubilize; and bacteria, viruses, and other microorganisms are destroyed. Echinacea also increases the levels of properdin, a serum protein that stimulates the alternate complement pathway.[2,3,26]

Effect on white blood cells

Echinacea elevates serum white blood cell counts when they are low.[2,3,27–30] In addition, studies have shown that echinacea polysaccharides bind to receptors on the surface of white blood cells and literally turn these cells on. The white blood cells most sensitive to echinacea are T lymphocytes, macrophages, and natural killer cells.

Effect on T lymphocytes

T lymphocytes, or T cells, are a type of white blood cell responsible for "cell-mediated immunity." Cell-mediated immunity refers to immune mechanisms not controlled or mediated by antibodies. Cell-mediated immunity is extremely important in providing resistance to infection by moldlike bacteria, yeast (including *Candida albicans*), fungi, parasites, and viruses (including herpes simplex, Epstein–Barr virus, and viruses that cause hepatitis). If you are suffering from an infection by these organisms, it's a good indication that your cell-mediated immunity is not functioning up to par. Cell-mediated immunity is also critical in protecting against the development of cancer, autoimmune disorders such as rheumatoid arthritis, and allergies. Not surprisingly, echinacea has been used to treat all of these conditions.

Echinacea promotes nonspecific T cell activation. When echinacea polysaccharides bind to the surface of T cells, the T cells increase their production of interferon and other immune potentiators. The result is enhanced T cell replication, macrophage activity, antibody binding, and increased numbers of circulating neutrophils.[2–4] Neutrophils are another type of white blood cell. Neutrophils actively phagocytize—that is, engulf and destroy—bacteria, tumor cells, and dead particulate matter. Neutrophils are especially important in preventing bacterial infection.

The nonspecific T cell activation by echinacea also increases the activity of another type of white blood cell—natural killer cells. They are called "natural killer cells" because they destroy cells that have become cancerous or infected with viruses. They are the body's first line of defense against cancer development.

The level or activity of natural killer cells in chronic fatigue syndrome is usually low.

Effect on macrophages

Macrophages are blood monocytes that have taken up residence in specific tissues such as the liver, spleen, and lymph nodes. From here these large cells filter the lymphatic fluid (or *lymph*), engulfing (or phagocytizing) foreign particles including bacteria and cellular debris. Macrophages and monocytes are, in essence, the garbage collectors of the body. Macrophages protect the body against invasion by microorganisms, as well as prevent damage to the lymphatic system.

Echinacea polysaccharides have also been shown to enhance macrophage phagocytosis and stimulate macrophages to produce a number of immune-potentiating compounds (e.g., tumor necrosis factor [TNF], interferon, and interleukin 1). Furthermore, macrophages have been shown to destroy tumor cells in tissue culture and inhibit *Candida albicans* infection in rats infected intravenously with a lethal dose (30,000 cells) of *Candida albicans*.[2,3,5,6,31] The interactions with macrophages are most likely responsible for much of the immune system enhancement of echinacea polysaccharides.

In addition to the polysaccharides, fat-soluble alkylamides and caffeic acid derivatives such as cichoric acid are thought to contribute to the immunostimulatory aspects of echinacea, especially alcoholic extracts.[3,32,33] Although most research has been devoted to the water-soluble components (i.e., the polysaccharides), the fat-soluble fraction enhances macrophage phagocytosis most potently.[3,32,33]

The carbon clearance test is often used to measure systemic macrophage activation. The method involves measuring, at timed intervals, the rate of disappearance of carbon granules from the blood following administration of a test substance. Root extracts of echinacea administered orally exert greater effects on phagocytic activity than does the aerial portion, with *Echinacea purpurea* > *E. angustifolia* > *E. pallida*.[3,32,33]

Antiviral properties

The fresh-pressed juice of the aerial portion of *E. purpurea*, along with alcoholic and aqueous extracts of the roots, possess antiviral activity. Some viruses inhibited in cell culture include influenza, herpes virus, and vesicular stomatitis virus.[3,34]

Although certain echinacea components (e.g., echinacoside, other caffeic acid derivatives, and polysaccharides) may block virus receptors on the cell surface, the antiviral effects may also be due to inhibition of hyaluronidase,[21,35] as the virus-inhibiting action of echinacea is significantly diminished when hyaluronidase is added to the cell cultures.[3] Remember, many organisms secrete the enzyme hyaluronidase (the spreading factor), which increases connective tissue permeability and allows the organism to become more invasive.[36]

From a clinical perspective, echinacea's inhibition of hyaluronidase coupled with its general immunostimulatory properties are probably more important than its direct antiviral activity. Echinacea's nonspecific antiviral action works by enhancing cytotoxic killing of virus-infected cells and the release of interferon. Interferons bind to cell surfaces, where it stimulates synthesis of intracellular proteins that block the transcription of viral RNA.

Antibacterial properties

The direct antibacterial activity of echinacea is quite mild. This is somewhat surprising, as echinacea has a long history of effective use in both internal and external bacterial infections. It is possible that it possesses some anti-infective properties that prevent bacterial adherence, although this has yet to be determined. Clearly, its clinical efficacy is due to its strong immune-potentiating actions.

Echinacea does possess some mild antibacterial action due largely to echinacoside, the complex caffeic acid derivative, found in highest concentrations in the root of *E. angustifolia*. Echinacoside and caffeic acid inhibit the growth of *Staphylococcus aureus*, *Corynebacterium diphtheria*, and *Proteus vulgaris*. Approximately 6.3 milligrams of echinacoside is equivalent to 10 Oxford units of penicillin.[2,3,10]

Anticancer activity

Echinacea obviously possesses indirect anticancer activity via its general immunoenhancing effects. Particularly important is its stimulation of macrophages to greater cytotoxic activity against tumor cells. (Z)-1,8-pentadecadiene, a lipid-soluble component found in the root of *E. angustifolia* and *E. pallida*, possesses, *in vivo*, significant direct anticancer activity.[37]

Clinical applications

Echinacea has long been used, with proven efficacy, to treat infections. Although injectable preparations are common, oral preparations are generally thought to yield similar or even better results.[3]

An exception to echinacea's general effectiveness in the treatment of infections may be the acquired immunodeficiency syndrome (AIDS). It is unclear at this time if echinacea should be recommended for AIDS treatment. Although this condition is associated with widespread depression of the immune system (presumably owing to the actions of the human immunodeficiency virus, HIV), stimulation of T cell replication as well as increasing levels of tumor necrosis factor (TNF) may also stimulate replication of the virus. While there are some anecdotal reports of echinacea's efficacy in HIV-infected individuals, more research is necessary to determine echinacea's effects in HIV.

Infections

Numerous clinical studies confirm echinacea's immune-enhancing actions. Various echinacea extracts or products have shown results in general infectious conditions, influenza, colds, upper respiratory tract infections, urogenital infections, and other infectious conditions.

The effect against *Candida albicans* noted in animal studies has been confirmed in several clinical studies.[2,3] A study by Coeugniet and Kuhnast,[38] featured in Table 8.1, demonstrated that the fresh-pressed juice of *E. purpurea* greatly accentuates the efficacy of a topical antimycotic agent (econazol nitrate), decreasing recurrence from 60.5 to 5–16.7 percent. They used standardized skin tests to show that this enhancement was due to echinacea's boosting of cell-mediated immunity.[38] Notice that the oral and injectable forms produced similar results.

The common cold

One of the most popular uses of echinacea is in the treatment of the common cold. Two recent studies offer considerable support for this clinical

Table 8.1 Treatment of recurrent candidiasis with the fresh-pressed juice of *Echinacea purpurea*: Rate of recurrence at 6 months[a]

Therapeutic scheme	No. of patients	Recurrence rate (%)
Topical antimycotic alone	43	60.5
Topical antimycotic + subcutaneous injection of fresh-pressed juice of *E. purpurea*	20	15.0
Topical antimycotic + intramuscular injection of fresh-pressed juice of *E. purpurea*	60	5.0
Topical antimycotic + intravenous injection of fresh-pressed juice of *E. purpurea*	20	15.0
Topical antimycotic + oral fresh-pressed juice of *E. purpurea*	60	16.7

[a]Data from Ref. 38.

application. In one study, 180 patients with influenza were given either an extract of *E. purpurea* root at a daily dose of 450 or 900 milligrams, or a placebo.[39] The 450-milligram dose was found to be no more effective than a placebo; however, the group taking the 900-milligram dose showed significant reduction of cold symptoms.

In the other study, 108 patients with colds received either an extract of the fresh-pressed juice of *E. purpurea* (4 milliliters twice daily) or placebo for 8 weeks.[40] The number of patients remaining healthy: echinacea, 35.2 percent; placebo, 25.9 percent. Length of time between infections: echinacea, 40 days; placebo, 25 days. When infections did occur in patients receiving echinacea, they were less severe and resolved more quickly. Patients showing evidence of a weakened immune system (CD4/CD8 ratio, <1.5) benefited most from echinacea.

Snake bite

Echinacea has quite a reputation among naturopathic physicians and native American healers for the treatment of snake bite. Echinacea's inhibition of hyaluronidase,[21] a component of snake venom, might account for much of its reputed efficacy; most snake venoms permeate the body by way of hyaluronidase, which breaks down connective tissue in the ground substance between cells.

Wound healing

Several uncontrolled clinical studies substantiate echinacea's wound-healing activities.[3,41] The largest (4,598 patients) demonstrated that a salve of the juice of the aerial portion of *E. purpurea* had an 85 percent overall success rate in the treatment of inflammatory skin conditions such as abscesses, folliculitis, wounds of all kinds, eczema, burns, herpes, and varicose ulcers of the leg.[3]

Arthritis

Echinacea's antiinflammatory activity helps alleviate rheumatoid arthritis: in an uncontrolled study performed by Seidel and Knobloch,[42] 15 drops of the fresh-pressed juice of *E. purpurea* three times daily resulted in a 21.8 percent decrease in inflammation. Although this improvement was less than that of cortisone (42 percent) and prednisone (49.2 percent), no side effects were noted with the echinacea—whereas cortisone and prednisone have well-known side effects.

Cancer

One of the detrimental effects of radiation and chemotherapy in cancer treatment is that they depress white blood cell levels. Echinacea may offset this depression. Several studies have noted the stimulatory effects of echinacea on white blood cell counts in patients receiving radiation for cancer therapy.[29,30] A study using the fresh-pressed juice of *E. purpurea* demonstrated that 85 percent of fifty-five patients showed a stabilization of white blood cell counts compared to the control group, which showed a steady decline in levels (starting value of 6,000 down to 2,500 after 45 days).[29] This strongly supports the use of echinacea by patients undergoing orthodox cancer treatments.

Commercial preparations

It should be clear by now that it's not easy to decide which echinacea preparation is best to use. Not only is it difficult to determine which species is most effective—the portion of the plant used and how it is prepared are also serious questions for debate. Dosage recommendations for all currently available forms are given below, along with a few observations regarding the "preparations controversy."

Another problem that needs to be addressed is quality control. Since 1904, many commercial sources of echinacea have contained adulterants and no echinacea. For example, it has been estimated that, owing to supplier errors in collection, more than 50 percent (and possibly as much as 90 percent at times) of the echinacea sold in the United States from 1908 through 1991 has actually been *Parthenium integrifolium* (Missouri snakeroot).[2,43] Some suggest this adulteration is due to confusion of the common names. Others point out that while *Parthenium integrifolium* looks quite different ". . . once the root is cut and sifted it has an uncanny resemblance to *E. angustifolia* or *E. pallida* roots, though it possess its own characteristic flavor and fragrance."[43] From a practical as well as clinical viewpoint, consumers, retailers, pharmacists, and physicians should require that suppliers adequately document their product; we should be assured that we are in fact buying echinacea, and be told which species it is!

The best species

No "best" *Echinacea* species can be recommended at this time, as different experimental models have at times yielded inconsistent results. Rather, the clinician must recognize the unique value of each species. Although *E. angustifolia* has long been considered the best species and to possess the greatest activity, some studies dispute this. For example, in one study *E. purpurea* demonstrated greater enhancement of phagocytosis.[33] In fact, in a recent study an aqueous extract of *E. angustifolia* did not demonstrate any impact on phagocytic function in rats, whether it was administered orally, intraperitoneally, or intravenously.[44] As *E. purpurea* is the easiest to grow commercially, it may become the most utilized in the United States as it is in Europe.

The best part of the plant to use

Most laboratory studies report that the root possesses the greatest immune-enhancing properties. However, most of the data in these studies is based on the use of fresh-pressed juice from the aerial portion of *E. purpurea*. Therefore, this question cannot be fully answered until more clinical research is done with root preparations.

The best solvents

Even a small amount of ethanol results in precipitation or breakdown of the immunoactive polysaccharides, indicating aqueous extracts may be best. However, an aqueous extract leaves behind valuable fat-soluble immune-enhancing alkylamides and caffeic acid derivatives. To optimize an extract's immune-enhancing effects, many manufacturers use low ethanol (10–20 percent) hydro/alcoholic mixtures. These extracts typically possess both water- and fat-soluble compounds.

The best preparations

Echinacea products are available in many different forms: crude plant in either ground or powdered form, freeze-dried, alcohol-based tinctures and liquid extracts, aqueous tinctures and liquid extracts, and dry powdered alcoholic or aqueous extracts. Although there is no consensus, many experts consider the fresh-pressed juice of *E. purpurea* to be the best preparation because it provides the greatest range of active compounds and has by far the greatest level of clinical support.

Some standardized preparations of the fresh-pressed juice of *Echinacea purpurea* are guaranteed to contain a minimum of 2.4 percent beta-1,2-fructofuranosides. Standardizing the product for these compounds guarantees that the plant was harvested in the blossom stage, the product was carefully prepared and suffered no enzymatic or microbiological degradation, and that the product is stabilized.

Dosage

The following recommendations are for the use of echinacea as a general immune stimulant during infection. Doses should be given three times daily:

- Dried root (or as tea): 1–2 grams
- Freeze-dried plant: 325–650 milligrams
- Juice of aerial portion of E. purpurea stabilized in 22 percent ethanol (preferably standardized to contain a minimum of 2.4 percent beta-1,2-fructofuranosides): 2–3 ml (½ to ¾ teaspoon)
- Tincture (1:5): 3–4 milliliters (¾ to 1 teaspoon)
- Fluid extract (1:1): 1–2 milliliters (¼ to ½ teaspoon)
- Solid (dry powdered) extract (6.5:1 or 3.5 percent echinacoside): 300 milligrams

Whether echinacea should be used on a long-term or continual basis really depends on your need. If you are a healthy individual with no apparent depression of the immune system, continual administration is certainly not indicated. However, as recent studies have shown in patients with impaired immune function, long-term administration can provide long-term benefit. The usual recommendation for long-term use is 8 weeks on followed by 1 week off.

Toxicity

Echinacea is not toxic when used at the recommended doses; no studies report acute or chronic toxicity reactions due to echinacea. The fresh-pressed juice of E. purpurea, given intravenously, has caused fever (a 0.5 to 1 degree C elevation in body temperature) on occasion. This reaction is presumably a result of secretion of interferon and interleukin 1 by activated macrophages.[2,3]

The LD_{50} (50 percent lethal dose) of intravenously administered fresh-pressed juice of E. purpurea has been determined to be 50 milliliters per kilogram body weight in mice and rats. The polysaccharides in E. purpurea (aerial portion) have an LD_{50} of 1,000–2,500 milligrams per kilogram when given peritoneally to mice. Chronic administration of the fresh-pressed juice of E. purpurea to rats at doses many times the human therapeutic dose gave no evidence of any toxic effects.[45] Mutagenic tests with the fresh-pressed juice of E. purpurea demonstrated no mutagenic activity.[2,3]

References

1. McGregor RL: The taxonomy of the genus *Echinacea* (Compositae). *Univ Kansas Sci Bull* **48**, 113–142, 1968.
2. Hobbs C: *The Echinacea Handbook*. Eclectic Medical Publications, Portland, OR, 1989.
3. Bauer R and Wagner H: *Echinacea* species as potential immunostimulatory drugs. *Econ Med Plant Res* **5**, 253–321, 1991.
4. Wagner V, *et al.*: Immunostimulating polysaccharides (heteroglycans) of higher plants. *Arzneimittel-Forsch* **35**, 1069–1075, 1985.
5. Stimpel M, *et al.*: Macrophage activation and induction of macrophage cytotoxicity by purified polysaccharide fractions from the plant *Echinacea purpurea*. *Infect Immu* **46**, 845–849, 1984.
6. Luettig B, *et al.*: Macrophage activation by the polysaccharide arabinogalactan isolated from plant cell cultures of *Echinacea purpurea*. *J Natl Cancer Inst* **81**, 669–675, 1989.
7. Tubaro A, *et al.*: Anti-inflammatory activity of a polysaccharide fraction of *Echinacea angustifolia* root. *J Pharm Pharmacol* **39**, 567–569, 1987.
8. Bauer R, Remiger P, and Wagner H: Alkylamides from the roots of *Echinacea angustifolia*. *Dtsch Apoth Ztg* **128**, 174–180, 1988.
9. Christ B and Muller KH: Zur serienmabigen Bestimmung dess Gehhaltes an Flavonol-derivaten in Drogen. *Arch Pharm* **293**(65), 1033–1042, 1960.
10. Stoll A, Renz J, and Brack A: Antibacterial substances. II. Isolation and constitution of echinacoside, a glycoside from the roots of *Echinacea angustifolia*. *Helv Chim Acta* **33**, 1877–1893m 1950.
11. Bauer R and Remiger P: Der Einsatz der HPLC bei der Standardisierung von Echinacea-Drogen *Arch Pharm* **322**, 324, 1989.
12. Bauer R, Reminger P, and Alstat E: Alkamides and caffeic acid derivatives from the roots of *Echinacea tennesseensis*. *Planta Medica* **56**, 533–534, 1990.
13. Neugebuaer H: The constituents of *Echinacea*. *Pharmazie* **4**, 137–140, 1949.
14. Heinzer F, Meusy JP, and Chavanne M: *Echinacea pallida* and *Echinacea purpurea*: Follow-up of weight development and chemical composition for the first two culture years. Paper presented at the 36th Annual Congress of the Society of Medicinal Plant Research, Freiburg, Germany, September 12–16, 1988.
15. Schulte KE, Ruecker G, and Perlick J: The presence of polyacetylene compounds in *Echinacea purpurea* and *Echinacea angustifolia*. *Arzneimittel-Forsch* **17**, 825–829, 1967.
16. Bauer R, Khan IA, and Wagner H: TLC and HPLC analysis of *Echinacea pallida* and *E. angustifolia* roots. *Planta Medica* **54**, 426–430, 1988.
17. Bauer R and Remiger P: TLC and HPLC analysis of *Echinacea pallida* and *E. angustifolia* roots. *Planta Medica* **55**, 367–371, 1989.
18. Roder E, *et al.*: Pyrrolizidine in *Echinacea angustifolia* DC, und *Echinacea purpurea* MOENCH-Isolierung und Analytik. *Dtsch Apoth Ztg* **124**, 2316–2318, 1984.
19. Vogel VJ: *American Indian Medicine*. University of Oklahoma Press, Norman, OK, 1970, pp. 356–357.
20. Felter H: *The Eclectic Materia Medica, Pharmacology and Therapeutics*. Eclectic Medical Publications, Portland, OR, 1983, pp. 347–351
21. Busing K: Hyaluronidasehemmung durch echinacin. *Arzneimittel-Forsch* **2**, 467–469, 1952.
22. Bonadeo I and Lavazza M: Echinacin B: Polisaccaride attivo dell' *Echinacea*. *Riv Ital Essenze Profumi* **53**, 281–295, 1971.
23. Tragni E, *et al.*: Evidence from two classic irritation tests for an anti-inflammatory action of a natural extract, Echinacina B. *Food Chem Toxicol* **23**, 317–319, 1985.
24. Koch FE and Uebel H: Experimentelle untersuchungen uber den einflur von *Echinacea purpurea* auf das hypophysennebennierenrinden-system. *Arzneimittel-Forsch* 133–137, 1953.
25. Wagner H, *et al.*: In vitro inhibition of arachidonate metabolism by some alkylamides and phenylated phenols. *Planta Medica* **55**, 566–567, 1989.
26. Mose J: Effect of echinacin on phagocytosis and natural killer cells. *Med Welt* **34**, 1463–1467, 1983.
27. Djonlagic H and Feiereis H: Leukopoese und alkalische leukozytenphosphatase im echinacin-test bei colities ulcerosa. *Z Gastroenterol* **1**, 19–22, 1975.
28. Foster S: *Echinacea. Nature's Immune Enhancer*. Healing Arts Press, Rochester, VT, 1991.
29. Pohl P: Therapy of radiation-induced leukopenia by Esberitox. *Med Klin* **64**, 1546–1547, 1969.
30. Chone B and Manidakis G: Echinacin-test zur leukozytenprovokation bei efict strahlentherapie. *Dtsch Med Wochenschr* **27**, 1406–1409, 1969.

31. Roesler J, *et al.*: Application of purified polysaccharides from cell cultures of the plant *Echinacea purpurea* to mice mediates protection against systemic infections with *Listeria monocytogenes* and *Candida albicans. Int J Immunopharmacol* **13**, 27–37, 1991.

32. Vomel V: Influence of a non-specific immune stimulant on phagocytosis of erythrocytes and ink by the reticuloendothelial system of isolated perfused rat livers of different ages. *Arzneimittel-Forsch* **34**, 691–695, 1984.

33. Bauer R, *et al.*: Immunological *in vivo* and *in vitro* examinations of *Echinacea* extracts. *Arzneimittel-Forsch* **38**, 276–281, 1988.

34. Wacker A and Hilbig W: Virus-inhibition by *Echinacea purpurea. Planta Medica* **33**, 89–102, 1978.

35. Koch F and Haase H: Eine Modifikation des spreading-testes im tierversuch, gleichzeitig ein beitrag zum wirkungsmechanismus von echinacin. *Arzneimittel-Forsch* **2**, 464–467, 1952.

36. Hopp E and Burn H: Ground substance in the nose in health and infection. *Ann Oto Rhino Laryngol* **65**, 480–489, 1956.

37. Voaden D and Jacobson M: Tumor inhibitors. 3. Identification and synthesis of an oncolytic hydrocarbon from American coneflower roots. *J Med Chem* **15**, 619–623, 1972.

38. Coeugniet EG and Kuhnast R: Recurrent candidiasis: Adjuvant immunotherapy with different formulations of Echinacin. *Therapiewoche* **36**, 3352–3358, 1986.

39. Braunig B, *et al.*: *Echinacea purpurea* radix for strengthening the immune response in flu-like infections. *Z Phytother* **13**, 7–13, 1992.

40. Schoneberger D: The influence of immune-stimulating effects of pressed juice from *Echinacea purpurea* on the course and severity of colds. Results of a double-blind study. *Forum Immunol* **8**, 2–12, 1992.

41. Kinkel HJ, Plate M, and Tullner HU: Effect of echinacin ointment in healing of skin lesions. *Med Klin* **79**, 580, 1984.

42. Seidel K and Knobloch H: Nachweis und vergleich der antiphlogistischen wirkung antirheumatischer medikamente. *Z Rheum* **16**, 231–238, 1957.

43. Awang DVC and Kindack DG: *Echinacea. Can Pharm J* **124**, 512–516, 1991.

44. Schumacher A and Friedberg KD: Analysis of the effect of *Echinacea angustifolia* on unspecified immunity of the mouse. *Arzneimittel-Forsch* **41**, 141–147, 1991.

45. Mengs U, Clare CB and Poiley JA: Toxicity of *Echinacea purpurea. Arzneimittel-Forsch* **41**, 1076–1081, 1991.

9
Ephedra

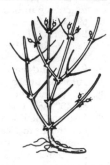

Key uses of ephedra:

- Asthma
- Hay fever
- Common cold
- Weight loss aid

General description

Ephedra species are erect, branching shrubs found in desert or arid regions throughout the world. *Ephedra sinica* (Chinese ephedra or Ma Huang) is found in Asia; *Ephedra distacha* (European ephedra) is found in Europe; *Ephedra trifurca* or *Ephedra viridis* (desert tea), *Ephedra nevadensis* (Mormon tea), and *Ephedra americana* (American ephedra) are found in North America; and *Ephedra gerardiana* (Pakistani ephedra) is found primarily in India and Pakistan. The 1½- to 4-foot shrubs typically grow on dry, rocky or sandy slopes. The many slender, yellow-green branches of ephedra have two very small leaf scales at each node. The mature, double-seeded cones are visible in the fall.

Chemical composition

Chemical analysis of the stems and branches of *Ephedra species* focuses on the alkaloid content. In *Ephedra sinica*, the total alkaloid content can reach 3.3 percent, with 40–90 percent of this being ephedrine and the remaining alkaloids being primarily pseudoephedrine and norpseudoephedrine. In *Ephedra gerardiana*, the alkaloid content usually varies from 0.8 to 1.4 percent, and is about half ephedrine and half other alkaloids (pseudoephedrine, N-methylephedrine, norpseudoephedrine, etc.). Mormon tea or *Ephedra nevadensis* contains no ephedrine.[1,2]

History and folk use

The medicinal use of *Ephedra sinica* in China dates from approximately 2800 B.C. Ma Huang refers to the stem and branch, whereas Ma Huanggen refers to the root and rhizome. Ma Huang was used primarily in the treatment of the common cold, asthma, hay fever, bronchitis, edema, arthritis, fever, hypotension, and urticaria.[1]

Ma Huanggen's effect is believed to oppose that of the stem and branches. Its use was limited to the treatment of profuse night sweating.[3]

Western medicine's interest in ephedra began in 1923, with the demonstration that the isolated alkaloid ephedrine possessed a number of pharmacological effects.[3] Ephedrine was synthesized in 1927 and since this time both ephedrine and pseudoephedrine have been used extensively in over-the-counter cold and allergy medications.[3]

Pharmacology

The pharmacology of ephedra centers around its ephedrine content. Ephedrine and pseudoephedrine have been extensively investigated and are widely used in prescription and other-the-counter medications for asthma, hay fever, and rhinitis.[3] In 1973, more than 20 million prescriptions contained either of these alkaloids. The pharmacology of ephedrine and pseudoephedrine is discussed below, followed by therapeutic applications of *Ephedra sinica*.

Ephedrine

Ephedrine's basic pharmacological action is similar to that of epinephrine (adrenaline), although ephedrine is much less active. Ephedrine also differs from epinephrine in its ability to be absorbed orally, its longer duration of action, and its more pronounced effect on the brain and central nervous system (CNS). The CNS effects of ephedrine are similar to those of amphetamines, but again much less potent.[3]

The cardiovascular effects of ephedrine are also similar to those of epinephrine, that is, ephedrine increases blood pressure, cardiac output, and heart rate, but lasts longer (about ten times longer). Like epinephrine, ephedra will also increase heart, brain, and muscle blood flow at the expense of kidney and intestinal blood flow.[3]

Bronchial muscle (the muscles of our airways), and uterine muscles are relaxed by ephedrine.[3]

Pseudoephedrine

Pseudoephedrine relaxes bronchial muscle like ephedrine, but exerts weaker effects on the heart and central nervous system. Pseudoephedrine is often recommended in preference to ephedrine in the treatment of chronic asthma, as it has fewer side effects.[3]

Pseudoephedrine has also demonstrated a significant antiinflammatory effect in various experimental models.[4,5] Other ephedra alkaloids, including ephedrine, also exhibit antiinflammatory activity, but at much lower potency.

Clinical applications

Ephedra is used to treat asthma, hay fever, the common cold, and as a weight loss aid. Each of these applications is discussed below.

Asthma and hay fever

Ephedra and its alkaloids are effective bronchodilators in the treatment of mild to moderate asthma and hay fever.[3] The peak bronchodilation effect occurs in 1 hour and lasts about 5 hours after adminstration.

Many believe that the therapeutic effect of ephedra will diminish if used for a long period of time, owing to a weakening of the adrenal glands caused by ephedrine. But, according to the American Pharmaceutical Association, "there is far more discussion of ephedrine tachyphylaxis [rapid decrease in effectiveness] or tolerance than is evidenced as a significant problem in the scientific literature."[6] A 1977 study of ephedrine therapy in asthmatic children, published in the Journal of the American Medical Association, concluded: "Ephedrine is a potent bronchodilator that, in appropriate doses, can be administered safely along with therapeutic doses of theophylline without the fear of progressive tolerance or toxicity."[7]

Nonetheless, many practitioners of natural medicine prescribe ephedra in combination with substances that support the adrenal glands, such as licorice (*Glycyrrhiza glabra*) and *Panax ginseng* and/or supplemental levels of vitamin C, magnesium, zinc, vitamin B_6, and pantothenic acid.

The old-time herbal treatment of asthma involves the use of ephedra in combination with herbal expectorants. Expectorants modify the quality and quantity of secretions from the respiratory tract, causing the user to spit up the secretions and ultimately improving respiratory tract function. Examples of commonly used expectorants include licorice (*Glycyrrhiza glabra*), grindelia (*Grindelia camporum*), euphorbia (*Euphorbia hirta*), sundew (*Drosera rotundifolia*), and senega (*Polygala senega*).

Weight loss aid

Ephedra preparations may be useful as a weight loss aid. Although ephedrine does suppress appetite, its main mechanism for promoting weight loss appears to be by increasing the metabolic rate of adipose tissue.[8,9] Its weight-reducing effects are greatest in those individuals with a low basal metabolic rate and/or decreased diet-induced thermogenesis.

Many people are predisposed to being overweight because their bodies lay down fat efficiently; other people go the other way—they burn fat efficiently. The reason for the difference has to do with how our bodies process the food we eat. A certain amount of the food we eat is converted immediately to heat. This effect is known as *diet-induced thermogenesis* (heat production). The degree of diet-induced thermogenesis is what determines whether an individual is likely to be obese. In lean individuals a meal may stimulate an up to 40 percent increase in heat production. In contrast, obese individuals often display only a 10 percent (or less) increase in heat production. In these people the food energy is stored instead of being converted to heat.

The degree of heat production—whether it be high or low—is determined by the sympathetic nervous system. This portion of the nervous system controls many body functions, including metabolism. In other words, the reason why many obese individuals have a "slow metabolism" is because of a lack of stimulation by the sympathetic nervous system. Ephedrine can activate the sympathetic nervous system, thereby increasing the metabolic rate and thermogenesis. This results in weight loss by addressing the underlying defect in metabolism.

The thermogenic effects of ephedrine can be enhanced by methylxanthines and salicylates. Herbs rich in these active ingredients can be used just like the isolated principles. Good methylxanthine sources include coffee (*Coffea arabica*), tea (*Camellia sinensis*), cola nut (*Cola nitida*), and guarana (*Paullinea cupana*). Natural salicylates can be found in members of the mint and oak families. The optimum dosage of the crude plant preparation or extract depends on the content of active ingredient. Standardized preparations may produce more dependable results.

In one animal study, ephedrine when used alone resulted in a loss of 14 percent in body weight and 42 percent in body fat; however, ephedrine used in combination with caffeine or theophylline resulted in a loss of 25 percent in body weight and 75 percent in body fat.[10] In contrast, when either caffeine or theophylline was used alone there was no significant loss in body weight. The animals in this study lost weight owing to the increased metabolic rate and fat cell breakdown promoted by ephedrine and enhanced by caffeine and theophylline.

Let's review some of the studies on ephedrine and weight loss.

Ephedrine only   Ephedrine as the sole weight loss agent has been the subject of several clinical studies.[11,12] The results have been inconsistent. For example, in one study, overweight individuals were given, three times daily, either a placebo (group I), 25 milligrams of ephedrine (group II), or 150 milligrams of ephedrine (group III) for 3 months. Dietary treatment consisted of 1,000 calories per day for females and 1,200 calories per day for males. Weight loss was similar in all groups. Patients in group III (ephedrine, 150 milligrams per day) showed significantly more side effects than the placebo group.

In another study, ten obese women were treated with diet therapy (1,000–1,400 calories per day) and either ephedrine (50 milligrams three times per day) or placebo for 2 months and then crossed over.[12] Weight loss was significantly greater during the ephedrine period (5.3 pounds) than during the placebo period (1.4 pounds).

The reason for these differences appears to be that ephedrine is effective primarily in those people with defects in diet-induced thermogenesis, and is ineffective in those without this defect. Overall, the results seem to indicate that ephedrine alone is not as effective in promoting weight loss compared to combination products, even when ephedrine is given at a high daily dosage (e.g., 150 milligrams per day).

Ephedrine with methylxanthines   As mentioned earlier, the effectiveness of ephedrine in weight loss is greatly enhanced when it is combined with caffeine and/or theophylline. Most of the recent studies have used a combination providing 20 milligrams of ephedrine and 200 milligrams of caffeine three times daily. Long-term studies have shown good safety and efficacy.[13,14]

In one of the largest studies, 180 overweight patients were treated by diet and either an ephedrine–caffeine combination (20 milligrams/200 milligrams), ephedrine alone (20 milligrams), caffeine alone (200 milligrams) or placebo three times a day for 24 weeks.[14] The mean weight loss was significantly greater in the group given the ephedrine–caffeine combination. Each member of the ephedrine–caffeine group lost, on average, 36 pounds in

24 weeks compared to 29 pounds for those in the placebo group. In the groups receiving ephedrine or caffeine only, weight loss was similar to that of the placebo group. Side effects (tremor, insomnia, and dizziness) were transient, and after 8 weeks of treatment there was no difference in side effects between the group receiving the ephedrine–caffeine combination and the placebo group. Both systolic and diastolic blood pressure fell similarly in all four groups, indicating the weight loss promoted by ephedrine and caffeine counteracts any increase in blood pressure these substances may promote.

Although more recent studies have used a daily dose of 60 milligrams of ephedrine and 600 milligrams of caffeine, these high doses may not be necessary. In one study, a daily dose of 22 milligrams ephedrine, 30 milligrams caffeine, and 50 milligrams theophylline was shown to greatly increase the basal metabolic rate and diet-induced thermogenesis.[15]

Ephedrine and aspirin   The thermogenic effects of ephedrine are further enhanced by aspirin.[16–19] In one study, the effect of ephedrine (30 milligrams) and aspirin (300 milligrams) on the acute thermogenic response to a liquid meal (250 kilocalories) was investigated in lean and obese women.[18] The resting metabolic rate was measured prior to each of the following treatments: meal only, meal plus ephedrine, or meal plus ephedrine and aspirin. Following the meal-only treatment, the mean increase in metabolic rate was 0.17 and 0.13 kilocalories per minute in the lean and obese groups, respectively. With the meal-plus-ephedrine treatment, the corresponding rises were 0.21 and 0.19 kilocalories per minute. And, following the meal plus ephedrine and aspirin the rise was 0.23 kilocalories per minute in both groups.

Another study looked at the safety and efficacy of a mixture of ephedrine (75–150 milligrams), caffeine (150 milligrams), and aspirin (330 milligrams), in divided premeal doses, compared to a placebo in twenty-four obese humans.[19] Dietary intake was not restricted. Overall weight loss in 8 weeks was 4.84 pounds for the combination group versus 1.5 pounds for the placebo group. Eight of thirteen placebo subjects returned 5 months later and received the combination treatment. After 8 weeks, mean weight loss with the combination treatment was 7 pounds versus 2.86 pounds for the period of time when they were on the placebo. Six subjects continued on the formula for 7 to 26 months. After 5 months on ephedrine–caffeine–aspirin, average weight loss in five of these subjects was 11.44 pounds. The sixth subject lost 145 pounds in 13 months by self-imposed caloric restriction in combination with taking the ephedrine–caffeine–aspirin combination. In all studies, no significant changes in heart rate, blood pressure, blood glucose, insulin, and cholesterol levels, and no differences in the frequency of side effects, were found between groups.

Dosage

The appropriate dose of ephedra depends on the alkaloid content. The average total alkaloid content of *Ephedra sinica* is 1 to 3 percent. For asthma and as a weight loss aid the dose of ephedra should contain an ephedrine content of 12.5–25.0 milligrams and be taken two to three times daily. For the crude herb this would require a dose of 500 to 1,000 milligrams three times per day. Standardized preparations are preferred as they are more dependable in terms of therapeutic activity. For example, *Ephedra sinica* extracts are available that have a standardized alkaloid content of 10 percent. The dosage of a 10 percent alkaloid content extract would be 125 to 250 milligrams three times daily.

Toxicity

Ephedra can produce the same side effects that ephedrine produces, that is, increased blood pressure, increased heart rate, insomnia, and anxiety.

The Food and Drug Administration (FDA) advisory review panel on nonprescription drugs recommended that ephedrine not be taken by patients with heart disease, high blood pressure, thyroid disease, diabetes, or difficulty in urination due to enlargement of the prostate. In addition, ephedrine should not be used by patients taking antihypertensives or antidepressants.

References

1. Chang HM and But PP: *Pharmacology and Applications of Chinese Materia Medica*, Vol. 2. World Scientific Publishing, Teaneck, NJ, 1987.
2. Duke JA: *Handbook of Medicinal Herbs*. CRC Press, Boca Raton, FL, 1985.
3. Gilman AG, Goodman AS, and Gilman A: *The Pharmacologic Basis of Therapeutics*. Macmillan, New York, 1980.
4. Hikino H, Konno C, Takata H, and Tamada M: Antiinflammatory principle of ephedra herbs. *Chem Pharm Bull* **28**, 2900–2904, 1980.
5. Kasahara Y, *et al.*: Antiinflammatory actions of ephedrines in acute inflammations. *Planta Medica* **54**, 325–331, 1985.
6. American Pharmaceutical Association: *Handbook of Nonprescription Drugs*, 8th Ed. American Pharmaceutical Association, Washington, DC, 1986.
7. Tinkelman DG and Avner SE: Ephedrine therapy in asthmatic children. *JAMA* **237**, 553–557, 1977.
8. Astrup A, *et al.*: The effect of chronic ephedrine treatment on substrate utilization, the sympatho-adrenal activity, and expenditure during glucose-induced thermogenesis in man. *Metabolism* **35**, 260–265, 1986.
9. Astrup A, *et al.*: Pharmacology of thermogenic drugs. *Am J Clin Nutr* **55**(Suppl 1), 246S–248S, 1992.
10. Dulloo AG and Miller DS: The thermogenic properties of ephedrine/methylxanthine mixtures: Animal studies. *Am J Clin Nutr* **43**, 388–394, 1986.
11. Pasquali R: A controlled trial using ephedrine in the treatment of obesity. *Int J Obes* **9**, 93–98, 1985.
12. Pasquali R and Casimirri F: Clinical aspects of ephedrine in the treatment of obesity. *Int J Obes* **17**(Suppl 1), S65–68, 1993.

13. Toubro S, *et al.*: Safety and efficacy of long-term treatment with ephedrine, caffeine and an ephedrine/caffeine mixture. *Int J Obes* **17**(Suppl 1), S69–72, 1993.
14. Astrup A, *et al.*: The effect and safety of an ephedrine/caffeine compound compared to ephedrine, caffeine and placebo in obese subjects on an energy restricted diet. A double blind trial. *Int J Obes* **16**, 269–277, 1992.
15. Dulloo AG and Miller DS: The thermogenic properties of ephedrine/methylxanthine mixtures: Human studies. *Int J Obes* **10**, 467–481, 1986.
16. Dulloo AG, Seydoux J, and Girardier L: Potentiation of the thermogenic antiobesity effects of ephedrine by dietary methylxanthines: Adenosine antagonism or phosphodiesterase inhibition? *Metabolism* **41**(11), 1233–1241, 1992.
17. Dulloo AG: Ephedrine, xanthines and prostaglandin-inhibitors: Actions and interactions in the stimulation of thermogenesis. *Int J Obes* **17**(Suppl 1), S35–40, 1993.
18. Horton TJ and Geissler CA: Aspirin potentiates the effect of ephedrine on the thermogenic response to a meal in obese but not lean women. *Int J Obes* **15**, 359–366, 1991.
19. Daly PA, *et al.*: Ephedrine, caffeine and aspirin: Safety and efficacy for treatment of human obesity. *Int J Obes* **17**(Suppl 1):S73–78, 1993.

10
Feverfew

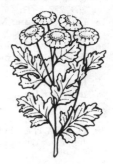

Key uses of feverfew:

- Migraine headaches (prevention and treatment)
- Fever
- Inflammation

General description

Feverfew (*Tanacetum parthenium*), a member of the sunflower family, grows in flower gardens throughout Europe and the United States. The round, leafy, branching stems bear alternate, bipinnate leaves with ovate, hoary-green leaflets. The flowers are small and daisy-like, with yellow disks and from ten to twenty white, toothed rays. The name *feverfew* is a corruption of the word *febrifuge*, used to signify its tonic and fever-dispelling properties.

Chemical composition

The major active chemicals in the plant are sesquiterpene lactones, principally parthenolide. The flowering herb also contains 0.02–0.07 percent essential oils (L-camphor, L-borneol, terpenes, and miscellaneous esters).[1,2]

History and folk use

Feverfew has been used for centuries as a febrifuge and for the treatment of migraines and arthritis. Other historical uses of feverfew have been in the treatment of anemia, earache, dysmenorrhea, dyspepsia, trauma, and intestinal parasites.[1] It has also been used as an abortifacient, and in gardens to control noxious pests (its pyrethrin component is an effective insecticide and herbicide).

Pharmacology

Feverfew has demonstrated some remarkable pharmacological effects in experimental studies. Its long history of use in the treatment of inflammatory conditions such as fever, arthritis, and migraine suggests that it acts like the more common, nonsteroidal antiinflammatory agents (NSAIDs), such as aspirin. Extracts of feverfew inhibit the manufacture of compounds that promote inflammation, including inflammatory prostaglandins, leukotrienes, and thromboxanes. Unlike aspirin and other NSAIDs, inhibition by feverfew is at the initial stage of synthesis and is more like that of cortisone than NSAIDs.[3]

Feverfew also has a favorable effect on the behavior of blood platelets[3,4]: it inhibits platelet aggregation and inhibits the secretion of inflammatory and allergic mediators such as histamine and serotonin. Parthenolide components also exert a tonic effect on vascular smooth muscle.[5]

Feverfew's combined action on smooth muscle and platelets is probably why it is effective in the prevention and treatment of migraine headaches.

Clinical applications

Feverfew has been used for centuries to relieve fever, migraines, and arthritis. The only condition with confirmed scientific documentation at the present time is in the prevention and treatment of migraine headache.

Migraine headache

In his book *The Family Herbal* (1772), physician John Hill noted, "In the worst headache this herb exceeds whatever else is known."[10] Recently, interest in feverfew as a treatment for migraine headache has increased tremendously. This renewed interest began in the 1970s in Great Britain, where increased public awareness of the herb led to scientific investigation. A 1983 survey found that 70 percent of 270 migraine sufferers who had eaten feverfew daily for prolonged periods claimed that the herb decreased the frequency and/or intensity of their attacks.[6] Many of these patients had been unresponsive to orthodox medicines. This prompted two clinical investigations of the therapeutic and preventive effects of feverfew in the treatment of migraine.

The first double-blind study was done at the London Migraine Clinic, and involved patients who reported being helped by feverfew.[6] Those patients who received the placebo (and as a result stopped using feverfew) experienced a significant increase in the frequency and severity of headache, nausea, and vomiting during the 6 months of the study, while patients taking feverfew showed no change in the frequency or severity of their symptoms. Two patients in the placebo group who had been in complete remission during self-treatment with feverfew leaves developed recurrence of incapacitating migraine and had to withdraw from the study. The resumption of self-treatment led to renewed remission of symptoms in both patients.

The second double-blind study was performed at the University of Nottingham.[7] The results of the study clearly demonstrated that feverfew was effective in reducing the number and severity of migraine attacks. In the study, seventy-two patients were randomly allocated to receive either one capsule of dried feverfew leaves (82 milligrams) daily or placebo. After 4 months patients were transferred to the other treatment for another 4 months. Treatment with feverfew was associated with a reduction in the mean number and severity of attacks and in the degree of vomiting; duration of single attacks was unaltered.

Rheumatoid arthritis

Inflammatory compounds released by white blood cells and platelets contribute greatly to the inflammation and cellular damage found in rheumatoid arthritis. The inhibition of the release of inflammatory particles by feverfew is much greater than that achieved by NSAIDs like aspirin.[4] This coupled with many of feverfew's other effects indicate that feverfew could greatly reduce inflammation in rheumatoid arthritis.

One double-blind, placebo-controlled study[8] demonstrated no apparent benefit from oral feverfew in rheumatoid arthritis. However, the dosage used was extremely small (76 milligrams of dried, powdered feverfew leaf, corresponding to two medium-sized leaves, per day); the level of parthenolide was not determined in the product; and the patients continued to take NSAIDs, a practice that has been suggested to reduce the efficacy of feverfew. Therefore, it is safe to conclude that the benefit of feverfew in rheumatoid arthritis has not yet been determined.

Dosage

The effectiveness of feverfew depends on adequate levels of parthenolide, the active principle. Unfortunately, a recent analysis of the parthenolide content of more than thirty-five different commercial preparations indicates a wide variation in the amount of parthenolide.[9] The majority of products contained no parthenolide or only traces.

The preparations used in successful clinical trials had a parthenolide content of 0.4 to 0.66 percent. To achieve the benefits noted in the migraine studies, the dosage of parthenolide must be similar. The dosage of feverfew used in the London Migraine Clinic study was one capsule containing 25 milligrams of the freeze-dried, pulverized leaves twice daily. In the Nottingham study it was one capsule containing 82 milligrams of dried powdered leaves once daily. Therefore, the daily dosage of parthenolide that may be effective in the prevention of a migraine headache is roughly 0.25 to 0.5 milligrams.

While these low dosages may be effective in preventing an attack, a higher dose (1–2 grams) is necessary during an acute attack.

Toxicity

The 6-month migraine studies[6,7] made no report of toxic reactions in patients taking feverfew. Feverfew has been used by large numbers of people for many years without reports of toxicity. Chewing the leaves, however, may result in aphthous ulcerations, and some sensitive persons will develop an exudative dermatitis from external contact.[10]

References

1. Duke JA: *Handbook of Medicinal Herbs*. CRC Press, Boca Raton, FL, 1985. p. 118.
2. Bohlmann F and Zdero C: Sesquiterpene lactones and other constituents from *Tanacetum parthenium*. *Phytochemistry* **21**, 2543–2549, 1982.
3. Makheja AM and Bailey JM: A platelet phospholipase inhibitor from the medicinal herb feverfew (*Tanacetum parthenium*). *Prostaglandins Leukotrienes Med* **8**, 653–660, 1982.
4. Heptinstall S, *et al.*: Extracts of feverfew inhibit granule secretion in blood platelets and polymorphonuclear leukocytes. *Lancet* **i**, 1071–1074, 1985.
5. Barsby RWJ, *et al.*: Feverfew and vascular smooth muscle: Extracts from fresh and dried plants show opposing pharmacological profiles, dependent upon sesquiterpene lactone content. *Planta Medica* **59**, 20–25, 1993
6. Johnson ES, *et al.*: Efficacy of feverfew as prophylactic treatment of migraine. *Br Med J* **291**, 569–573, 1985.
7. Murphy JJ, Heptinstall S, and Mitchell JRA: Randomized double-blind placebo-controlled trial of feverfew in migraine prevention. *Lancet* **ii**, 189–192, 1988.

8. Pattrick M, *et al.*: Feverfew in rheumatoid arthritis: a double blind, placebo controlled study. *Ann Rheum Dis* **48**, 547–549, 1989.
9. Heptinstall S, *et al.*: Parthenolide content and bioactivity of feverfew (*Tanacetum parthenium* (L.) Schultz-Bip.). Estimation of commercial and authenticated feverfew products. *J Pharm Pharmacol* **44**, 391–395, 1992.
10. Awang DVC: Feverfew. *Can Pharm J* **122**, 266–270, 1989.

11
Garlic

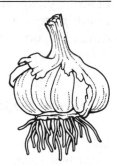

Key uses of garlic:

- Cancer prevention
- Diabetes
- High blood pressure
- High cholesterol
- Infection

General description

Garlic (*Allium sativum*), a member of the lily family, is a perennial plant that is cultivated worldwide. The garlic bulb is composed of individual cloves enclosed in a white skin. It is the bulb, either fresh or dehydrated, that is used as a spice or medicinal herb.

Chemical composition

Garlic contains a volatile oil (0.1–0.36 percent) composed of sulfur-containing compounds: allicin, diallyl disulfide, diallyl trisulfide, and others. The garlic oil is obtained by steam distillation of the crushed fresh bulbs.[1] These volatile compounds are generally considered to be responsible for most of the pharmacological properties of garlic. Other constituents of garlic include alliin (*S*-allyl-L-cysteine sulfoxide), *S*-methyl-L-cysteine sulfoxide, protein (16.8 percent, dry weight basis), high concentrations of trace minerals (particularly selenium), vitamins, glucosinolates, and enzymes (alliinase, peroxidase, and myrosinase).[1,2]

The pungent odor of garlic is caused mainly by allicin. Allicin forms when the enzyme alliinase reacts with the compound alliin. The essential oil of garlic yields approximately 60 percent of its weight in allicin after exposure to alliinase. Because the enzyme is inactivated by heat, cooked garlic produces less odor than raw garlic, and is not nearly as powerful in physiological effect.[1]

History and folk use

Garlic has long been used to treat a wide variety of conditions. Sanskrit records document the use of garlic remedies approximately 5,000 years ago, while the Chinese have been using it for at least 3,000 years. The Codex Ebers, an Egyptian medical papyrus dating from about 1550 B.C., mentions garlic as an effective remedy for a variety of ailments, including hypertension, headache, bites, worms, and tumors. Hippocrates, Aristotle, and Pliny cited numerous therapeutic uses for garlic. In general, garlic has been used throughout the world to treat coughs, toothache, earache, dandruff, hypertension, atherosclerosis, hysteria, diarrhea, dysentery, diphtheria, vaginitis, and many other conditions.[1–3]

Stories, verse, and folklore (such as its alleged ability to ward off vampires) give historical documentation to garlic's power. Sir John Harrington in *The Englishman's Doctor*, written in 1609, summarized garlic's virtues and faults[3]:

> Garlic then have power to save from death
> Bear with it though it maketh unsavory breath,
> And scorn not garlic like some that think
> It only maketh men wink and drink and stink.

In 1721, during a widespread plague in Marseilles, four condemned criminals were recruited to bury the dead. The gravediggers proved to be immune to the disease. Their secret was a concoction they drank, consisting of macerated garlic in wine. This became known as *vinaigre des quatre voleurs* (four thieves' vinegar), and it is still available in France today.

Garlic's antibiotic activity was noted by Pasteur in 1858. Garlic was used by Albert Schweitzer in Africa for the treatment of amebic dysentery, and as an antiseptic in the prevention of gangrene during World Wars I and II.

Pharmacology

Garlic has a wide range of well-documented effects; it can be used as an antimicrobial agent, for immune enhancement, for cancer prevention, and for its cardiovascular effects. The following subsections focus on these properties.

Antimicrobial activity

Garlic exerts broad-spectrum antimicrobial activity against many genera of bacteria, virus, worms, and fungi, as summarized in several works.[4-6] These findings seem to support the historical use of garlic in the treatment of a variety of infectious conditions.

Antibacterial activity

As far back as 1944, studies have demonstrated that both garlic juice and allicin inhibited the growth of *Staphylococcus, Streptococcus, Bacillus, Brucella,* and *Vibrio* species at low concentrations.[7,8] In more recent studies using serial dilution and filter paper disk techniques, fresh and vacuum-dried powdered garlic preparations were found to be effective antibiotic agents against many bacteria, including *Staphylococcus aureus,* alpha- and beta-hemolytic *Streptococcus, Escherichia coli, Proteus vulgaris, Salmonella enteritidis, Citrobacter* species, *Klebsiella pneumoniae,* and mycobacteria.[4-6,9,10] These studies compared the antimicrobial effects of garlic with those of commonly used antibiotics, including penicillin, streptomycin, chloramphenicol, erythromycin, and tetracyclines. Besides confirming garlic's well-known antibacterial effects, the studies demonstrated this herb's efficacy in inhibiting the growth of some bacteria that had become resistant to one or more of the antibiotics.

Antifungal activity

Garlic has demonstrated significant antifungal activity in many *in vitro* and *in vivo* studies.[4,11-16] From a clinical perspective, its inhibition of *Candida albicans* is most significant—both animal and test tube (*in vitro*) studies have shown garlic to be more potent than nystatin, gentian violet, and six other reputed antifungal agents.[4,12-14]

I offer the following as an illustration of just how powerful garlic's antifungal action can be. In one study at a major Chinese hospital, garlic therapy alone was used effectively in the treatment of cryptococcal meningitis, one of the most serious fungal infections imaginable.[15]

Anthelmintic effects

Garlic extracts exert anthelmintic activity against common intestinal parasites including *Ascaris lumbricoides* (roundworm) and hookworm.[17,18]

Antiviral effects

Garlic's antiviral effects have been demonstrated by its protection of mice from infection with intranasally inoculated influenza virus, and by its enhancement of neutralizing antibody production when given with influenza vaccine.[19]

In vitro, fresh garlic, allicin, and other sulfur components of garlic killed herpes simplex types 1 and 2, parainfluenza virus type 3, vaccinia virus, vesicular stomatitis virus, and human rhinovirus type 2.[20] The order of virucidal activity was as follows: ajoene > allicin > allyl methyl thiosulfinate > methyl allyl thiosulfinate. Ajoene is found in oil-macerates of garlic, but not in fresh garlic extracts. No activity was detected when alliin, deoxyalliin, diallyl disulfide, and diallyl trisulfide were tested. Fresh garlic extract was virucidal against all viruses tested; but the virucidal activity of commercial products depended how they were prepared. Those products producing the highest level of allicin and other thiosulfinates had the best virucidal activity.[20]

Immune enhancing and anticancer effects

Garlic possesses important immune-enhancing and anticancer properties. The famous Greek physician Hippocrites prescribed the eating of garlic as a treatment for cancer. On the basis of animal research and some human studies, this recommendation may have been extremely wise. Several garlic components display significant immune-enhancing as well as anticancer effects.[21–23]

Human studies showing garlic's immune-enhancing and anticancer effects are largely based on population studies.[21–24] From these studies it appears that there is an inverse relationship between cancer rates and garlic consumption; that is, cancer rates are lowest where garlic consumption is greatest. For example, in China, a study comparing populations in different regions found that death from gastric cancer in regions where garlic consumption was high was significantly less than in regions with lower garlic consumption.[24]

Garlic extracts and allicin have displayed potent antitumor effects in animal studies.[25–34] Human studies show that garlic inhibits the formation of nitrosamines (powerful cancer-causing compounds formed during digestion).[35,36]

Cardiovascular effects

Garlic protects against heart disease and strokes by intervening in the process of atherosclerosis at many steps. As there is substantial clinical information on garlic's beneficial effects on the cardiovascular system, the pharmacology is discussed in Clinical Applications (following).

Other effects

Garlic extract exerts significant antiinflammatory activity in experimental models of inflammation.[2,17] This activity is probably a result of garlic's inhibition of the formation of inflammatory compounds.

Garlic (and onions) have often been used in the treatment of diabetes. Allicin has been shown to have significant hypoglycemic action. This effect is thought to be due to increased hepatic metabolism and/or increased release of insulin and/or insulin-sparing effect.[37] The latter mechanism appears to be the major factor, as allicin and other sulfhydryl compounds in garlic and onions compete with insulin (also a disulfide protein) for insulin-inactivating compounds, which results in an increase in free insulin.

Garlic possesses diuretic, diaphoretic, emmenagogue, and expectorant action.[1,9] It is also a carminative, antispasmodic, and digestant, making it useful in cases of flatulence, nausea, vomiting, colic, and indigestion.[17,38]

Clinical applications

The modern use of garlic has focused on its ability to lower cholesterol and blood pressure in the attempt to reduce the risk of dying prematurely from a heart attack or stroke. The majority of studies showing a positive effect of garlic and garlic preparations are those that delivered a sufficient dosage of allicin. Since allicin is the component in garlic that is responsible for its easily identifiable odor, some manufacturers have developed highly sophisticated methods in an effort to provide the full benefits of garlic—they provide "odorless" garlic products concentrated for alliin because alliin is relatively "odorless" until it is converted to allicin in the body. Products concentrated for alliin and other sulfur components provide all of the benefits of fresh garlic, but are more "socially acceptable."

Based on a great deal of clinical research, the dosage of a commercial garlic product should provide a daily dose of at least 10 milligrams alliin or a total allicin potential of 4,000 micrograms.

In addition to the use of garlic preparations, garlic consumption as a food should be encouraged, despite its odor, in patients with high cholesterol levels, ischemic heart disease, hypertension, diabetes, candidiasis, asthma, infections (particularly respiratory tract infections), and gastrointestinal complaints.

Table 11.1 Effects of garlic and onion consumption on serum lipids under carefully matched diets

Garlic/onion consumption	Cholesterol (mg/dl)	Triglyceride (mg/dl)
Garlic (50 g/week), onion (600 g/week)	159	52
Garlic (10 g/week), onion (200 g/week)	172	75
No garlic or onions	208	109

High cholesterol level

Garlic offers significant protection against heart disease and strokes.[39–43] Foremost is its ability to improve cholesterol levels. According to the results of numerous double-blind, placebo-controlled studies in patients with initial cholesterol levels greater than 200 mg/dl, supplementation with commercial preparations providing a daily dose of at least 10 milligrams of alliin or a total allicin potential of 4,000 micrograms can lower total serum cholesterol levels by about 10 to 12 percent. In addition, low-density lipoprotein (LDL) cholesterol will decrease by about 15 percent, high-density lipoprotein (HDL) cholesterol levels will usually increase by about 10 percent, and triglyceride levels will typically drop 15 percent.[43–47]

Although the effect of supplemental garlic preparations effects on cholesterol levels is not phenomenal, the combination of lowered LDL and increased HDL can greatly improve the ratio of LDL to HDL—a significant goal in trying to prevent heart disease and strokes. In addition, garlic preparations standardized for alliin content exert several other beneficial effects in preventing heart disease and strokes (discussed below).

In addition to taking a garlic supplement, individuals with high cholesterol levels should eat more garlic and onions, as increased dietary garlic and onion consumption can also lower cholesterol levels.[39–42,48] In a 1979 population study, researchers studied three populations of vegetarians in the Jain community in India, who consumed differing amounts of garlic and onions.[49] Numerous favorable effects on blood lipids, as shown in Table 11.1, were observed in the group that consumed the largest amount of garlic and onions. Blood fibrinogen (discussed below) levels were highest in the group eating no onions or garlic. The study is quite significant because the subjects had nearly identical diets, except in terms of garlic and onion consumption.

Blood pressure-lowering activity

Garlic has demonstrated hypotensive action in both experimental animals and humans.[39–42,50–52] It has been shown to decrease systolic pressure by

20–30 mm Hg and diastolic pressure by 10–20 mm Hg in people with high blood pressure.[52] The mode of action of garlic as an antihypertensive appears to be related to its sulfur content and lipid-lowering properties.

Platelet aggregation inhibition

Excessive platelet aggregation (clumping together) is linked very strongly to atherosclerosis, heart disease, and strokes. Garlic preparations standardized for alliin content, as well as garlic oil, inhibit platelet aggregation.[39–42,53] In one study, 120 patients with increased platelet aggregation were given either 900 milligrams per day of a dried garlic preparation containing 1.3 percent alliin or a placebo for 4 weeks.[53] In the garlic group, spontaneous platelet aggregation disappeared, the microcirculation of the skin increased by 47.6 percent, plasma viscosity decreased by 3.2 percent, diastolic blood pressure dropped from an average of 74 to 67 mm Hg, and fasting blood glucose concentration dropped from an average of 89.4 to 79 milligrams per deciliter.

Fibrinolytic activity

Epidemiological studies have suggested that fibrinogen is a major, primary risk factor for cardiovascular disease.[54] Fibrinogen is an "acute-phase" protein involved in the blood-clotting system. However, it plays many other important roles, including several that promote atherosclerosis: these roles include its acting as a cofactor in platelet aggregation, determining the viscosity of blood, and stimulating the migration and proliferation of smooth muscle cells in the the inner tissue (intima) of the artery walls.

Early clinical studies stimulated detailed population studies on the possible link between fibrinogen and cardiovascular disease. The first such study was the Northwick Park heart study in the United Kingdom.[54] This large study involved 1,510 men aged 40 to 64 years, who were randomly recruited and tested for a range of clotting factors, including fibrinogen. At the 4-year follow-up the association between cardiovascular deaths and fibrinogen levels was stronger than that for cholesterol. This association has been confirmed in five other prospective epidemiological studies.[54]

The clinical significance of these findings can be summarized as follows:

1. Fibrinogen levels should be determined and monitored in patients with or at high risk for coronary heart disease or stroke.
2. Garlic and other natural therapies (e.g., omega-3 oils, bromelain, and capsicum) designed to promote fibrinolysis may offer significant benefit in the prevention of heart attacks, strokes, and other thromboembolic events.

Garlic preparations standardized for alliin content, garlic oil, and both fried and raw garlic have been shown in human studies[55,56] to increase serum fibrinolytic activity significantly. This increase occurs within the first 6 hours after ingestion and continues for up to 12 hours.

Prevention of low-density lipoprotein oxidation

There is growing evidence that LDL oxidation plays a significant role in the development of atherosclerosis. Accordingly, substances that prevent oxidation of LDL should slow down atherosclerosis. Vitamin E, vitamin C, and beta-carotene have been shown to offer protection against LDL oxidation and heart disease via their antioxidant effects. To test garlic's possibilities, a study was conducted[57] to determine if garlic might lessen the risk of atherosclerotic disease by reducing lipoprotein oxidation.

Garlic is known to exert antioxidant activity, but until recently there were no studies examining its effects on LDL oxidation. Healthy human volunteers given 600 milligrams per day of a garlic preparation providing 7.8 milligrams of alliin for 2 weeks had a 34 percent lower susceptibility to lipoprotein oxidation compared to controls.[57] These results are quite significant, given the short amount of time it took to produce coupled with the importance of reducing lipoprotein oxidation.

Dosage

The modern use of garlic features commercial preparations designed to offer the benefits of garlic without the odor. The marketplace is swamped with garlic products, with each manufacturer claiming their product is the best.

Preparations standardized for alliin content provide the greatest assurance of quality. However, American consumers must be aware of the subtle techniques manufacturers of garlic products use to disguise the quality of their products.

For example, many manufacturers will claim a very high "total allicin potential." However, on closer examination of the label the words "at time of manufacture" can be found in very small print. What this means, basically, is that the product is not stable and the manufacturer does not guarantee the level of alliin at the most critical time—when the product is actually used. The level of alliin or the total allicin potential at time of manufacture is totally meaningless. Make sure that the level of alliin and the total allicin potential is clearly stated and that the product is stable.

The commercial product should provide a daily dose of at least 10 milligrams of alliin or a total allicin potential of 4,000 micrograms. This amount is equal to approximately 1 clove (4 grams) of fresh garlic.

Toxicity

For the vast majority of individuals, garlic is nontoxic at the dosages commonly used. For some, however, it can cause irritation to the digestive tract, while others are apparently unable to detoxify allicin and other sulfur-containing components effectively. Prolonged feeding of large amounts of raw garlic to rats results in anemia, weight loss, and failure to grow.[58] Although the exact toxicity of garlic has yet to be definitively determined, side effects are rare at the dosage recommended above.

References

1. Leung A: *Encyclopedia of Common Natural Ingredients Used in Food, Drugs, and Cosmetics.* John Wiley & Sons, New York, 1980, pp. 176–178.
2. Raj KP and Parmar RM: Garlic—condiment and medicine. *Indian Drugs* 15, 205–210, 1977.
3. Block E: The chemistry of garlic and onions. *Sci Am*, March 1985, pp. 114–118.
4. Adetumbi MA and Lau BH: *Allium sativum* (garlic)—a natural antibiotic. *Med Hypothesis* 12, 227–237, 1983.
5. Koch HP: Garlicin—fact or fiction? *Phytother Res* 7, 278–280, 1993.
6. Hughes BG and Lawson L: Antimicrobial effects of *Allium sativum* L. (Garlic), *Allium ampeloprasum* L. (elephant garlic), and *Allium cepa* L. (onion), garlic compounds and commercial garlic supplement products. *Phytother Res* 5, 154–158, 1991.
7. Huddleson IF, *et al.*: Antibacterial substances in plants. *J Am Vet Med Assoc* 105, 394–397, 1944.
8. Cavallito CJ and Bailey JH: Allicin, the antibacterial principle of *Allium sativum*. I. Isolation, physical properties and antibacterial action. *J Am Chem Soc* 66, 1950–1951, 1944.
9. Sharma VD, *et al.*: Antibacterial property of *Allium sativum* Linn.: In vivo and in vitro studies. *Indian J Exp Biol* 15, 466–468, 1977.
10. Elnima EI, *et al.*: The antimicrobial activity of garlic and onion extracts. *Pharmazie* 38, 747–748, 1983.
11. Amer M, Taha M, and Tosson Z: The effect of aqueous garlic extract on the growth of dermatophytes. *Int J Dermatol* 19, 285–287, 1980.
12. Moore GS and Atkins RD: The fungicidal and fungistatic effects of an aqueous garlic extract on medically important yeast-like fungi. *Mycologia* 69, 341–348, 1977.
13. Sandhu DK, Warraich MK, and Singh S: Sensitivity of yeasts isolated from cases of vaginitis to aqueous extracts of garlic. *Mykosen* 23, 691–698, 1980.
14. Prasad G and Sharma VD: Efficacy of garlic (*Allium sativum*) treatment against experimental candidiasis in chicks. *Br Vet J* 136, 448–451, 1980.
15. Hunan Hospital: Garlic in cryptococcal meningitis. A preliminary report of 21 cases. *Chin Med J* 93, 123–126, 1980.
16. Fromtling R and Bulmer G: In vitro effect of aqueous extract of garlic (*Allium sativum*) on the growth and viability of *Cryptococcus neoformans*. *Mycologia* 70, 397–405, 1978.
17. Vahora SB, Rizwan M, and Khan JA: Medicinal uses of common Indian vegetables. *Planta Medica* 23, 381–393, 1973.
18. Bastidas GJ: Effect of ingested garlic on *Necator americanus* and *Ancylostoma canium*. *Am J Trop Med Hyg* 18, 920–923, 1969.

19. Nagai K: Experimental studies on the preventive effect of garlic extract against infection with influenza virus. *Jpn J Infect Dis* **47**, 321, 1973.
20. Weber ND, *et al.*: In vitro virucidal effects of *Allium sativum* (garlic) extract and compounds. *Planta Medica* **58**, 417–423, 1992.
21. Lau B, *et al.*: *Allium sativum* (garlic) and cancer prevention. *Nutr Res* **10**, 937–948, 1990.
22. Dorant E, *et al.*: Garlic and its significance for the prevention of cancer in humans: A critical review. *Br J Cancer* **67**, 424–429, 1993.
23. Dausch JG and Nixon DW: Garlic: A review of its relationship to malignant disease. *Prev Med* **19**, 346–361, 1990.
24. You WC, *et al.*: *Allium* vegetables and reduced risk of stomach cancer. *J Natl Cancer Inst* **81**, 162–164, 1989.
25. Choy YM, *et al.*: Effect of garlic, Chinese medicinal drugs and amino acids on growth of Erlich ascites tumor cells in mice. *Am J Chin Med* **11**, 69–73, 1982.
26. Weisberger AS and Pensky J: Tumor inhibition by a sulfhydryl-blocking agent related to an active principle of garlic (*Allium sativum*). *Cancer Res* **18**, 1301–1308, 1958.
27. Lin X, Liu J, and Milner J. Dietary garlic powder suhe in vivo formation of DNA adducts induced by N-nitroso compounds in liver and mammary tissues. *FASEB J* **6**, A1392, 1992.
28. Nagabhushan M, *et al.*: Anticarcinogenic action of diallyl sulfide in hamster buccal pouch and forestomach. *Cancer Lett* **6**, 207–216, 1992.
29. Meng C and Shyu K: Inhibition of experimental carcinogenesis by painting with garlic extract. *Nutr Cancer* **14**, 207–217, 1990.
30. Niukian K, *et al.*: Effects of onion extract on the development of hampster buccal pouch carcinomas as expressed in tumor burden. *Nutr Cancer* **9**, 171–176, 1987.
31. Wargovich MJ: Diallyl sulfide, a flavor compound of garlic, inhibits diamethylhydrazine-induced colon cancer. *Carcinogenesis* **3**, 487–489, 1987.
32. Belman S: Onion and garlic oils inhibit tumor promotion. *Carcinogenesis* **4**(8), 1063–1065, 1983.
33. Criss WE, *et al.*: Inhibition of tumor growth with low dietary protein and with dietary garlic extracts. *Fed Proc* **41**, 281, 1982.
34. Kroning F. Garlic as an inhibitor for spontaneous tumors in mice. *Acta Unio Int Cancrum* **20**, 855, 1964.
35. Mei X, *et al.*: The blocking effect of garlic on the formation of N-nitrosoproline in the human body. *Acta Nutr Sin* **11**, 144–145, 1989.
36. Xing M, *et al.*: Garlic and gastric cancer—the effect of garlic on nitrite and nitrate in gastric juice. *Acta Nutr Sin* **4**, 53–55, 1982.
37. Bever BO and Zahnd GR: Plants with oral hypoglycemic action. *Q J Crude Drug Res* **17**, 139–196, 1979.
38. Barowsky H and Boyd LJ: The use of garlic (Allistan) in gastrointestinal disturbances. *Rev Gastroenterol* **11**, 22–26, 1944.
39. Norwell DY and Tarr RS: Garlic, vampires, and CHD. *Osteopath Ann* **11**, 546–549, 1983.
40. Lau BH, Adetumbi MA, and Sanchez A: *Allium sativum* (garlic) and atherosclerosis: A review. *Nutr Res* **3**, 119–128, 1983.
41. Kendler BS: Garlic (*Allium sativum*) and onion (*Allium cepa*): A review of their relationship to cardiovascular disease. *Prev Med* **16**, 670–685, 1987).
42. Ernst E: Cardiovascular effects of garlic (*Allium sativum*): A review. *Pharmatherapeutica* **5**, 83–89, 1987.
43. Kleijnen J, *et al.*: Garlic, onions and cardiovascular risk factors: A review of the evidence from human experiments with emphasis on commercially available preparations. *Br J Clin Pharmacol* **28**, 535–544, 1989.
44. Warshafsky S, Kamer RS, and Sivak SL: Effect of garlic on total serum cholesterol. *Ann Intern Med* **119**, 599–605, 1993.
45. Jain AK, *et al.*: Can garlic reduce levels of serum lipids? A controlled clinical study. *Am J Med* **94**, 632–635, 1993.
46. Rotzch W, *et al.*: Postprandial lipaemia under treatment with *Allium sativum*. Controlled double-blind study in healthy volunteers with reduced HDL_2-cholesterol levels. *Arzneimittel-Forsch* **42**, 1223–1227, 1992.
47. Mader FH: Treatment of hyperlipidemia with garlic-powder tablets. *Arzneimittel-Forsch* **40**, 1111–1116, 1990.
48. Bordia A: Effect of garlic on blood lipids in patients with coronary heart disease. *Am J Clin Nutr* **34**, 2100–2103, 1981.
49. Sainani GS, *et al.*: Effect of dietary garlic and onion on serum lipid profile in the Jain community. *Indian J Med Res* **69**, 776–780, 1979; Sainani GS, *et al.*: Dietary garlic, onion and some coagulation parameters in Jain community. *J Assoc Physicians India* **27**, 707–712, 1979.

50. Malik ZA and Siddiqui S: Hypotensive effect of freeze-dried garlic (*Allium sativum*) sap in dog. *J Pak Med Assoc* **31**, 12–13, 1981.
51. Petkov V: Plants with hypotensive, antiatheromatous and coronary dilating action. *Am J Chin Med* **7**, 197–236, 1979.
52. Foushee DB, Ruffin J, and Banerjee U: Garlic as a natural agent for the treatment of hypertension: A preliminary report. *Cytobios* **34**, 145–162, 1982.
53. Kiesewetter H, *et al.*: Effect of garlic on thrombocyte aggregation, microcirculation, and other risk factors. *Int J Clin Pharmacol Ther Toxicol* **29**, 151–155, 1991.
54. Ernst E: Fibrinogen: An important risk factor for atherothrombotic diseases. *Ann Med* **26**, 15–22, 1994.
55. Chutani SK and Bordia A: The effect of fried versus raw garlic on fibrinolytic activity in man. *Atherosclerosis* **38**, 417–421, 1981.
56. Legnani C, *et al.*: Effects of dried garlic preparation on fibrinolysis and platelet aggregation in healthy subjects. *Arzneimittel-Forsch* **43**, 119–121, 1993.
57. Phelps S and Harris WS: Garlic supplementation and lipoprotein oxidation susceptibility. *Lipids* **28**, 475–477, 1993.
58. Nakagawa S, *et al.*: Effect of raw and extracted-aged garlic juice on growth of young rats and their organs after perioral administration. *J Toxicol Sci* **5**, 91–112, 1980.

12
Ginger

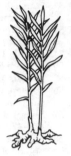

Key uses of ginger:

- Nausea and vomiting
- Motion sickness
- Arthritis
- Migraine headaches

General description

Ginger (*Zingiber officinale*) is an erect perennial herb with thick tuberous rhizomes (underground stems) from which the above-ground (aerial) stem grows to a height of 2–4 feet. Grasslike leaves, 6–12 inches long and ¾ inch wide, shoot off from the aerial stem. Wild ginger produces a beautiful flower, but cultivated ginger rarely flowers. Although ginger is native to southern Asia, it is now extensively cultivated throughout the tropics (e.g., India, China, Jamaica, Haiti, and Nigeria). Jamaica is the major producer, with exports to all parts of the world amounting to more than 2 million pounds annually.

The knotted and branched rhizome, commonly called the "root," is the portion of ginger used for culinary and medicinal purposes. Extracts and the oleoresin are produced from dried unpeeled ginger, as peeled ginger loses much of its essential oil content.[1,2] Ginger oil is produced from the fresh ginger via steam distillation.

Chemical composition

The following compounds have been isolated from ginger: starch (up to 50 percent); protein (ca. 9 percent); lipids (6–8 percent) composed of tri-

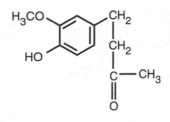

Figure 12.1 Gingerol

glycerides, phosphatidic acid, lecithins, and free fatty acids; a protease (2.26 percent); volatile oils (1–3 percent), the principal components of which are sesquiterpenes (bisabolene, zingiberene, and zingiberol) and various "pungent" principles, aromatic ketones known collectively as gingerols (Figure 12.1); vitamins (especially niacin and vitamin A); and resins.[1,2]

The pungent principles are thought to be the most pharmacologically active components of ginger. Gingerol and its derivatives can be found in concentrations as high as 33 percent in ginger oleoresin. The fresh oleoresin will have a higher percentage of the more pungent gingerol, as gingerol can be dehydrated during storage to form shogaol (Figure 12.2) or have its fatty acid moiety cleaved to form zingerone (Figure 12.3). The oleoresin is made by extracting the oily and resinous materials with the aid of a solvent (alcohol, hexane, or acetone).

History and folk use

Ginger has been used for thousands of years in China for medicinal purposes. Chinese records dating from the fourth century B.C. indicate that it was used to treat numerous conditions: stomachache, diarrhea, nausea, cholera, hemorrhage, rheumatism, and toothaches.[1] It was used by Eclectic physicians in this country in the late 1800s as a carminative, diaphoretic, appetite stimulant, and local counterirritant.[3]

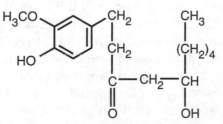

Figure 12.2 Shogaol

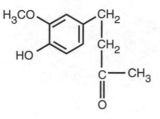

Figure 12.3 Zingerone

Ginger is widely used as a spice, especially in Asian and Indian dishes. It is also used in many baked goods, beverages (ginger ale), candy, liqueurs, and cosmetic products (perfumes, soaps, creams, etc.).

Pharmacology

Ginger possesses numerous pharmacological properties, the most relevant being its antioxidant effects; inhibition of prostaglandin, thromboxane, and leukotriene synthesis; inhibition of platelet aggregation; cholesterol-lowering actions; choleretic effects; cardiotonic effects; gastrointestinal actions; thermogenic properties; and antibiotic activities.

Antioxidant effects

Ginger's strong antioxidant properties led to an investigation of its ability to prevent the development of rancidity in meat products.[4] Ginger was shown to prolong the shelf life of fresh, frozen, and precooked pork patties. Since the use of many synthetic antioxidants is prohibited by law, ginger may one day be used commercially to extend the shelf life of meats and other foods.

In another study, curcumin from turmeric was found to be about thirty times more potent than zingerone in preventing lipid peroxidation.[5]

Effects on prostaglandin metabolism

Numerous constituents in ginger are potent inhibitors of prostaglandin and leukotriene synthesis.[6–8] The most potent components appear to be the pungent principles, although the aqueous extract has also demonstrated inhibition. Inhibition of prostaglandin and leukotriene formation could help explain ginger's historical use as an antiinflammatory agent; fresh ginger contains a protease whose effect on inflammation may be similar to that of other plant proteases (e.g., bromelain, ficin, and papain).[1]

Effects on platelets

Ginger, like garlic and onions, inhibits platelet aggregation (see page 127 for discussion). However, ginger's effects may be far more powerful. In a comparative study,[9] an aqueous extract of ginger was shown to exert greater inhibitory effects on platelet aggregation than aqueous garlic and onion extracts. Ginger also inhibited thromboxane formation and proaggregatory prostaglandins more effectively than onion and garlic. Ginger, but not onion or garlic, also significantly reduced platelet lipid peroxide formation.

The superiority of ginger over onions was also demonstrated in a controlled study.[10] Female volunteers given either 70 grams of raw onions or 5 grams of raw ginger demonstrated that ginger has a pronounced effect in lowering platelet thromboxane production, while onion actually produced a mild elevation (pooled results).

Cholesterol-lowering and hepatic effects

Ginger has been shown to reduce significantly serum and hepatic cholesterol levels in cholesterol-fed rats by impairing cholesterol absorption as well as by stimulating the conversion of cholesterol to bile acids.[11–13] In addition, ginger has also been shown to increase bile secretion.[14] Therefore, ginger works to lower cholesterol by promoting its excretion and impairing its absorption.

Cardiotonic properties

Gingerol has shown potent cardiotonic activity (positive ionotropic and chronotropic effects) on isolated guinea pig left atria.[15,16] These effects are a result of acceleration of calcium uptake by the heart muscle.

Individuals with heart problems or high blood pressure are probably better off using fresh ginger rather than dried preparations. This recommendation is based not only on the fact that gingerol is the more potent cardiotonic, but also because shogaol produces a blood pressure-elevating effect in animals.[17] Gingerol is found predominantly in fresh ginger, while shogaol is rarely found in fresh ginger.

Analgesic effects

Ginger has demonstrated analgesic effects in experimental studies in animals.[18] This effect is thought to be a result of shogaol inhibiting the release of substance P, in a fashion similar to capsaicin, the pungent principle of capsicum (see pp. 71–75 for discussion).

Gastrointestinal smooth muscle effects

One interesting aspect of ginger is its ability to simultaneously improve gastric motility while exerting antispasmodic effects. This is consistent with its use as a gastrointestinal tonic. A lipophilic ginger extract was shown to enhance gastric motility as evidenced by increased intestinal transport of a charcoal meal fed to rats,[19] and various fat-soluble components (such as galanolactone) of ginger have demonstrated antagonism of serotonin receptor sites.[20] This latter mechanism may be responsible for ginger's antispasmodic effects on visceral and vascular smooth muscle. Ginger has been shown to inhibit diarrhea.[21]

Antiulcer effects

Ginger demonstrates significant antiulcer effects in a variety of animal models.[22–24] Ginger prevents ulcer formation due to ethanol, indomethacin, aspirin, and other common ulcer-causing compounds. The pungent principles appear to be responsible for this effect. Interestingly, in one study, roasted ginger demonstrated inhibition of ulcer formation in three gastric ulcer models while dry ginger had no such effect.[25]

Thermogenic properties

Ginger is noted for its apparent ability to warm the body and has historically been used as a diaphoretic. In animal studies, ginger has been shown to help maintain body temperature and inhibit serotonin-induced hypothermia.[21,26]

Crude extracts and the pungent components of ginger increase oxygen consumption, perfusion pressure, and lactate production in the perfused rat hind limb.[27] These effects signify increased thermogenesis. Gingerol is the most potent thermogenic component of ginger. A human study demonstrated that consuming a ginger sauce (containing unspecified amounts of ginger principles) with a meal produced no significant effect on metabolic rate.[28] However, there were two problems with this study: (1) the concentration of gingerol in the preparation used was probably low or zero and (2) the effective concentration range of gingerol for its thermogenic effects is quite narrow.

Given ginger's historical use as a "warming" substance, these scientific investigations appear to support its use as a diaphoretic and thermogenic aid, although confirmation in humans is still lacking.

Antibiotic activity

Ginger, shogaol, and zingerone have been shown to inhibit strongly the growth of *Salmonella typhi*, *Vibrio cholerae*, and *Tricophyton violaceum*, while aqueous extracts at 2.5, 5, and 25 percent concentration are effective against *Trichomonas vaginalis*.[29]

Clinical applications

Ginger is widely used as a condiment for its unique flavors, but from the above-described pharmacology it obviously has important medicinal effects as well. In general, like many other culinary herbs and spices such as garlic and onions, ginger provides many health-promoting effects. Specifically, ginger provides benefit to many body systems, including the digestive (particularly liver, and gallbladder) and cardiovascular systems.

Historically, the majority of complaints for which ginger was used concerned the gastrointestinal system. A clue to ginger's efficacy in alleviating gastrointestinal distress is offered in several recent double-blind studies on motion sickness, hyperemesis gravidum, and postoperative nausea and vomiting. Human studies have also shown a positive effect in cases of arthritis and migraine headaches.

Motion sickness

Ginger was first shown to be effective in treating motion sickness by Mowrey and Clayson in 1982.[30] In their study, ginger (940 milligrams) was shown to be far superior to Dramamine (100 milligrams) in relieving symptoms of nausea and vomiting. Since this initial study several better-designed follow-up studies have studied the effectiveness of ginger as a motion sickness medication.

The inclusion of ginger in motion sickness trials prompted the National Aeronautics and Space Administration (NASA) to fund a study at Louisiana State University.[31] This study compared ginger, both fresh and dry powdered, to scopolamine by measuring the number of head movements subjects in a rotating chair could make before reaching an end point of motion sickness (i.e., vomiting). Ginger was not shown to produce any protection against motion sickness in this model or in two additional protocols (vestibular stimulation only and combined vestibular–visual stimulation).[31] However, in a perhaps more real-life test, ginger (1 gram) given to naval cadets, unaccustomed to sailing in heavy seas, was shown to reduce cold sweating and the tendency to vomit compared to a placebo in a double-blind trial.[32]

Mowrey and Clayson[31] proposed that the antimotion sickness effects of ginger were due to local gastrointestinal tract effects rather than central nervous system effects. Although ginger's mechanism of action in alleviating gastrointestinal distress has yet to be fully explained, there is evidence to support this hypothesis. Ginger has been shown to inhibit partially the excessive gastric motility characteristic of motion sickness.[31] Providing further support for a gastric versus a central nervous system mechanism of action, one study clearly demonstrated that neither the inner ear (vestibular) nor the visual system, both of which are of critical importance in the occurrence of motion sickness, was influenced by ginger (1 gram).[33] However, other results suggest that ginger may dampen vestibular impulses to the autonomic centers of the brain.[34]

The overall effectiveness of ginger in motion sickness has yet to be determined. Issues raised by these studies include the variability in the quality of commercial ginger preparations and the time required for ginger to produce its effects. Commercial preparations vary widely in chemical composition and often contain adulterants; in the ginger study conducted at sea,[32] ginger reduced symptoms of cold sweating and vomiting only after 4 hours. In other words, it appears that ginger may prove to be more effective when well-defined preparations are given at least 4 hours prior to experiencing stressful motion.

Nausea and vomiting

Ginger's antiemetic action has been studied in hyperemesis gravidum, the most severe form of pregnancy-related nausea and vomiting. This condition usually requires hospitalization. In a double-blind randomized cross-over trial, 250 milligrams of ginger root powder administered four times a day brought about a significant reduction in both the severity of the nausea and the number of attacks of vomiting in nineteen of twenty-seven cases of early pregnancy (less than 20 weeks).[35] These clinical results, along with ginger's safety and the relative small dose required, support the use of ginger in nausea and vomiting in pregnancy, particularly in view of the problems (e.g., teratogenicity) with antiemetic drugs. Ginger is becoming a well-accepted prescription even in orthodox obstetrical practices.

The antiemetic action of ginger was also observed in women who had undergone major gynecological surgery. In a double-blind study, 500 milligrams of dry powdered ginger root was shown to reduce significantly the incidence of nausea compared to placebo; the effects of ginger were similar to those of the drug metoclopramide.[36]

Inflammatory conditions

Ginger's ability to inhibit the formation of inflammatory prostaglandins, thromboxanes, and leukotrienes, along with its strong antioxidant activities and protease component, suggest a possible benefit in inflammatory conditions. To test this hypothesis, a preliminary clinical study was conducted on seven patients with rheumatoid arthritis, in whom conventional drugs had provided only temporary or partial relief.[37] One patient took 50 grams per day of lightly cooked ginger while the remaining six took either 5 grams of fresh or 0.1–1 gram of powdered ginger daily. All patients reported substantial improvement, including pain relief, increased joint mobility, and decreased swelling and morning stiffness.

In the follow-up to this study, twenty-eight patients with rheumatoid arthritis, eighteen with osteoarthritis, and ten with muscular discomfort who had been taking powdered ginger for periods ranging from 3 months to 2.5 years were evaluated.[38] On the basis of clinical observations, Srivastava and Mustafa reported that 75 percent of the arthritis patients and 100 percent of the patients with muscular discomfort experienced relief in pain or swelling. The recommended dosage was 500 to 1,000 milligrams per day, but many patients took three to four times this amount. Patients taking the higher dosages also reported quicker and better relief.

Ginger has also been reported to be beneficial in migraine headache.[39] Given ginger's pharmacological activities on platelet function and inflammation, this recommendation makes sense.

Dosage

There remain many questions concerning the best form of ginger and the proper dosage. Most research studies have utilized 1 gram of dry powdered ginger root. Practically speaking, this is a small dose of ginger. For example, ginger is commonly consumed in India at a daily dose of 8 to 10 grams. Furthermore, although most studies have used powdered ginger root, fresh (or possibly freeze-dried) ginger root at an equivalent dosage may yield even better results because it contains higher levels of gingerol as well as the active protease.

In the treatment of nausea and vomiting due to motion sickness, pregnancy, or surgery a dosage of 1 to 2 grams of dry powdered ginger per day may be effective. This would be equivalent to approximately 10 grams or one-third of an ounce of fresh ginger root, roughly a ¼ inch slice. For inflammatory conditions such as rheumatoid arthritis, the dosage should be double this amount.

Toxicity

Some individuals consuming high doses, that is, greater than the equivalent of 6 grams of dried powdered ginger alone on an empty stomach, may experience some gastrointestinal discomfort. Administration of 6 grams of dried powdered ginger has been shown to increase the exfoliation of gastric surface epithelial cells in human subjects.[40] This may cause some gastric distress and ultimately could lead to ulcer formation. Therefore, it is recommended that doses on an empty stomach be less than 6 grams.

Ginger does not appear to be toxic. Although ginger extracts and several components in ginger have been shown to possess potent mutagenic activity, ginger also contains several equally potent antimutagenic substances.[41-42] The significance of this mutagenicity (the study was conducted in *Escherichia coli*, not the Ames test) has not been entirely determined, but the long historic use and lack of carcinogenic effect or toxicity in animals suggest that it is not a problem.

In acute toxicity tests in mice, ginger extract administered as a lavage was tolerated up to 2.5 grams per kilogram with no mortality or side effects during a 7-day trial period.[43] Increasing the dosage to 3.0–3.5 grams per kilogram resulted in a 10–30 percent mortality. In comparison, 600 milligrams of aspirin per kilogram produced mortality in 25 percent, stomach ulcers in 40 percent, and hypothermia in 60 percent.

References

1. Leung A: *Encyclopedia of Common Natural Ingredients Used in Food, Drugs, and Cosmetics.* John Wiley & Sons, New York, 1980, pp.184–186.
2. Tyler V, Brady L, and Robbers J: *Pharmacognosy*, 8th Ed. Lea & Febiger, Philadelphia, 1981, pp. 156–157.
3. Felter H: *The Eclectic Materia Medica, Pharmacology and Therapeutics.* Eclectic Medical Publications, Portland, OR, 1983, p. 702.
4. Lee YB, Kim YS, and Ashmore CR: Antioxidant property in ginger rhizome and its application to meat products. *J Food Sci* **51**, 20–23, 1986.
5. Reddy AC and Lokesh BR: Studies on spice principles as antioxidants in the inhibition of lipid peroxidation of rat liver microsomes. *Mol Cell Biochem* **111**, 117–124, 1992.
6. Kiuchi F, *et al.*: Inhibition of prostaglandin and leukotriene biosynthesis by gingerols and diarylheptanoids. *Chem Pharm Bull* **40**, 387–391, 1992.

7. Kiuchi F, Shibuyu M, and Sankawa U: Inhibitors of prostaglandin biosynthesis from ginger. *Chem Pharm Bull* **30**, 754–757, 1982.

8. Srivastava KC: Isolation and effects of some ginger components on platelet aggregation and eicosanoid biosynthesis. *Prostaglandins Leurotrienes Med* **25**, 187–198, 1986.

9. Srivastava K: Effects of aqueous extracts of onion, garlic and ginger on the platelet aggregation and metabolism of arachidonic acid in the blood vascular system: In vitro study. *Prostaglandins Leukotrienes Med* **13**, 227–235, 1984.

10. Srivastawa KC: Effect of onion and ginger consumption on platelet thromboxane production in humans. *Prostaglandins Leukotrienes Essent Fatty Acids* **35**, 183–185, 1989.

11. Gujral S, Bhumra H, and Swaroop M: Effect of ginger (*Zingebar officinale* Roscoe) oleoresin on serum and hepatic cholesterol levels in cholesterol fed rats. *Nutr Rep Int* **17**, 183–189, 1978.

12. Giri J, Sakthi Devi TK, and Meerarani S: Effect of ginger on serum cholesterol levels. *Indian J Nutr Diet* **21**, 433–436, 1984.

13. Srinivasan K and Sambaiah K: The effect of spices on cholesterol-7-alpha-hydroxylase activity and the serum and hepatic cholesterol levels in the rat. *Int J Vitam Nutr Res* **61**, 364–369, 1991.

14. Yamahara J, *et al.*: Cholagogic effect of ginger and its active constituents. *J Ethnopharmacol* **13**, 217–225, 1985.

15. Shoji N, *et al.*: Cardiotonic principles of ginger (*Zingiber officinale* Roscoe). *J Pharm Sci* **10**, 1174–1175, 1982.

16. Kobayashi M, *et al.*: Cardiotonic action of [8]-gingerol, an activator of the Ca^{++}-pumping adenosine triphosphatase of sarcoplasmic reticulum, in guinea pig arterial muscle. *J Pharmacol Exp Ther* **246**, 667–673, 1988.

17. Suekawa M, Aburada M, and Hosoya E: Pharmacological studies on ginger. II. Pressor action of (6)-shogoal in anesthetized rats, or hindquarters, tail and mesenteric vascular beds of rats. III. Effect of spinal destruction on (6)-shagoal-induced pressor response in rats. *J Pharmacobio-Dyn* **9**, 842–860, 1986.

18. Onogi T, *et al.*: Capsaicin-like effect of (6)-shogoal on substance P-containing primary afferents of rats: A possible mechanism of its analgesic action. *Neuropharmacology* **31**, 1165–1169, 1992.

19. Yamahara J, *et al.*: Gastrointestinal motility enhancing effect of ginger and its active constituents. *Chem Pharm Bull* **38**, 430–431, 1990.

20. Huang QR, *et al.*: Anti-5-hydroxytryptamine effect of galanolactone, diterpinoid isolated from ginger. *Chem Pharm Bull* **39**, 397–399, 1991.

21. Huang Q, *et al.*: The effect of ginger on serotonin induced hypothermia and diarrhea. *Yakugaku Zasshi* **110**, 936–942, 1990.

22. Al Yahya MA, *et al.*: Gastroprotective activity of ginger, *Zingiber officinale* Rosc., in albino rats. *Am J Chin Med* **17**, 51–56, 1989.

23. Yamahara J, *et al.*: The anti-ulcer effect in rats of ginger constituents. *J Ethnopharmacol* **23**, 299–304, 1988.

24. Yamahara J, *et al.*: Stomachic principles in ginger. II. Pungent and anti-ulcer effects of low polar constituents isolated from ginger, the dried rhizome of *Zingiber officinale* Roscoe cultivated in Taiwan. The absolute stereostructure of a new diarylheptanoid. *J Pharm Soc Jpn* **112**, 645–655, 1992.

25. Wu H, *et al.*: Effect of dry ginger and roasted ginger on experimental gastric ulcers in rats. *China J Chin Mat Med* **15**, 278–280, 317–318, 1990.

26. Kano Y, Zong QN, and Komatsu K: Pharmacological properties of galenical preparation. XIV. Body temperature retaining effect of the Chinese traditional medicine, "goshuyu-to" and component crude drugs. *Chem Pharm Bull* **39**, 690–692, 1991.

27. Elderhsaw TPD, *et al.*: Pungent principles of ginger (*Zingiber officinale*) are thermogenic in the perfused rat hind limb. *Int J Obes* **16**, 755–763, 1992.

28. Henry CJK and Piggott SM: Effect of ginger on metabolic rate. *Hum Nutr Clin Nutr* **41C**, 89–92, 1987.

29. Chang HM and But PPH: *Pharmacology and Applications of Chinese Materia Medica*, Vol. 1. World Scientific, Philadelphia, 1986, pp. 366–369.

30. Mowrey D and Clayson D: Motion sickness, ginger, and psychophysics. *Lancet* **i**, 655–657, 1982.

31. Stewart JJ, *et al.*: Effects of ginger on motion sickness susceptibility and gastric function. *Pharmacology* **42**, 111–120, 1991.

32. Grontved A, *et al.*: Ginger root against seasickness—a controlled trial on the open sea. *Acta Otolaryngol* **105**, 45–49, 1988.

33. Holtman S, *et al.*: The anti-motion sickness mechanism of ginger. *Acta Otolaryngol* **108**, 168–174, 1989.

34. Grontved A and Hentzer E: Vertigo-reducing effect of ginger root. *OTO Rhinolaryngology* **48**, 282–286, 1986.

35. Fischer-Rasmussen W, *et al.*: Ginger treatment of hyperemesis gravidarum. *Eur J Obstet Gynecol Reprod Biol* **38**, 19–24, 1990.

36. Bone ME, *et al.*: Ginger root—a new antiemetic. The effect of ginger root on postoperative nausea and vomiting after major gynecological surgery. *Anaesthesia* **45**, 669–671, 1990.
37. Srivastava KC and Mustafa T: Ginger (*Zingiber officinale*) and rheumatic disorders. *Med Hypothesis* **29**, 25–28, 1989.
38. Srivastava KC and Mustafa T: Ginger (*Zingiber officinale*) in rheumatism and musculoskeletal disorders. *Med Hypothesis* **39**, 342–348, 1992.
39. Mustafa T and Srivastava KC: Ginger (*Zingiber officinale*) in migraine headaches. *J Ethnopharmacol* **29**, 267–273, 1990.
40. Desai HG, Kalro RH, and Choksi AP: Effect of ginger and garlic on DNA content of gastric aspirate. *Ind J Med Res* **92**, 139–141, 1990.
41. Nakamura H and Yamamoto T: Mutagen and antimutagen in ginger, *Zingiber officinale*. *Mutat Res* **103**, 119–126, 1982.
42. Nagabhushan M, Amonkar AJ, and Bhide SV: Mutagenicity of gingerol and shogaol and antimutagenicity of zingerone in salmonella/microsome assay. *Cancer Lett* **36**, 221–233, 1987.
43. Macolo N, *et al.*: Ethnopharmacologic investigation of ginger (*Zingiber officinale*). *J Ethnopharmacol* **27**, 129–140, 1989.

13
Ginkgo biloba

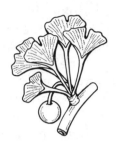

Key uses of *Ginkgo biloba*:

- Cerebral vascular insufficiency (insufficient blood flow to the brain)
- Dementia
- Depression
- Impotence
- Inner ear dysfunction (vertigo, tinnitus, etc.)
- Multiple sclerosis
- Neuralgia and neuropathy
- Peripheral vascular insufficiency (intermittent claudication, Raynaud's disease,etc.)
- Premenstrual syndrome
- Retinopathy (macular degeneration, diabetic retinopathy, etc.)
- Vascular fragility

General description

Ginkgo biloba is a deciduous tree that lives as long as 1,000 years and may grow to a height of 100 to 122 feet and a diameter of 3 to 4 feet. The ginkgo has short horizontal branches with short shoots bearing fan-shaped leaves that measure 5 to 10 centimeters across. Because the leaf resembles those of maidenhair fern, the ginkgo has been called the "maidenhair tree." Ginkgo bears a foul-smelling, inedible fruit and an edible, ivory-colored inner seed that is sold in marketplaces in the orient. Extracts from the leaves of the ginkgo tree are used medicinally.

Chemical composition

The active components of ginkgo leaves are the ginkgo flavone glycosides or ginkgo heterosides (flavonoid molecules to which are attached sugars unique to the ginkgo), several terpene molecules unique to ginkgo (ginkgolides and bilobalide), and organic acids.[1]

The *Ginkgo biloba* extract (GBE) marketed in Europe under the trade names Tanakan, Rökan, Ginkgobil, Kaveri, and Tebonin is a well-defined, complex product prepared from the green leaves. Extracts identical to these preparations are available in the United States as food supplements. The culturing, harvesting, and extracting techniques have been thoroughly standardized and require careful control.

Ginkgo biloba extract is standardized to contain 24 percent flavonoid glycosides, as these molecules represent a convenient analytical reference group. Although the flavonoid glycosides play a major role in the pharmacological activity of GBE, other components are also important. The three major backbone flavonoids of the *Ginkgo biloba* flavonols are quercetin, kaempferol, and isorhamnetine (Figure 13.1). The sugar (glucoside) components include glucose and rhamnose, which are present as single sugars or as disaccharides (two sugar molecules attached to each other).

Other significant flavonoid components of GBE include proanthocyanidins (see Grape Seed Extract, Chapter 16).

The major terpene molecules of GBE, which account for 6 percent of the extract, are the ginkgolides and bilobalide (Figure 13.2). These substances are unique to ginkgo and are not found in any other plants.

Compound	R	R'	R''
Kaempferol	H	OH	H
Quercetin	OH	OH	H
Isorhamnetine	OH_3	OH	H

Figure 13.1 The major backbone flavonoids of GBE

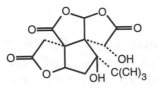

Figure 13.2 Bilobalide

Other constituents of GBE include a number of organic acids. These compounds contribute valuable properties to the extract by making the (usually water-insoluble) flavonoid and terpene molecules of ginkgo water soluble.

History and folk use

Ginkgo biloba is the world's oldest living tree species. The sole surviving species of the family Ginkgoaceae, the ginkgo tree can be traced back more than 200 million years to the fossils of the Permian period and for this reason is often referred to as the "living fossil."

Once common in North America and Europe, the ginkgo was almost destroyed during the Ice Age in all regions of the world except China, where it is has long been cultivated as a sacred tree.

In the late seventeenth century, Engelbert Kaempfer, a German physician and botanist, became the first European to discover and catalog the ginkgo tree. The flavonoid kaempferol is named after Kaempfer. In 1771, Linnaeus named the tree *Ginkgo biloba*.

The ginkgo tree was brought to America in 1784, to the garden of William Hamilton near Philadelphia. The ginkgo is now planted throughout much of the United States as an ornamental tree. Partly because the ginkgo is the most resistant of tree species to insects, disease, and pollution, it is frequently planted along streets in cities.[1]

The medicinal use of *Ginkgo biloba* can be traced back to the oldest Chinese materia medica (2800 B.C.). Traditional Chinese medicine prescribes ginkgo leaves for their ability to "benefit the brain," relieve the symptoms of asthma and coughs, and help the body eliminate filaria.

Ginkgo leaf extracts are now among the leading prescription medicines in both Germany and France, where they account for 1.0 and 1.5 percent, respectively, of total prescription sales. In 1989 alone, more than 100,000 physicians worldwide wrote more than 10 million prescriptions for GBE.

Pharmacology

The standardized concentrated extract of *Ginkgo biloba* leaves (24 percent ginkgo heteroside content) has demonstrated remarkable pharmacological effects. Interestingly, the total extract is more active than its single isolated components.[1,2] This suggests synergism between the various components of GBE—an explanation that is well supported in more than 300 clinical and experimental studies utilizing the extract.[1-4]

Tissue effects

Ginkgo biloba extract exerts a profound, widespread influence on tissue, including membrane-stabilizing, antioxidant, and free radical-scavenging effects. *Ginkgo biloba* extract also enhances the utilization of oxygen and glucose.[1-3]

Cellular membranes provide the first line of defense in maintaining the integrity of the cell. Largely composed of fatty acids (phospholipids), cellular membranes also serve as fluid barriers, exchange sites, and electrical capacitors. These membranes are fragile and vulnerable to damage, especially the lipid peroxidation induced by oxygenated free radicals. *Ginkgo biloba* extract is an extremely effective inhibitor of lipid peroxidation of cellular membranes.[1,2]

Red blood cells provide excellent models for evaluating the effects of substances on membrane functions. Red blood cell studies utilizing GBE have demonstrated that in addition to directly stabilizing membrane structures and scavenging free radicals, GBE also enhances membrane transport of potassium into (and sodium out of) the cell by activating the sodium pump. In essence, GBE leads to better membrane polarization. This is particularly important in excitable tissues, such as nerve cells.[1,2]

Nerve cell effects

The membrane-stabilizing and free radical-scavenging effects of GBE are perhaps most evident in the brain and nerve cells. Brain cells contain the highest percentage of unsaturated fatty acids in their membranes of any cells in the body, making them extremely susceptible to free radical damage.

The brain cell is also extremely susceptible to hypoxia. Unlike most other tissues, the brain has very little energy reserve. Its functions require large amounts of energy in the form of a constant supply of glucose and oxygen. Diminished circulation to the brain sets off a chain of reactions that disrupt membrane function and energy production and ultimately lead to cellular death.

Ginkgo biloba extract is remarkable in its ability to prevent metabolic disturbances in experimental models of insufficient blood supply to the brain.[1,2,5-8] It accomplishes this by enhancing oxygen utilization and increasing cellular uptake of glucose, thus restoring energy production.

All of the above-mentioned metabolic effects are in addition to GBE's ability to reestablish effective tissue perfusion. Particularly interesting is GBE's ability to normalize the circulation in the areas most affected by microembolization, namely the hippocampus and striatum.[1,2]

Additional nervous tissues actions of GBE are discussed in Clinical Applications (below). Briefly, GBE promotes an increased nerve transmission rate, improves synthesis and turnover of brain neurotransmitters, and normalizes acetylcholine receptors in the hippocampus (the area of the brain most affected by Alzheimer's disease).[1,2]

Vascular effects

The mechanisms of GBE's vascular effects have been investigated utilizing a number of *in vivo* and *in vitro* techniques.[1,2] Isolated vessel techniques allow the effects of GBE on different parts of the vascular system (e.g., arterial, arteriolar, microcirculatory, venular, and venous components) to be isolated, while *in vivo* studies provide information on the total circulatory phenomena (i.e., GBE's ability to increase the perfusion rate to various regions).

In general, GBE exerts its vascular effects primarily on the lining of the blood vessels (vascular endothelium) and the system that regulates blood vessel tone. Its vasodilating action is explained by direct stimulation of the release of endothelium-derived relaxing factor (EDRF) and prostacyclin (a beneficial prostaglandin). In addition, GBE inhibits an enzyme that causes relaxation of the blood vessels.[1,2]

Gingko biloba extract stimulates greater tone in the venous system, thus aiding the dynamic clearing of toxic metabolites that accumulate during ischemia (times of insufficient oxygen supply).[1,2]

Gingko biloba extract normalizes circulation by producing tonic effects. These effects are much more apparent in an ischemic vascular area than in a normally perfused area.[9] However, despite intense investigation, many of GBE's tonic effects on vascular components are still largely unexplained. It is truly remarkable that a substance can simultaneously combat the phenomena resulting from vascular spasm and, with the same efficiency, restore circulation to areas subject to vasomotor paralysis.

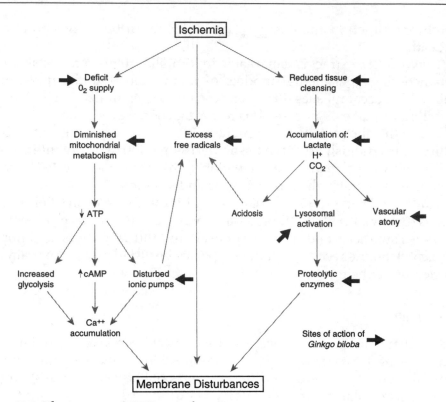

Figure 13.3 The impact of GBE on ischemia

The importance of this dual action is becoming more apparent in cerebral insufficiency as single-direction drugs (i.e., *vasodilators*), can often aggravate the condition by preferentially dilating the healthy areas, thereby deflecting blood and oxygen away from the ischemic area (Figure 13.3).

Platelet effects

Gingko biloba extract and isolated ginkgolides have profound effects on platelet function, including inhibition of platelet aggregation, inhibition of platelet adhesion, and degranulation (release of allergic and inflammatory components).[3] These effects appear to be due to direct membrane and anti-oxidant effects, increased synthesis of prostacyclin, and the antagonism of a substance known as platelet-activating factor (PAF).

Gingko biloba extract and the ginkgolides have been shown to be potent inhibitors of PAF.[3,9,10] Platelet-activating factor is a potent stimulator of platelet aggregation and degranulation. It is also involved in many inflammatory and allergic processes including neutrophil activation, increasing vascular permeability, smooth muscle contraction including bronchoconstriction, and reduction in coronary blood flow. *Gingko biloba* extract and ginkgolides compete with PAF for binding sites and inhibit the various events induced by PAF.[1,2,9,10] These actions may be responsible for many of the clinical effects of GBE.

Absorption and distribution of Ginkgo biloba extract

The pharmacokinetics (absorption, distribution, and elimination) of *Ginkgo biloba* have been studied using radiolabeled extracts in rats.[1–3] Following oral administration, at least 60 percent of the radiolabeled extract was absorbed. Because blood levels peaked after 1.5 hours, upper gastrointestinal tract absorption was suspected.

The flavonoids appear to have an affinity for organs rich in connective tissues, such as the aorta, eyes, skin, and lungs. Levels of radioactivity in these tissues are two to three times higher than in blood and decrease little over the course of time. Retained specific activity in the heart is twice that found in the skeletal muscles. Of the glands, the adrenals retained the greatest level of radioactivity.

At 72 hours, the hippocampus and the striated bodies show radioactivity five times greater than in the blood. This deposition pattern parallels the improvement in circulation observed following administration of GBE to rats experiencing blood clot-induced ischemia. Other areas of the brain such as the cerebral cortex, brain stem, and cerebellum do not show such high levels of radioactivity.

Clinical applications

Ginkgo biloba extract's primary clinical application has been in the treatment of vascular insufficiency. In more than fifty double-blind clinical trials, patients with chronic cerebral (brain) arterial insufficiency and patients with peripheral arterial insufficiency have responded favorably to GBE. As described above, GBE exerts an extraordinary array of pharmacological activities, which implies a broad spectrum of possible clinical applications; this implication is borne out by the frequent reports of new applications of GBE.

Cerebral vascular insufficiency and impaired mental performance

Cerebral vascular insufficiency is extremely common among the elderly of developed countries, owing to the high prevalence of atherosclerosis (hardening of the arteries). In well-designed studies, GBE has displayed a statistically significant regression of the major symptoms of cerebral vascular insufficiency and impaired mental performance. These symptoms include short-term memory loss, vertigo, headache, ringing in the ears, lack of vigilance, and depression.[1-4,11-18]

The significant regression of these symptoms following treatment with GBE suggests that vascular insufficiency may be the major causative factor accounting for these so-called "age-related cerebral disorders," rather than a true degenerative process.

A recent review surveyed the quality of research in more than forty clinical studies on GBE in the treatment of cerebral insufficiency.[4] The results of the analysis indicate that GBE is effective in reducing all symptoms of cerebral insufficiency, including impaired mental function (senility) and the quality of research was comparable to Hydergine, an FDA-approved drug used in the treatment of cerebral vascular insufficiency and Alzheimer's disease. Eight studies were noted as being extremely well designed and are summarized in Table 13.1.[11-18]

It appears that by increasing cerebral blood flow, and therefore oxygen and glucose utilization, GBE offers relief of these presumed "side effects" of aging and may offer significant protection against their development. Furthermore, *Ginkgo biloba*'s antiaggregatory effect on platelets offers additional protection against stroke. This has been supported in a clinical study of poststroke patients, which demonstrated that GBE improved blood and blood viscosity.[19]

As well as improving blood supply to the brain, experimental and clinical studies show that GBE increases the rate at which information is transmitted at the nerve cell level.[20-22] The memory-enhancing effects of GBE are not limited to the elderly. In one double-blind study, the reaction time in healthy young women performing a memory test was improved significantly after the administration of GBE.[22]

Alzheimer's disease

Ginkgo biloba extract shows great benefit in many cases of senility, including Alzheimer's disease.[1-4,20,23] In addition to GBE's ability to increase the functional capacity of the brain via the mechanisms described above, it has also been shown to normalize the acetylcholine receptors in the hippocampus of aged animals, to increase cholinergic transmission, and to address many of the other major elements of Alzheimer's disease.[1,2]

Although preliminary studies in established Alzheimer's patients are quite promising, at this time it appears that GBE is most effective in delaying mental deterioration in the early stages of Alzheimer's disease.

If mental deficit is due to vascular insufficiency or depression and not Alzheimer's disease, GBE is usually effective in reversing the deficit.[1-4]

Tinnitus (ringing in the ear)

Permanent severe tinnitus is extremely difficult to treat. Previous studies have shown contradictory results following the administration of GBE (24 percent ginkgo flavone glycosides) in the treatment of tinnitus. For example, in Meyer's study,[24] GBE improved the condition of all patients. However, in Coles's study,[25] in which twenty-one patients with tinnitus took GBE for 12 weeks, the results were mixed: eleven reported no change, four reported slight to very slight improvement, and five reported their tinnitus was worse. The explanation for these differing results lies in the fact that the patients in Meyer's study had recent-onset tinnitus, whereas eighteen of Coles's patients had had tinnitus for at least 3 years.

The most recent study of GBE in tinnitus utilized a two-part design: the first part was open, with no placebo control; the second part was a double-blind, placebo-controlled cross-over study.[26] The eighty patients in the open study had been referred to the Department of Audiology (Sahlgren's Hospital, Göteborg, Sweden) for treatment of permanent severe tinnitus. Twenty patients reporting a positive effect to *Ginkgo biloba* extract (14.6 milligrams twice daily) after 2 weeks were recruited for the double-blind study. Patients were given either the GBE or placebo for 2 weeks and then crossed over into the other group. Evaluation indicated that six patients preferred GBE, seven preferred placebo, and seven had no preference.

On the surface, this study would seem to indicate that GBE is not effective in the treatment of permanent severe tinnitus. However, closer examination reveals that the GBE treatment was bound to fail: First, the dosage used (14.6 milligrams twice daily or 29.2 milligrams daily) was far less than the standard dosage of 40 milligrams three times daily (or roughly four times the daily dosage used in the study). Second, in studies of patients with cerebral vascular insufficiency it is well established that GBE often takes at least 2 weeks before benefit becomes apparent: the longer GBE is used, the more obvious the benefit. In a condition such as permanent severe tinnitus, 2 to 4 weeks is simply not enough time. However, given the small, insufficient dosage it probably would not have mattered if the subjects had been studied for a longer period of time.

The degree to which GBE is of benefit in the treatment of permanent severe tinnitus remains to be determined, but given the excellent safety profile of GBE it is certainly worth a try.

Cochlear deafness

Ischemia is usually the underlying factor in acute cochlear deafness. *Ginkgo biloba* extract has been shown to improve recovery in cases of acute cochlear

Table 13.1 Characteristics of well-conducted controlled trials

Trial	Indication Duration of symptoms Average age	Daily dose/ Duration of treatment
Schmidt,[11] 1991	Cerebral insufficiency 26 months 59 years	150 mg/12 weeks
Bruchert,[12] 1991	Cerebral insufficiency 46 months 69 years	150 mg/12 weeks
Meyer,[13] 1986	Tinnitus, dizziness, hearing impairment 4–5 months 50 years	16 mg (4 ml)/3 months
Taillandier,[14] 1986	Cerebral insufficiency 5 years 82 years	160 mg/12 months

Haguenauer,[15] 1986	Vertiginous syndrome and
	  tinnitus, headaches,
	  nausea, hearing loss
	21 weeks
	50 years
		160 mg/3 months

Vorberg,[16] 1989	Cerebral insufficiency 21 months 70 years	112 mg/12 weeks
Eckmann,[17] 1990	Cerebral insufficiency 32 months 55 years	160 mg/6 weeks
Wesnes,[18] 1987	Mild idiopathic cognitive impairment 71 years	120 mg/12 weeks

1. No.* randomized 2. No. analyzed	Endpoints	Results
1. 50/49 2. 50/49	1. 12 symptoms; OS(4) 2. Overall assessment doctor; OS(3) 3. Overall assessment patient; OS(3)	1. Significant differences for 8 of 12 2. 72% vs 8% improved 3. 70% vs 14% improved
1. 156/157 2. 110/99	1. 12 symptoms; OS(4) 2. Overall assessment doctor; OS(3) 3. Overall assessment patient; OS(3)	1. Significant differences for 8 of 12 2. 71% vs 32% improved 3. 83% vs 53% improved
1. 58/45 (?) 2. 55/45 (?)	1. Symptoms; OS(4) 2. Overall assessment; days to improvement or cure	1. Significant difference for intensity; positive trend for discomfort 2. 70 days vs 119 days
1. 101/109 2. 80/86	1. Scale for geriatric patients (17 items); change from random- ization after 3 months 2. After 6 months 3. After 9 months 4. After 12 months	1. 10% vs 4% 2. 15% vs 4% 3. 15% vs 8% 4. 17% vs 8%
1. 35/35 2. 34/33	1. Symptoms; VAS and others 2. Overall assessment doctor; OS(5)	1. Vertigo: 75% vs 18% beneficial change 2. 47% vs 18% symptoms disappeared
1. 50/50 2. 49/47	6 symptoms; OS(4)	1. Concentration: 54% vs 19% improved 2. Memory: 52% vs 17% improved 3. Anxiety: 48% vs 17% improved 4. Dizziness: 61% vs 23% improved 5. Headache: 65% vs 24% improved 6. Tinnitus: 37% vs 12% improved
1. 30/30 2. 29/29	12 symptoms; OS(4)	Significant differences for 11 of 12 symp- toms after 4 and 6 weeks
1. 28/30 2. 27/27	1. Cognitive test battery 2. Behavioral rating scale 3. VAS mood 4. Overall assessment doctor and patient	1. Significant differences for combined scores 2. No differences 3. No significant differences 4. No differences, nearly all patients improved

*Ginkgo/placebo
OS(4) = 4-point ordinal scale; VAS = visual analog scale

deafness due to unknown factors or due to sound trauma or pressure (barotrauma).[27]

Senile macular degeneration and diabetic retinopathy

Ginkgo biloba extract appears to address, quite effectively, the underlying factors in senile macular degeneration, the most common cause of blindness in adults. In double-blind studies, GBE demonstrated a statistically significant improvement in long-distance visual acuity in both macular degeneration and diabetic retinopathy.[1,2,28]

Ginkgo biloba extract has demonstrated impressive protective effects against free radical damage to the retina in experimental studies. Furthermore, GBE has been shown to prevent diabetic retinopathy in diabetic rats, suggesting it may have a protective effect in human diabetics as well.[1,2]

Peripheral arterial insufficiency

Peripheral arterial disease has as its primary lesion the same cholesterol-containing plaque that is responsible for other conditions associated with atherosclerosis, for example, coronary artery disease and cerebral vascular insufficiency.

In peripheral arterial insufficiency, the arterial obstruction or narrowing causes a reduction in blood flow during exercise or at rest. Clinical symptoms are caused by the consequent ischemia. The most common symptom is a pain on exertion—intermittent claudication. The pain usually occurs in the calf and is described as a cramp or tightness, or severe fatigue. The pain is usually bilateral. The pain is caused not only by reduced oxygen delivery, but also by an increase in the production of toxic metabolites and cellular free radicals. These free radicals accumulate and react with the lipid constituents of the cell membrane.

Pain at rest indicates serious reduction in resting blood flow. It is an obvious sign of severe disease. The pain may be localized to one or more toes, or it may have a stocking-type distribution. The pain is usually described as burning or gnawing and is generally worse at night. A purple color or pallor of the extremity is usually apparent. In moderate to severe narrowing of the artery, the skin can become dry, scaly, and shiny. The hair may disappear, and the toenails may become brittle, ridged, and deformed.

The standard medical approach to peripheral vascular disease and intermittent claudication includes avoidance of tobacco (which causes vasoconstriction), a regular exercise program consisting of walking, and/or a prescription for pentoxifylline (Trental). Surgery is also an option, although most patients with intermittent claudication need not take this risk.[29]

Trental has emerged as the "drug of choice" in the standard medical treatment of intermittent claudication.[30] Seventeen placebo-controlled trials have shown that Trental increases the total and pain-free walking distance achieved by patients with intermittent claudication. However, the level of improvement (approximately 65 percent for pain-free walking distance) is less than that achieved with exercise or with *Ginkgo biloba* extract.

In nine double-blind, randomized clinical trials of GBE versus placebo in two matched groups of patients with peripheral arterial insufficiency of the leg, GBE was shown to be quite active and superior to placebo (eight studies) and equal to pentoxifylline (one study).[1-3,31-36] Not only were measurements of pain-free walking distance (75 to 110 percent) and maximum walking distance (52.6 to 119 percent) dramatically increased, but plethysmographic and Doppler ultrasound measurements demonstrated increased blood flow through the affected limb; blood lactate levels also dropped.[6-15]

The demonstration that *Ginkgo biloba* extract improves limb blood flow as well as walking tolerance (in studies following strict methodology and with sufficient patients for reliable evaluation) indicates that GBE is far superior to pentoxifylline and standard medical therapy in the treatment of peripheral arterial insufficiency. This includes other peripheral vascular disorders such as diabetic peripheral vascular disease, Raynaud's disease, acrocyanosis, and postphlebitis syndrome.

The longer GBE is used, the greater the benefit. The following table summarizes a 2-year trial of GBE (160 milligrams per day) in the treatment of peripheral arterial disease (Fontaine stage IIb). Pain-free walking distance increased by 300 percent.[1]

Parameter	Time of measurement	
	Week 0	Week 104
Pain-free walking distance (m)	62.9	172.4
Total walking distance (m)	113.8	384.0
Rest flow (ml/100 ml/min)	1.6	2.7
Peak flow (ml/100 ml/min)	3.7	6.9
Doppler measurement after strain (mm Hg)	46.5	72.6

The usual daily dosage of GBE is 120 milligrams (40 milligrams three times a day); however, some of the studies employed a dosage of 160 milligrams per day, including the study summarized in the table above.

Ginkgo biloba phytosome in peripheral vascular insufficiency

Ginkgo biloba extract bound to phosphatidylcholine forms what is called a *phytosome*. The creation of GBE phytosome requires the combination of one part GBE extract with two parts phosphatidylcholine to produce a completely new molecule composed of a central GBE component encased by two phosphatidylcholine molecules. GBE phytosomes may provide significant advantages over unbound GBE. The major advantage is the improvement in absorption from the gastrointestinal tract. The phosphatidylcholine molecules envelop the GBE molecules in a way that improves absorption, and also protects the GBE molecules from being degraded by digestion. In addition to greater absorption, there is improved utilization and incorporation into biological membranes. Once delivered to the tissue, the GBE phytosome exerts much greater antioxidant effects compared to unbound GBE.

Preliminary (unpublished) studies in patients with intermittent claudication and Raynaud's disease indicate that GBE phytosome exerts greater clinical benefit than unbound GBE.[37] In a clinical trial involving patients with intermittent claudication (Fontaine stage IIb), the overall improvement in walking distance after 12 weeks of therapy with GBE (40 milligrams three times daily) was 90 percent. In comparison, the group receiving GBE phytosome (60 milligrams three times daily) demonstrated a 120 percent improvement. In a study on Raynaud's disease, GBE phytosome demonstrated a 40 to 60 percent improvement in symptoms compared to unbound GBE.

Impotence

Most cases of impotence (erectile dysfunction) are due to impaired blood flow to erectile tissue. Recent evidence indicates that *Ginkgo biloba* extract may be extremely beneficial in the treatment of erectile dysfunction due to lack of blood flow.[38] Sixty patients with proven erectile dysfunction, and who had not responded to papaverine injections of up to 50 milligrams, were treated with *Ginkgo biloba* extract in a dose of 60 milligrams per day for 12 to 18 months. The penile blood flow was reevaluated by duplex sonography every 4 weeks.

The first signs of improved blood supply were seen after 6 to 8 weeks. After 6 months of therapy 50 percent of the patients had regained potency; in 20 percent a new trial of papaverine injection was successful; 25 percent of the patients showed improved blood flow, but papaverine was still not successful; 5 percent remained unchanged.

According to the results of this preliminary study, *Ginkgo biloba* extract appears to be very effective in the treatment of erectile dysfunction due to lack of blood flow. The improved arterial inflow to erectile tissue is assumed to be due to GBE's enhancement of blood flow through both arteries and veins without any change in systemic blood pressure.

It should be noted that ginkgo's effects are more apparent with long-term therapy, and better results may be obtained with a 120-milligram per day dose in order to take full advantage of ginkgo's effect in improving blood flow.

Premenstrual syndrome and idiopathic cyclic edema

Premenstrual syndrome (PMS) is often characterized by fluid retention, vascular congestion, increased capillary permeability, and breast tenderness. A recent double-blind, placebo-controlled study sought to determine the effectiveness of GBE in the treatment of these symptoms.[39] The population studied was a group of 165 women between the ages of 18 and 45 years who had suffered from these congestive symptoms for at least three cycles. The patients were then assigned to receive either the ginkgo extract (80 milligrams twice daily) or placebo from day 16 of one menstrual period to day 5 of the next. Researchers concluded, on the basis of extensive symptom evaluation by the patients and physicians, that the ginkgo extract was effective against the congestive symptoms of PMS, particularly breast pain or tenderness. Patients taking the ginkgo extract also noted improvements in neuro-psychological assessments. These results indicate that *Ginkgo biloba* extract may hold some promise in the treatment of PMS.

Antidepressant effects

Double-blind studies demonstrating GBE's ability to improve general mood in patients suffering from cerebral vascular insufficiency led researchers to begin investigating the antidepressive effects of GBE. In a recent double-blind study, forty elderly patients (age ranged from 51 to 78 years) diagnosed with depression, and who had not benefited fully from standard antidepressant drugs, were given either 80 milligrams of GBE three times daily or a placebo.[40] By the end of the fourth week of study, the average total score (on the Hamilton Depression Scale) achieved by the GBE-treated group fell from 14 to 7. At the end of the 8-week study, the total score of the GBE group had dropped to 4.5. In comparison, the placebo group dropped from 14 to only 13.

The results of this study can be interpreted as suggesting that GBE may offer significant benefit as an antidepressant on its own or in combination with standard drug therapy (tricyclics and tetracyclics were used in the study). In addition, it is important to point out that the dosage used in the study (80 milligrams three times daily) is higher than the standard dosage of 40 milligrams three times daily.

Antiallergic properties

Mixtures of ginkgolides, as well as the *Ginkgo biloba* extract standardized to contain 24 percent ginkgo flavone glycosides, have shown clinical effects in allergic conditions owing to their inhibition of platelet-activating factor (PAF)—a key chemical mediator in asthma, inflammation, and allergies.[9,10]

One double-blind placebo study investigated the ability of a mixture of ginkolides to block the effects of PAF injected into the skin.[9] Normally, PAF injection causes the immediate formation of a hive (classic wheal-and-flare reaction). However, if the ginkgolide mixture (120 milligrams) was given prior to PAF injection, it effectively counteracted the wheal-and-flare reaction. Specifically, the ginkgolide reduced the flare (reddened) area by a mean of 62.4 percent and the wheal (hive) volume by a mean of 60 percent.

Mixtures of ginkgolides, as well as purified ginkgolides, are investigational drugs in several European countries. The hope is that they will be shown to be clinically effective in asthma, eczema, and other allergies, as well as in many other conditions in which PAF plays a central role.[9,10]

Future applications of *Ginkgo biloba* extract

Experimental studies as well as some preliminary clinical evidence indicate that GBE may be of benefit in cases of angina, congestive heart failure, and in acute respiratory distress syndrome. Its action on inhibiting platelet activating factor may also make it useful in the treatment of conditions other than allergies, including various types of shock, thrombosis, graft protection during organ transplantation, multiple sclerosis, and burns.[1,2]

Dosage

Most of the clinical research on *Ginkgo biloba* has utilized a standardized extract, containing 24 percent ginkgo heterosides (flavone glycosides), at a dosage of 40 milligrams three times a day. However, some studies have used a slightly higher dosage of 80 milligrams three times daily.

It is difficult to devise a dosage schedule using other forms of ginkgo, owing to the extreme variation in the content of active compounds in dried leaf and crude extracts. Whatever form of ginkgo is used, it appears to be essential that it be standardized for content and activity. For example, a standard 1:5 tincture obtained from crude ginkgo leaf with the highest possible flavonoid content would require 1 ounce of the tincture per day to provide a dosage level equivalent to that of the standardized extract.

Clinical research clearly shows that GBE should be taken consistently for at least 12 weeks in order to be effective. Although most people report benefits within 2 to 3 weeks, some may take longer to respond.

Toxicity

Ginkgo biloba extract is extremely safe and side effects are uncommon. In 44 double-blind studies involving 9,772 patients taking GBE, the number of side effects reported was extremely small. The most common side effect, gastrointestinal discomfort, occurred in only twenty-one cases, followed by headache (seven cases) and dizziness (six cases).[2-4]

In contrast to the tolerance of the leaf extract, contact with or ingestion of the fruit pulp has produced severe allergic reactions.[41] Contact with the fruit pulp causes erythema and edema, with the rapid formation of vesicles accompanied by severe itching. The reaction resembles an allergic reaction to the poison ivy–oak–sumac group, suggesting cross-reactivity between *Ginkgo biloba* fruit and this family. Ingestion of as little as two pieces of fruit pulp has been reported to cause severe gastrointestinal irritation from the mouth to the anus.

References

1. DeFeudis FV (ed.): Ginkgo biloba *Extract (EGb 761): Pharmacological Activities and Clinical Applications.* Elsevier, Paris, 1991.
2. EW Funfgeld (ed.): *Rokan (Ginkgo biloba). Recent Results in Pharmacology and Clinic.* Springer-Verlag, New York, 1988.
3. Kleijnen J and Knipschild P: *Ginkgo biloba. Lancet* **340**, 1136–9, 1992.
4. Kleijnen J and Knipschild P: *Ginkgo biloba* for cerebral insufficiency. *Br J Clin Pharmacol* **34**, 352–358, 1992.
5. Schaffler VK and Reeh PW: Double-blind study of the hypoxia-protective effect of a standardized *Ginkgo biloba* preparation after repeated administration in healthy volunteers. *Arzneimittel-Forsch* **35**, 1283–1286, 1985.
6. Chatterjee SS and Gabard B: Studies on the mechanism of action of an extract of *Ginkgo biloba*, a drug for the treatment of ischemic vascular diseases. *Naunyn-Schmiedeberg's Arch Pharmacol* **320**, R52, 1982.
7. Le Poncin, *et al.*: Effect of *Ginkgo biloba* on changes induced by quantitative cerebral microembolization in rats. *Arch Int Pharmacodyn Ther* **243**, 236–244, 1980.
8. Karcher L, Zagerman P, and Krieglstein J: Effect of an extract of *Ginkgo biloba* on rat brain energy metabolism in hypoxia. *Naunyn-Schmiedeberg's Arch Pharmacol* **327**, 31–35, 1984.
9. Koltai M, *et al.*: Platelet activating factor (PAF). A review of its effects, antagonists and possible future clinical implications (Part I). *Drugs* **42**(1), 9–29, 1991.

10. Koltai M, et al.: Platelet activating factor (PAF). A review of its effects, antagonists and possible future clinical implications (Part II). *Drugs* **42**(2), 174–204, 1991.
11. Schmidt U, Rabinovici K, and Lande S: Einfluss eines *Ginkgo biloba* Specialextraktes auf doe befomdlickeit bei zerebraler Onsufficizienz. *Muench Med Wochenschr* **133**(Suppl 1), S15–18, 1991.
12. Bruchert E, Heinrich SE, and Ruf-Kohler P: Wirksamkeit von LI 1370 bei alteren Patienten mit Himleistungsschwache. Multizentrische doppelblindstudie des fachverbandes Deutscher Allegemeinaezte. *Muench Med Wochenschr* **133**(Suppl 1), S9–114, 1991.
13. Meyer B: Etude multicentrique randomisee a double insu face au placebo due traitment des acouphenes par l'extrait de *Gingko biloba*. *Presse Med* **15**, 1562–1564, 1986.
14. Taillandier J, et al.: Traitment des troubles du vidillissement cerebral pal l'extrait *Ginkgo biloba*. *Presse Med* **15**, 1583–1587, 1986.
15. Haguenauer JP, et al.: Traitment des troubles de l'equilibre par l'extrait *Ginkgo biloba*. *Press Med* **15**, 1569–1572, 1986.
16. Vorberg G, Schmidt U, and Schenk N: Wirksamkeit eines neuen *Ginkgo biloba* extraktes bei 100 patienten mit zerebraler insuffizienz. *Herg Gefasse* **9**, 936–941, 1989.
17. Eckmann F: Himleistungssstorungen—behandlung mit *Ginkgo biloba* extrakt. *Forsch Med* **108**, 557–560, 1990.
18. Wesnes K, et al.: A double-blind placebo-controlled trial of Tanakan in the treatment of idiopathic cognitive impairment in the elderly. *Hum Psychopharmacol* **2**, 159–169, 1987.
19. Anadere I, Chmiel H, and Witte S: Hemorrheological findings in patients with completed stroke and the influence of *Ginkgo biloba* extract. *Clin Hemorheol* **4**, 411–420, 1985.
20. Gessner B, Voelp A, and Klasser M: Study of the long-term action of a *Ginkgo biloba* extract on vigilance and mental performance as determined by means of quantitative pharmaco-EEG and psychometric measurements. *Arzneimittel-Forsch* **35**, 1459–1465, 1985.
21. Hofferberth B: Effect of *Ginkgo biloba* extract on neurophysiological and psychometric measurement in patients with cerebro-organic syndrome—a double-blind study versus placebo. *Arzneimittel-Forsch* **39**, 918–922, 1989.
22. Hindmarch I and Subhan Z: The psychopharmacological effects of *Ginkgo biloba* extract in normal healthy volunteers. *Int J Clin Pharmacol Res* **4**, 89–93, 1984.
23. Funfgeld EW: A natural and broad spectrum nootropic substance for treatment of SDAT—the *Ginkgo biloba* extract. In: *Alzheimer's Disease and Related Disorders* (Iqbal K, Sisniewski HM, and Winblad B, eds.). Alan Liss, New York, 1989, pp. 1247–1260.
24. Meyer B: A multicenter randomized double-blind study of *Ginkgo biloba* extract versus placebo in the treatment of tinnitus. In: *Rokan (Ginkgo biloba): Recent Results in Pharmacology and Clinic* (Funfgeld EW, ed.). Springer-Verlag, New York, 1988, pp. 245–250.
25. Coles RRA: Trial of an extract of *Ginkgo biloba* (EGB) for tinnitus and hearing loss. *Clin Otolaryngol* **13**, 501–504, 1988.
26. Holgers KM, Axelsson A, and Pringle I: *Ginkgo biloba* extract for the treatment of tinnitus. *Audiology* **33**, 85–92, 1994.
27. Bascher V and Steinert W: Differential diagnosis of sudden deafness and therapy with high dose infusions of *Ginkgo biloba* extract. In: *Vertigo, Nausea, Tinnitus, and Hypoacusia in Metabolic Disorders* (Clausen CF, Kirtane MV, and Schlitter K eds.). Elsevier, Amsterdam, 1988, pp. 575–582.
28. Lanthony P and Cosson JP: Evolution de la vision des couleurs dand la retinopathie diabetique debutante traitee par extrait de *Ginkgo biloba*. *J Fr Ophtalmol* **11**, 671–674, 1988.
29. De Felice M, Gallo P, and Masotti G: Current therapy of peripheral obstructive arterial disease. The non-surgical approach. *Angiology* **41**, 1–11, 1990.
30. Ernst E: Pentoxifylline for intermittent claudication. A critical review. *Angiology* **45**, 339–345, 1994.
31. Schneider B: *Ginkgo biloba* extract in peripheral arterial diseases. Meta-analysis of controlled clinical studies. *Arzneimittel-Forsch* **42**, 428–436, 1992.
32. Thomson GJ, et al.: A clinical trial of *Gingko biloba* extract in patients with intermittent claudication. *Int Angiol* **9**, 75–78, 1990.
33. Saudreau F, et al.: Efficacy of *Ginkgo biloba* extract in the treatment of lower limb obliterative artery disease at stage III of the Fontaine classification. *J Mal Vasc* **14**, 177–182, 1989.
34. Rudofsky VG: The effect of *Ginkgo biloba* extract in cases of arterial occlusive disease. A randomized placebo controlled double-blind cross-over study. *Forschr Med* **105**, 397–400, 1987.
35. Bauer U: *Ginkgo biloba* extract in the treatment of arteriopathy of the lower limbs. Sixty-five week study. *Presse Med* **15**, 1546–1549, 1986.
36. Bauer U: Six-month double-blind randomized clinical trial of *Ginkgo biloba* extract versus placebo in two parallel groups in patients suffering from peripheral arterial insufficiency. *Arzneimittel-Forsch* **34**, 716–721, 1984.

37. Preliminary studies conducted under the direction of Dr. Ezio Bombardelli and Dr. Paulo Morrazoni (Milan, Italy).
38. Sikora R, *et al.*: *Ginkgo biloba* extract in the therapy of erectile dysfunction. *J Urol* **141**, 188A, 1989.
39. Tamborini A and Taurelle R: Value of standardized *Ginkgo biloba* extract (Egb 761) in the management of congestive symptoms of premenstrual syndrome. *Rev Fr Gynecol Obstet* **88**, 447–457, 1993.
40. Schubert H and Halama P: Depressive episode primarily unresponsive to therapy in elderly patients: Efficacy of *Ginkgo biloba* (Egb 761) in combination with antidepressants. *Geriatr Forsch* **3**, 45–53, 1993.
41. Becker LE and Skipworth GB: Ginkgo-tree dermatitis, stomatitis, and proctitis. *JAMA* **231**, 1162–1163, 1975.

14

Goldenseal and other berberine-containing plants

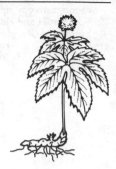

Key uses of berberine-containing plants:

- Infections of mucous membranes
- Parasitic infections of the gastrointestinal tract
- Inflammation of the gallbladder
- Cirrhosis of the liver

General description

The plants goldenseal (*Hydrastis canadensis*), barberry (*Berberis vulgaris*), Oregon grape (*Berberis aquifolium*), and goldthread (*Coptis chinensis*) share similar indications and effects due to their high content of berberis alkaloids. The chief berberis alkaloid, berberine, has been extensively studied in both experimental and clinical settings. Its pharmacological effects are reviewed below. The general description, history and folk use, chemical composition, and specific clinical indications for each plant are presented here. The pharmacology of the plants is primarily discussed collectively in terms of the activity of berberine.

Goldenseal

Goldenseal is native to eastern North America and cultivated in Oregon and Washington. It is a perennial herb with a knotty yellow rhizome from which arises a single leaf and an erect hairy stem. In early spring, it bears two five- to nine-lobed rounded leaves near the top, which are terminated by a single greenish-white flower. The parts used are the dried rhizome and roots.

Barberry

The common barberry is a deciduous spiny shrub that may reach 5 meters in height. Native to Europe, it has been naturalized in eastern North America. The parts used are the barks of the stem and root.

Oregon grape

The Oregon grape is an evergreen spineless shrub, 1 to 2 meters in height, native to the Rocky Mountains from British Columbia to California. The parts used are the rhizome and roots.[1,2]

Goldthread

Goldthread is a perennial herb native to China. The parts used are the rhizomes and root.

Chemical composition

Goldenseal

Alkaloids isolated from goldenseal root include hydrastine (1.5–4.0 percent), berberine (0.5–6.0 percent), berberastine (2.0–3.0 percent), canadine, canadaline, hydrastinine, and other related alkaloids. Other constituents include meconin, chlorogenic acid, phytosterins, and resins.[1,2]

Barberry

Barberry, like goldenseal, contains several alkaloids in the bark of its roots: jatrorrhizine, berberine, berberubine, berbamine, bervulcine, palmatine, columbamine, and oxyacanthine. It also contains chelidonic, citric, malic, and tartaric acids.[1,2]

Oregon grape

Oregon grape root contains the alkaloids berbamine, berberine, canadine, corypalmine, hydrastine, isocorydine, mahonine, and oxyacanthine. Resins and tannins have also been reported.[1,2]

Goldthread

Goldthread root contains berberine (5–8 percent) and other alkaloids similar to those found in goldenseal.[3]

History and folk use

Goldenseal

A native to North America, goldenseal was used extensively by the American Indians as an herbal medication and clothing dye. Its medicinal use centered around its ability to soothe the mucous membranes that line the respiratory, digestive, and genitourinary tracts in inflammatory conditions induced by allergy or infection. The Cherokee and other Indian tribes also used goldenseal in disorders of the eye and skin.[1,2]

Barberry

Barberry is native to most of Europe, and very similar species are found in North Africa and Asia. Barberry's historical use is as an antidiarrheal agent, bitter tonic, reducer of fever, and antihemorrhagic.[1,2]

Oregon grape

Oregon grape's historical and folk use is similar to that of goldenseal. In addition, Oregon grape was used in the treatment of chronic skin conditions such as acne, psoriasis, and eczema.[1,2]

Goldthread

In China, goldthread was used by practitioners of traditional medicine to "drain fire." Like goldenseal, it was used primarily to treat infectious conditions. Some specific uses included fever, dysentery, gastrointestinal infection, furuncles, boils, and eye infections.[3]

Pharmacology

The medicinal value of goldenseal, barberry, Oregon grape, and goldthread is thought to be due to their high content of isoquinoline alkaloids, of which berberine has been the most widely studied. Berberine has demonstrated antibiotic, immunostimulatory, anticonvulsant, sedative, hypotensive, uterotonic, choleretic, and carminative activity. Berberine's pharmacological activities support the historical use of the berberine-containing herbs.

Antibiotic activity

Perhaps the most celebrated of berberine's effects has been its antibiotic activity. Berberine exhibits a broad spectrum of antibiotic activity. Berberine has shown antibiotic activity against bacteria, protozoa, and fungi, including *Staphylococcus* species, *Streptomyces* species, *Chlamydia* species, *Corynebacterium diphtheria, Escherichia coli, Salmonella typhi, Vibrio cholerae, Diplococcus pneumoniae, Pseudomonas* species, *Shigella dysenteriae, Entamoeba histolytica, Trichomonas vaginalis, Neisseria gonorrhoeae* and *N. meningitidis, Treponema pallidum, Giardia lamblia, Leishmania donovani,* and *Candida albicans.*[1–10]

Its action against some of these pathogens (disease-producing organisms) is actually stronger than that of antibiotics commonly used in the treatment of diseases these pathogens cause. Berberine-containing plants should be considered in infectious processes involving the above-mentioned organisms. Berberine's action in inhibiting *Candida*, as well as pathogenic bacteria, prevents the overgrowth of yeast that is a common side effect of antibiotic use.

Antiinfective activity

Investigators decided to investigate berberine's ability to inhibit the adherence of group A streptococci to host cells, since the therapeutic effect of berberine appeared to be greater than its direct antibiotic effects.[11] Recent studies have shown that certain antimicrobial agents can block the adherence of microorganisms to host cells at doses much lower than those needed to kill cells or to inhibit cell growth.

Berberine inhibits the adhesion of streptococci to host cells by several modes of action. First, berberine causes streptococci to lose lipoteichoic acid; lipoteichoic acid is the major substance responsible for the adhesion of bacteria to host tissues. Second, berberine prevents the adhesion of fibronectin to streptococci, and elutes already-bound fibronectin.

The significance of the results of this study are quite profound. It raises many questions and forces researchers as well as practitioners to look at the treatment of bacterial infections in a new light. Is it better to utilize a substance with bactericidal or bacteriostatic actions rather than a substance that prevents the adherence of bacteria to host cells? Is the true value of botanicals with "antiinfective" actions a multifactorial effect on all aspects of infections, from immune stimulation to antimicrobial and antiadherence actions?

Simply stated, the results of the study indicated that berberine interferes with infections due to group A streptococci not only by inhibiting streptococcal growth, but also by blocking these organisms to host cells. The study implies berberine-containing plants may be ideal in the treatment of "strep throat," a condition historically treated with goldenseal by American naturopathic physicians. Berberine's action in inhibiting *Candida albicans* prevents the overgrowth of yeast that is a common side effect of antibiotic use.

Immunostimulatory activity

Berberine has been shown to increase the blood supply to the spleen.[12] This improved blood supply may promote optimal activity of the spleen. The spleen is responsible for filtering the blood and for releasing compounds that potentiate immune function. Berberine also activates macrophages.[13] These cells are responsible for engulfing and destroying bacteria, viruses, tumor cells, and other particulate matter.

The combined effect of improving blood supply to the spleen and increasing macrophage activity translates into improved filtration of the blood and is consistent with the historical use of berberine-containing plants as "blood purifiers."

Fever-lowering action

Historically, berberine-containing plants, especially goldthread, have been used as febrifuges. Berberine has produced an antipyretic effect three times as potent as that of aspirin in rats.[14] However, while aspirin suppresses fever through its action on prostaglandins, berberine appears to lower fever by enhancing the immune system's ability to handle fever-producing compounds produced by microorganisms.

Anticancer effects

Berberine exhibits potent anticancer activity directly by killing tumor cells and indirectly via stimulating white blood cells.[13,15,16] The most impressive effect was noted in a study demonstrating antitumor activity against human and rat malignant brain tumors.[15] Several experimental approaches were used in the study. *In vitro* studies were performed on a series of six human malignant brain tumor cell lines and rat 9L brain tumor cells. Berberine used alone at a dose of 150 micrograms per milliliter showed an average cell "kill rate" of 91 percent. This kill rate was over twice that of 1,3-bis(2-chloro-ethyl)-1-nitrosourea (BCNU), the standard chemotherapeutic agent for brain tumors, which had a cell kill rate of 43 percent. Studies in rats harboring solid 9L brain tumors also showed berberine has antitumor effects. Rats treated with berberine, 10 milligrams per kilogram, had a 81 percent cell kill rate. However, the combination treatment, berberine and BCNU, exhibited additive effects in killing cancer cells. These results indicate that berberine may prove to be more effective than BCNU or, at the very least, a valuable therapeutic addition in the treatment of difficult brain cancers.

Clinical applications

The broad antimicrobial effects of berberine combined with its antiinfective and immune-stimulating actions support the historical use of berberine-containing plants in infections of the mucous membranes, that is, the linings of the oral cavity, throat, sinuses, bronchi, genitourinary tract, and gastrointestinal tract. Berberine-containing plants may also be useful as an adjunct to standard cancer therapy.

Infectious diarrhea

Berberine has shown significant success in the treatment of acute diarrhea in several clinical studies. It has been found effective against diarrheas caused by *Escherichia coli* (traveler's diarrhea), *Shigella dysenteriae* (shigellosis), *Salmonella paratyphi* (food poisoning), *B.*, *Klebsiella*, *Giardia lamblia* (giardiasis), and *Vibrio cholerae* (cholera).[17-27] Studies in hamsters and rats have shown that berberine also has significant activity against *Entamoeba histolytica*, the causative agent of amebiasis.[7,8]

It appears that berberine is effective in treating the majority of common gastrointestinal infections. Clinical studies have produced results with berberine comparable to those of standard antibiotics in most cases. In fact, in several studies results were better.

For example, in a study of sixty-five children below 5 years of age with acute diarrhea caused by *Escherichia coli*, *Shigella*, *Salmonella*, *Klebsiella*, or *Faecalis aerogenes*, those given berberine tannate (25 milligrams every 6 hours) responded better compared to those receiving standard antibiotic therapy.[22]

In another study, forty children (age, 1–10 years) infected with the parasite *Giardia* received either berberine (5 milligrams per kilogram body weight each day), the drug metronidazole (10 milligrams per kilogram body weight each day), or a placebo of vitamin B syrup in three divided doses.[7] After

6 days, 48 percent of patients treated with berberine were symptom free and, on stool analysis, 68 percent were *Giardia* free. In the metronidazole (Flagyl) group, 33 percent of patients were without symptoms and, on stool analysis, all were *Giardia* free. In comparison, 15 percent of patients on placebo were asymptomatic and, on stool analysis, 25 percent were *Giardia* free. These results indicate that berberine was actually more effective than metronidazole in relieving symptoms at half the dose, but was less effective than the drug in clearing the organism from the intestines.

And finally, in a study of 200 adult patients with acute diarrhea the subjects were given standard antibiotic treatment with or without berberine hydrochloride (150 milligrams per day). Results of the study indicated that the patients receiving berberine recovered more quickly.[24] An additional thirty cases of acute diarrhea were treated with berberine alone. Berberine arrested diarrhea in all of these cases with no mortality or toxicity.

Despite these results, the best approach may be to use berberine-containing plants along with standard antibiotic therapy, because of the serious consequences of ineffectively treated infectious diarrhea.

Much of berberine's effectiveness is undoubtedly due to its direct antimicrobial activity; however, it also blocks the action of toxins produced by certain bacteria.[28–30] This toxin-blocking effect is most evident in diarrheas caused by enterotoxins (e.g., *Vibrio cholerae* and *Escherichia coli*), cholera, and traveler's diarrhea.[25–28]

Cholera is a serious disorder that needs standard therapy; however, traveler's diarrhea is usually self-limiting. Good results with berberine in the treatment of traveler's diarrhea have been obtained. In one study, patients with traveler's diarrhea randomly received berberine sulfate (400 mg) in a single dose or served as controls.[27] In treated patients, the mean stool volumes were significantly less than those of controls during three consecutive 8-hour periods after treatment. By 24 hours after treatment, significantly more treated patients stopped having diarrhea as compared to controls (42 versus 20 percent).

For those planning to travel to an underdeveloped country or an area of poor water quality or sanitation, the prophylactic use of berberine-containing herbs during, and 1 week prior to and after visiting, may be useful.

Trachoma

Water extracts of berberine-containing plants have often been employed in a variety of eye complaints, including infectious processes. In recent times, berberine has shown remarkable effect in the treatment of trachoma.[31,32] Trachoma is an infectious eye disease caused by the organism *Chlamydia trachomatis*, and is a major cause of blindness and impaired vision in under-developed countries. It affects approximately 500 million people worldwide and is severe enough to cause blindness in 2 million people worldwide.

The drug sulfacetamide is currently the most widely used anti-trachoma drug. In clinical trials comparing berberine (0.2 percent) and sulfacetamide (20.0 percent solution), sulfacetamide showed the best improvement (decrease in conjunctival discharge, edema, and pupillary reactions), but the conjunctival scrapings of all patients receiving sulfacetamide were still positive for *Chlamydia trachomatis*. These patients had a high rate of recurrence of symptoms. In contrast, patients treated with the berberine solution showed very mild ocular symptoms, which disappeared more gradually, but their conjunctival scrapings were always negative for *Chlamydia trachomatis*. These patients did not suffer relapse even 1 year after treatment, which suggests that berberine is probably curative for trachoma.[31,32]

Berberine's effect is believed to be due to stimulation of some host defense mechanism, rather than simply a direct action on the organism. As the berberine concentration used in these studies was 100 times less than the concentration of sulfacetamide, and berberine is much less expensive, it may be more cost effective than other treatments for trachoma. Berberine (0.2 percent solution) is appropriate therapy for many types of conjunctivitis.

Liver disorders

Berberine has been shown in several clinical studies to stimulate the secretion of bile (choleretic effect) and bilirubin.[33,34] In 225 patients with chronic cholecystitis (inflammation of the gallbladder), oral doses of 5 to 20 milligrams of berberine three times a day before meals caused, over a period of 24–48 hours, a disappearance of clinical symptoms, a decrease in bilirubin level, and an increase in the bile volume of the gallbladder.

Berberine has also been shown to correct metabolic abnormalities in patients with liver cirrhosis.[35]

Cancer

Berberine and and another alkaloid found in berberine-containing plants, berbamine, have been shown to exert beneficial effects in cancer therapy. In fact, berbamine has been used in China since 1972 in the treatment of depressed white blood cell (WBC) counts due to chemotherapy and/or radiation.

In one study,[36] 405 patients with WBC counts <4,000 were given 150 milligrams of berbamine daily (50 milligrams orally three times daily) for

1–4 weeks. Berbamine was viewed as "significantly effective" if the WBC count rose to >4,000 after 1 week or rose by more than 1,000 after 2 weeks; "effective" if the WBC count rose to >4,000 after 2 weeks or rose by more than 1,000 after 4 weeks; and "ineffective" if there was no change in the WBC count after 4 weeks of treatment. The overall results for the 405 patients: significantly effective in 163 cases (40.2 percent), effective in 125 cases (38.8 percent), and ineffective in 117 cases (29 percent). The total effective rate was 71 percent. However, when the WBC count before therapy was related to overall effectiveness, the effective rate was only 54.8 percent in thirty-one cases in which the WBC cell count was less than 1,000, and 82.7 percent in cases in which the WBC count was between 3,100 and 3,800.[36]

Dosage

As no detailed clinical studies have determined which berberine-containing herb to use for specific conditions, the following is offered only as a guideline based on experimental studies and historical use. However, the plants can be viewed as interchangeable.

Goldenseal indications

Infective, congestive, and inflammatory states of the mucous membranes; digestive disorders; gastritis; peptic ulcers; colitis; anorexia; and painful menstruation

Barberry indications

Gallbladder disease, including gallstones; and as a less expensive form of berberine in the treatment of the conditions listed above for goldenseal

Oregon grape indications

Chronic skin diseases and in the conditions listed above for goldenseal

Goldthread indications

Infective, congestive, and inflammatory states of the mucous membranes; fever; and infectious disorders of the skin

The dose should be based on berberine content. As goldenseal preparations vary widely in quality, standardized extracts are preferred. The following doses should be taken three times a day:

- Dried root or as infusion (tea): 2–4 grams
- Tincture (1:5): 6–12 milliliters (1½ to 3 teaspoons)
- Fluid extract (1:1): 2–4 milliliters (½ to 1 teaspoon)
- Solid (powdered dry) extract (4:1 or 8–12 percent alkaloid content): 250–500 milligrams

Toxicity

Berberine and berberine-containing plants are generally nontoxic at the recommended dosages; however, berberine-containing plants are not recommended for use during pregnancy and higher dosages may interfere with vitamin B metabolism.

The oral LD_{50} (50 percent lethal dose) in rats for berberine was greater than 1,000 milligrams per kilogram body weight, indicating the toxicity is extremely low.[37]

References

1. Duke JA: *Handbook of Medicinal Herbs*. CRC Press, Boca Raton, FL, 1985, pp. 78, 238–239, 287–288.
2. Leung AY: *Encyclopedia of Common Natural Ingredients Used in Food, Drugs, and Cosmetics*. John Wiley & Sons, New York, 1980, pp. 52–53, 189–190.
3. Chang HM and But PPH: *Pharmacology and Applications of Chinese Materia Medica*, Vol. 2. World Scientific, Teaneck, NJ, 1987, pp. 1029–1040.
4. Hahn FE and Ciak J: Berberine. *Antibiotics* 3, 577–588, 1976.
5. Amin AH, Subbaiah TV, and Abbasi KM: Berberine sulfate: Antimicrobial activity, bioassay, and mode of action. *Can J Microbiol* 15, 1067–1076, 1969.
6. Johnson CC, Johnson G, and Poe CF: Toxicity of alkaloids to certain bacteria. *Acta Pharmacol Toxicol* 8, 71–78, 1952.
7. Kaneda Y, *et al.*: In vitro effects of berberine sulfate on the growth of *Entamoeba histolytica, Giardia lamblia* and *Tricomonas vaginalis. Ann Trop Med Parasitol* 85, 417–425, 1991.
8. Subbaiah TV and Amin AH: Effect of berberine sulfate on *Entamoeba histolytica. Nature (London)* 215, 527–528, 1967.
9. Ghosh AK: Effect of berberine chloride on *Leishmania donovani. Indian J Med Res* 78, 407–416, 1983.
10. Majahan VM, Sharma A, and Rattan A: Antimycotic activity of berberine sulphate: An alkaloid from an Indian medicinal herb. *Sabouraudia* 20, 79–81, 1982.
11. Sun D, Courtney HS, and Beachey EH: Berberine sulfate blocks adherence of *Streptococcus pyogenes* to epithelial cells, fibronectin, and hexadecane. *Antimicrob Agents Chemother* 32, 1370–1374, 1988.
12. Sabir M and Bhide N: Study of some pharmacologic actions of berberine. *Indian J Physiol Pharm* 15, 111–132, 1971.
13. Kumazawa Y, *et al.*: Activation of peritoneal macrophages by berberine alkaloids in terms of induction of cytostatic activity. *Int J Immunopharmacol* 6, 587–592, 1984.
14. Sabir M, Akhter MH, and Bhide NK: Further studies on pharmacology of berberine. *Indian J Physiol Pharmacol* 22, 9–23, 1978.

15. Rong-xun Z, et al.: Laboratory studies of berberine used alone and in combination with 1,3-bis(2-chloroethyl)-1-nitrosourea to treat malignant brain tumors. *Chin Med J* **103**, 658–665, 1990.

16. Nishino H, et al.: Berberine sulfate inhibits tumor-promoting activity of teleocidin in two-stage carcinogenesis on mouse skin. *Oncology* **43**, 131–134, 1986.

17. Gupta S: Use of berberine in the treatment of giardiasis. *Am J Dis Child* **129**, 866, 1975.

18. Bhakat MP, et al.: Therapeutic trial of berberine sulphate in non-specific gastroenteritis. *Indian Med J* **68**, 19–23, 1974.

19. Kamat SA: Clinical trial with berberine hydrochloride for the control of diarrhoea in acute gastroenteritis. *J Assoc Physicians India* **15**, 525–529, 1967.

20. Desai AB, Shah KM, and Shah DM: Berberine in the treatment of diarrhoea. *Indian Pediatr* **8**, 462–465, 1971.

21. Sharma R, Joshi CK, and Goyal RK: Berberine tannate in acute diarrhea. *Indian Pediatr* **7**, 496–501, 1970.

22. Sack RB and Froehlich JL: Berberine inhibits intestinal secretory response of *Vibrio cholerae* toxins and *Escherichia coli* enterotoxins. *Infect Immun* **35**, 471–475, 1982.

23. Choudry VP, Sabir M, and Bhide VN: Berberine in giardiasis. *Indian Pediatr* **9**, 143–146, 1972.

24. Kamat SA: Clinical trial with berberine hydrochloride for the control of diarrhoea in acute gastroenteritis. *J Assoc Physicians India* **15**, 525–529, 1967.

25. Khin-Maung-U, et al.: Clinical trial of berberine in acute watery diarrhoea. *Br Med J* **291**, 1601–1605, 1985.

26. Gupte S: Use of berberine in treatment of giardiasis. *Am J Dis Child* **129**, 866, 1975.

27. Rabbani GH, et al.: Randomized controlled trial of berberine sulfate therapy for diarrhea due to enterotoxigenic *Escherichia coli* and *Vibrio cholerae*. *J Infect Dis* **155**, 979–984, 1987.

28. Akhter MH, Sabir M, and Bhide NK: Possible mechanism of antidiarrhoeal effect of berberine, *Indian J Med Res* **70**, 233–241, 1979.

29. Tai YH, Feser JF, Mernane WG, and Desjeux JF: Antisecretory effects of berberine in rat ileum. *Am J Physiol* **241**, G253–G258, 1981

30. Swabb EA, Tai YH, and Jordan L: Reversal of cholera toxin-induced secretion in rat ileum by luminal berberine. *Am J Physiol* **241**, G248–G252, 1981.

31. Babbar OP, et al.: Effect of berberine chloride eye drops on clinically positive trachoma patients. *Indian J Med Res* **76**(Suppl), 83–88, 1982.

32. Mohan M, et al.: Berberine in trachoma. *Indian J Opthalmol* **30**, 69–75, 1982.

33. Preininger V: The pharmacology and toxicology of the papaveraceae alkaloids. *Alkaloids* **15**, 207–251, 1975.

34. Chan MY: The effect of berberine on bilirubin excretion in the rat. *Comp Med East West* **5**, 161–168, 1977.

35. Watanabe A, Obata T, and Nagashima H: Berberine therapy of hypertyraminemia in patients with liver cirrhosis. *Acta Med Okayama* **36**, 277–281, 1982.

36. Liu CX, et al.: Studies on plant resources, pharmacology and clinical treatment with berbamine. *Phytother Res* **5**, 228–230, 1991.

37. Hladon B: Toxicity of berberine sulfate. *Acta Pol Pharm* **32**, 113–120, 1975.

15
Gotu kola

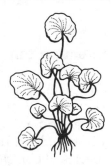

Key uses of *Gotu kola*:

- Cellulite
- Wound healing
- Varicose veins
- Scleroderma

General description

Gotu kola (*Centella asiatica*), or centella is an herbaceous perennial plant native to India, China, Indonesia, Australia, the South Pacific, Madagascar, and southern and middle Africa. This slender, creeping plant flourishes in and around water. Although it grows best in damp, swampy areas, centella is often observed growing along stone walls or other rocky, sunny areas at elevations of approximately 2,000 feet in India and Ceylon.[1]

Depending on the environment, the form and shape of centella can change dramatically. In shallow water, centella will form floating leaves while in dry locations, the leaves are small and thin, and numerous roots are formed.[1]

Typically, the constantly growing roots give rise to reddish stolons. The round-to-reniform, smooth-surfaced leaves, found on furrowed petioles, can reach a width of 3 centimeters and a length of 15 centimeters. The leaf margin may be smooth, crenate, or slightly lobed. Usually three to six red flowers arise in a sessile manner or on very short pedicels in axillary umbels at the end of 2- to 8-millimeter long peduncles. The fruit, formed throughout the growing season, is approximately 5 millimeters long with seven to nine ribs and a curved, strongly thickened pericarp.[1]

Historically, the entire plant is used medicinally, with harvesting occurring at any time during the year.[1]

Chemical composition

The primary pharmacologically active constituents of *Centella asiatica* are known to be triterpenoid compounds.[2] However, centella samples from India, Sri Lanka, and Madagascar apparently do not contain the same constituents.[3,4] In India, three (and possibly more) chemically different subspecies of *Centella asiatica* have been found.[5]

The concentration of triterpenes in centella can vary between 1.1 and 8 percent, with most samples yielding a concentration between 2.2 and 3.4 percent.[5]

Figure 15.1 diagrams the major triterpenoid components of *Centella asiatica*—asiatic acid, madecassic acid, asiaticoside, and madecassoside. The Madagascar variety is most commonly used to produce standardized extracts and yields triterpene concentrations of asiatic acid (29 to 30 percent), madecassic acid (29 to 30 percent), asiaticoside (40 percent), and madecassoside (1 to 2 percent).[2]

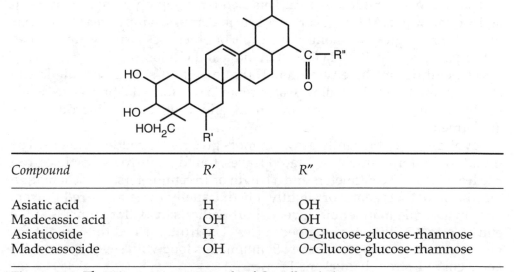

Compound	R′	R″
Asiatic acid	H	OH
Madecassic acid	OH	OH
Asiaticoside	H	O-Glucose-glucose-rhamnose
Madecassoside	OH	O-Glucose-glucose-rhamnose

Figure 15.1 The triterpene compounds of *Centella asiatica*

Centella also contains a green, strongly volatile oil composed of an unidentified terpene acetate (which accounts for 36 percent of the total oil), camphor, cineole, and other essential oils. Centella oil also contains glycerides of fatty acids, various plant sterols such as campesterol, stigmasterol, and sitosterol, and various polyacetylene compounds.[1,2]

Other notable compounds isolated from centella include the flavonoids kaempferol, quercetin, and their glycosides, *myo*-inositol, sugars, a bitter substance (vellarin), amino acids, and resins.[1,2]

History and folk use

Centella has been utilized as a medicine in India since prehistoric times and is thought to be identical to the plant mandukaparni, listed in the *Susruta Samhita*. Centella was also used extensively as a medicine, both internally and externally, by the people of Java and other islands of Indonesia. The medicinal use of centella in India and Indonesia centered around its ability to heal wounds and relieve leprosy.[1]

In the nineteenth century, centella and its extracts were incorporated into the Indian pharmacopeia, where in addition to being recommended for wound healing, it was recommended in the treatment of skin conditions such as leprosy, lupus, varicose ulcers, eczema, and psoriasis. It was also used to treat diarrhea, fever, amenorrhea, and diseases of the female genitourinary tract.[1]

In China, the leaves are prescribed for turbid leukorrhea and toxic fevers, while the shoots are used for boils and fevers. The plant is also used in the treatment of fractures, contusions, strains, and snakebites.[1] Centella was also used in China to delay senescence. One of the reported "miracle elixirs of life," centella's reputation as a promoter of longevity stems from the report of Chinese herbalist, LiChing Yun, who reportedly lived 256 years. LiChing Yun's longevity was supposedly a result of his regular use of an herbal mixture chiefly composed of centella.[6,7]

Centella asiatica was first accepted as a drug in France in the 1880s. Since then, extracts of centella have been used in the treatment of many of the same conditions listed above, along with those described below in Clinical Applications.

Centella, or gotu kola, has aroused much curiosity in American consumers. Many confuse gotu kola with kolanuts and assume gotu kola's rejuvenating activity is nothing more than the stimulant effect of caffeine. However, gotu kola is not related to the kolanut (*Cola nitida* or *Cola acuminata*), nor does it contain any caffeine.

Pharmacology

Centella asiatica, specifically the triterpenes, exerts remarkable wound-healing activity. Although the exact mechanism of action has not yet been fully determined, a number of interesting observations have been made.

In one of the early pharmacological investigations of centella, Boiteau and Ratsimamanga demonstrated that asiaticoside substantially hastened the healing of experimentally induced wounds.[8] Additional studies on the mechanisms of action of centella's enhancment of wound healing have shown that asiaticoside given orally, by intramuscular injection, or by implantation to rats, mice, guinea pigs, and rabbits produces the following effects:

- Stimulates hair and nail growth[1,8–10]
- Increases the development and maintainence of blood vessels into connective tissue[1,8–10]
- Increases the formation of mucin and structural components such as hyaluronic acid and chondroitin sulfate[1,8–10,12]
- Increases the tensile integrity of the dermis[1,8–10]
- Increases keratinization of epidermis through stimulation of germinal layer of the skin[1,10,12–14]
- Exerts a balancing effect on connective tissue[1,10]

The outcome of centella's complex actions is a balanced multiphasic effect on cells and tissues participating in the process of healing, particularly connective tissues. Enhanced development of normal connective tissue matrix is perhaps the prime therapeutic action of *Centella asiatica*.

Clinical applications

Obviously, from the brief description of centella's pharmacological activity given above, it is a valuable agent for the healing of wounds. Table 15.1[14–75] is an abridged list of documented clinical applications of *Centella asiatica*. The more popular uses of this valuable plant are discussed below.

Burns

The standardized extract from *Centella asiatica* has been effectively used in the treatment of patients with second- and third-degree burns caused by boiling water, electrical current, or gas explosion. Daily local application and/or intramuscular injections of the extract produced excellent results if the treatment was begun immediately after the accident. The extract prevented or

Table 15.1 Clinical applications of *Centella asiatica*

Conditions	References
Anal fissure	15
Bladder ulcers	16, 17
Burns	18, 19
Cellulite	20–25
Cirrhosis	26–28
Dermatitis	20, 29
Fibrocystic breast	30
Hemorrhoids	31
Keloids	32–34
Leprosy	14, 19, 35, 36
Lupus erythematosus	37
Mental retardation	38
Mycosis fungiodes	37
Peptic ulcer	39, 40
Perineal lesions	41
Periodontal disease	42
Retinal detachment	43
Scleroderma	44–47
Skin ulcers	48–55
Surgical wounds	8, 43, 49, 56–61
Tuberculosis	8, 62
Venous disorders	63–75
Wound healing	8, 43, 49, 56–61

limited the shrinking and swelling of the skin caused by skin infection, and it inhibited scar formation, increased healing, and decreased fibrosis.[18,19]

Cellulite

Standardized extracts of *Centella asiatica* have demonstrated good results in the treatment of cellulite in a number of clinical studies.[10,20–25] Bourguignon[20] observed the action of the extract on several types of cellulite in 65 patients who had undergone other therapies without success. Over a period of 3 months, very good results were produced in 58 percent of the patients and satisfactory results in 20 percent. Other investigations have shown a similar success rate (approximately 80 percent).[21–24]

The effect of centella in the treatment of cellulite appears to be related to its ability to enhance connective tissue structure and reduce sclerosis by acting directly on fibroblasts.

Cirrhosis of the liver

The therapeutic use of an extract of *Centella asiatica* in alcohol-induced cirrhosis (six patients), cirrhosis of unknown etiology (two patients), and chronic hepatitis has been reported.[26] In the cirrhosis patients, improvement in the histological findings and regression of inflammatory infiltration was observed. No effect was observed in the patients with chronic hepatitis. Other reports have supported the use of centella in fibrotic conditions of the liver.[27,28]

Keloids

The standardized extract of *Centella asiatica* has demonstrated impressive clinical results in the treatment of keloids and hypertrophic scars.[32-34] Its mechanism of action appears to be multifaceted, but is basically due to reducing the inflammatory phase of scar formation while simultaneously enhancing the maturation phase of scar formation.

Keloids and hypertrophic scars are characterized by a prolonged inflammatory phase, which may go on for months or even years without progressing to the maturation phase. The inflammatory phase is characterized on biopsy by large numbers of immature, swollen collagen bundles intermingled with inflammatory debris, while the maturation phase is characterized by mature fibrocytes, normal collagen fibers, and few inflammatory cell elements.

In one study, 227 patients with keloids or hypertrophic scars were treated by oral administration of a standardized centella extract (effective dose, 60 to 90 milligrams). The centella extract was used alone in 139 patients (the curative group) and 88 used the extract along with surgical scar revision (preventive group).[32]

In the curative group, 116 patients (82 percent) were found after 2 to 18 months to have benefited from the extract, either by relief of their symptoms or by disappearance of the inflammatory phase. In a double-blind substudy of 46 of the 139 patients, 22 of 27 receiving the extract improved while only 9 of 19 given a placebo improved.

In the preventive group, the centella extract also demonstrated significant positive effect. The therapeutic course in these patients was started a few weeks prior to surgery. If a positive response was observed, the patient was brought to surgery and kept on the centella extract for 3 months. (This method of preselection allowed the researchers to offer other forms of therapy to unresponsive patients.) Clinical improvement was observed in seventy-two of the eighty-eight patients (79 percent).

Leprosy

Several investigators have reported impressive clinical results using *Centella asiatica* and its extracts (oral, intramuscular, and/or topical) in the treatment of leprosy in both uncontrolled and controlled studies.[14,19,35,36] Therapeutic response is comparable to that of dapsone, the standard allopathic drug used in the treatment of leprosy.

In addition to its wound-healing activity, it appears that oxyasiaticoside, an oxidized form of asiaticoside, inhibits the growth of *Mycobacterium leprae in vitro* and *in vivo* by dissolving the waxy coating of the tubercle bacillus.[8]

Improving mental function

A significant increase in the mental abilities of thirty developmentally disabled children treated with *Centella asiatica* has been reported.[38] After a 12-week period, the children were more attentive and better able to concentrate on assigned tasks.

Centella's triterpenes have demonstrated mild tranquilizing, antistress, and antianxiety action via enhancement of cholinergic mechanisms.[76] Presumably this mechanism is responsible for the enhancement of mental function as well.

Scleroderma

The standardized extract of *Centella asiatica* has been tested in several trials in the treatment of scleroderma (including systemic sclerosis).[44–47] In addition to decreasing skin induration, patients have noticed a lessening of arthralgia and improved finger motility. Presumably the positive therapeutic response is a result of centella's balancing effect on connective tissue, thereby preventing the excessive collagen synthesis observed in scleroderma.

In one study of 13 female patients with scleroderma, oral administration of 20 milligrams of centella extract given three times weekly was very successful in 3 of 13, successful in 8 of 13, and unsuccessful in only 2 of 13.[47] Improvement consisted of decreased skin hardening, reduced joint pain, and improved finger mobility.

It has been more than 20 years since this study and other studies were performed. Given the positive results attained at an extremely low dose, it is unfortunate that more research has not been done.

Disorders of veins

Numerous studies have demonstrated that standardized extracts of *Centella asiatica* are effective in the treatment of varicose veins and venous insufficiency. This appears to be due to centella's ability to enhance the connective tissue structure of the connective tissue sheath that surrounds the vein, reduce hardening of the vein, and improve blood flow through the vein.[1,10,63–75]

Significant improvement in symptomatology (such as feelings of heaviness in the lower legs, numbing and tingling sensations, and night cramps), physical findings (edema, spider veins, leg ulcers, vein distensibility, etc.), and functional capacity (improved blood flow) was observed in approximately 80 percent of patients in the clinical trials.[1,10,63–75]

Wound healing

Standardized extracts of *Centella asiatica* have been shown, in a large number of clinical studies, to greatly aid wound repair.[1,8,10,43,48–61] The types of wounds healed include surgical wounds such as episiotomies and ear–nose–throat surgeries, skin ulcers due to arterial or venous insufficiency, traumatic injuries to the skin, gangrene, skin grafts, and perineal lesions produced during childbirth.

Dosage

The majority of clinical studies on *Centella asiatica* utilized proprietary formulas available in Europe (e.g., Madecassol, TECA, and Centelase). These standardized extracts contain asiaticoside (40 percent), asiatic acid (29 to 30 percent), madecassic acid (29 to 30 percent), and madecassoside (1 to 2 percent).

Since the concentration of triterpenes in centella can vary between 1.1 and 8 percent, it is difficult to calculate an appropriate dosage when simply using the crude plant material. However, since most samples yield a concentration between 2.2 and 3.4 percent, approximately 2 to 4 grams of crude plant material per day would contain an appropriate quantity of triterpenes, although it is not known if this correlates with the clinical efficacy of the standardized extracts.

Daily dosages for the various forms are as follows:

- Standardized extract (40 percent asiaticoside, 29–30 percent asiatic acid, 29–30 percent madecassic acid, and 1–2 percent madecassoside): 60 to 120 milligrams per day

- Crude dried plant leaves: 2 to 4 grams per day
- Tincture (1:5): 10 to 20 milliliters per day
- Fluid extract (1:1): 2.0 to 4.0 milliliters per day

Toxicity

Centella asiatica and its extracts are very well tolerated, especially orally.[1] However, the topical application of a salve containing centella has been reported to cause contact dermatitis, although quite infrequently.[1]

While the oral administration of asiaticoside at a dose of 1 gram per kilogram body weight has not proved toxic in toxicology studies, the toxic dose of asiaticoside by intramuscular application to mice and rabbits is reported as 40 to 50 milligrams per kilogram body weight.[1]

Asiaticoside has been implicated as a possible skin carcinogen when repeated applications are used.[77] Studies to determine if centella extracts are toxic to fetal development in rabbits have proved negative.[32]

References

1. Kartnig T: Clinical applications of *Centella asiatica* (L.) Urb. *Herbs Spices Med Plants* **3**, 146–73, 1988.
2. Castellani C, Marai A, and Vacchi P: The *Centella asiatica*. *Boll Chim Farm* **120**, 570–605, 1981.
3. Battacharya SC: Constituents of *Centella asiatica*. I. Examination of the Ceylonese variety. *J Indian Chem Soc* **33**, 579–586, 1956.
4. Battacharya SC: Constituents of *Centella asiatica*. I. Examination of the Indian variety. *J Indian Chem Soc* **33**, 893–898, 1956.
5. Rao PS and Seshadri TR: Variation in the chemical composition of Indian samples of *Centella asiatica*. *Curr Sci* **38**, 77–79, 1969.
6. Duke JA: *Handbook of Medicinal Herbs*. CRC Press, Boca Raton, FL, 1985.
7. Tyler V, Brady L, and Robbers J: *Pharmacognosy*, 8th Ed. Lea & Febiger, Philadelphia, 1981.
8. Boiteau P and Ratsimamanga AR: Asiaticoside extracted from *Centella asiatica*, its therapeutic uses in the healing of experimental or refractory wounds, leprosy, skin tuberculosis, and lupus. *Therapie* **11**, 125–149, 1956.
9. Boiteau P, Nigeon-Dureuil M, and Ratsimamanga AR: Action of asiaticoside on reticuloendothelial tissue. *Acad Sci Compt Rend* **232**, 760–762, 1951.
10. Monograph: *Centella asiatica*. Indena S.p.A., Milan, Italy, 1987.
11. Abou-Chaar CI: New drugs from higher plants recently introduced into therapeutics. *Lebanese Pharm J* **8**, 15–37, 1963.
12. Lawrence JC: The morphological and pharmacological effects of asiaticoside upon skin *in vitro* and *in vivo*. *Eur J Pharmacol* **1**, 414–424, 1967.
13. Lawrence JC: The effect of asiaticoside on guinea pig skin. *J Invest Dermatol* **49**, 95–96, 1967.
14. May A: The effect of asiaticoside on pig skin in organ culture. *Eur J Pharmacol* **4**, 177–181, 1968.
15. Bensaude A: The treatment of anal fissure. *Phleobologie* **33**, 683–688, 1980.
16. Aziz-Fam A: Use of titrated extract of *Centella asiatica* (TECA) in bilharzial bladder lesions. *Int Surg* **58**, 451–452, 1973.
17. Etrebi A, Ibrahim A, and Zaki K: Treatment of bladder ulcer with asiaticoside. *J Egypt Med Assoc* **58**, 324–327, 1975.
18. Gravel JA: Oxygen dressings and asiaticoside in the treatment of burns. *Laval Med* **36**, 413–415, 1965.
19. Boiteau P and Ratsimamanga AR: Important cicatrizants of vegetable origin and the biostimulins of Filatov. *Bull Soc Sci Bretagne* **34**, 307–315, 1959.

20. Bourguignon D: Study of the action of titrated extract of *Centella asiatica*. *Gaz Med Fr* **82**, 4579–4583, 1975.
21. Bonnett GF: Treatment of localized cellulitis with asiaticoside Madecassol. *Prog Med* **102**, 109–110, 1974.
22. Grosshans E and Keller F: Cellulite: Reality or imposter? *J Med Strasbourg* **14**, 563–567, 1983.
23. Keller F and Grosshans E: Cellulitis: Reality or fraud? *Med Hyg* **41**, 1513–1518, 1983.
24. Tenailleau A: On 80 cases of cellulitis treated with the standard extract of *Centella asiatica*. *Quest Med* **31**, 919–924, 1978.
25. Carraro Pereira I: Treatment of cellulitis with *Centella asiatica*. *Folha Med* **79**, 401–404, 1979.
26. Darnis F, *et al.*: Use of a titrated extract of *Centella asiatica* in chronic hepatic disorders. *Semin Hosp Paris* **55**, 1749–1750, 1979.
27. El Zawahry MD, Khalil AM, and El Banna MH: Madecassol, a new therapy for hepatic fibrosis. *Bull Soc Int Chir (Belgium)* **34**, 296–297, 1975.
28. El Zawahry MD, Khalil AM, and El Banna MH: Madecassol, a new therapy for hepatic fibrosis. *Bull Soc Int Chir (Belgium)* **34**, 573–577, 1975.
29. Fincato M: On the treatment of cutaneous lesions with extract of *Centella asiatica*. *Minerva Chir* **15**, 1235–1238, 1960.
30. Sterkers Desagnat M, Philbert M, and Moreau L: Medical treatments for benign disease of the breast. *Therapeutique* **51**, 121–124, 1975.
31. Guarnerio F, *et al.*: Treatment of hemorrhoids with *Centella asiatica*. *G Ital Angiol* **6**, 46–52, 1986.
32. Bosse JP, *et al.*: Clinical study of a new antikeloid drug. *Ann Plast Surg* **3**, 13–21, 1979.
33. Basset A, *et al.*: Treatment of keloids with Madecassol. *Bull Soc Fr Dermatol Syph* **77**, 826–827, 1970.
34. Ippolito F: Medical treatment of keloids. *G Ital Dermatol* **112**, 377–381, 1977.
35. Chakrabarty T and Deshmukh S: *Centella asiatica* in the treatment of leprosy. *Sci Culture* **42**, 573, 1976.
36. Chudhuri S, *et al.*: Use of a common Indian herb "Mandukaparni" in the treatment of leprosy. *J Indian Med Assoc* **70**, 177–180, 1978.
37. Wolram VS: Erfahrungern mit Maddecassol bei der behandlung ulzereroserser hautveranderungen. *Wien Med Wochenschr* **115**, 439–442, 1965.
38. Appa Rao MVR, Srinivasan K, and Koteswara RTL: The effect of *Centella asiatica* on the general mental ability of mentally retarded children. *Indian J Pschiatry* **19**, 54–59, 1977.
39. Kyoo WC: Medical treatment of peptic ulcer. *J Korean Med Assoc* **23**, 31–35, 1980.
40. Pergola F: Treatment of peptic ulcer with a titrated extract of *Centella asiatica*. *Med Chir Dig* **36**, 445–448, 1974.
41. Baudon-Glanddier B: Perineal lesions and asiaticoside. *Gaz Med Fr* **70**, 2463–2464, 1963.
42. Benedicenti A, Galli D, and Merlini A: The clinical therapy of periodontal disease: The use of potassium hydroxide and the water-alcohol extract of *Centella asiatica* in combination with laser therapy in the treatment of severe periodontal disease. *Parodontol Stomatol* **24**, 11–26, 1985.
43. Abou-Shousha ES and Khalil HA: Effect of asiaticoside (Madecassol) on the healing process in cataract surgical wounds and retinal detachment operations (clinical and experimental study). *Bull Ophthalmol Soc Egypt* **60**, 451–470, 1967.
44. Bletry O: Comment on the treatment of scleroderma. *Gaz Med Fr* **87**, 1989–1990, 1980.
45. Fontan I, *et al.*: Localized scleroderma. *Concours Med* **109**, 498–504, 1987.
46. Sasaki S, *et al.*: Experimental and clinical effects of asiaticoside (Madecassol) on fibroblasts, granulomas, and scleroderma. *Jpn J Clin Dermatol* **25**, 585–593, 1971.
47. Sasaki S, *et al.*: Studies on the mechanism of action of asiaticoside (Madecassol) on experimental granulation tissue and cultured fibroblasts and its clinical application in systemic scleroderma. *Acta Diabetol Lat* **52**, 141–150, 1972.
48. Balina LM, *et al.*: Clinical results of an asiaticoside in cutaneous ulcerous lesions. *Diabetes Med* **33**, 1693–1696, 1961.
49. Bazex J, Nogue J, and Peyrot J: Periulcerous eczema type cutaneous reaction during and after ulcers of the leg. *Rev Med Toulouse* **18**, 171–174, 1982.
50. Dulauney MM: Postphlebitic leg ulcers and indications for therapy. *Bordeaux Med* **12**, 1807–1810, 1979.
51. Hanna LK, Amin L, and El Serafy I: Trophic ulcers and their treatment with Madecassol. *Afr Med* **8**, 315–318, 1969.
52. Huriez CL: Action of the titrated extract of *Centella asiatica* on cicatrization of leg ulcers (10 mg tablets). Apropos of 50 cases. *Lille Med* **17**(Suppl 3), 574–579, 1972.
53. Sarteel AM and Merlen JF: Treatment of leg ulcers. *Phlebologie* **36**, 375–379, 1983.
54. Thiers H, *et al.*: Asiaticoside, the active principle of *Centella asiatica*, in the treatment of cutaneous ulcers. *Lyon Med* **197**, 385–389, 1957.
55. Vittori F: The treatment of ulcus cruris. *J Med Lyon* **63**, 429–432, 1982.

56. Castellani C, *et al.*: Asiaticoside and cicatrization of episiotomies. *Bull Fed Soc Gynecol Obstet* **18**, 184–186, 1966.
57. Collonna d'Istria J: Research on the healing action of Madecassol in cervical and laryngeal surgery after ionizing radiations. *J Fr Otorhinolaryngol* **19**, 507–510, 1970.
58. O'Keeffe P: A trial of asiaticoside on skin graft donor areas. *Br J Plast Surg* **27**, 194–195, 1974.
59. Pignataro O and Teatini GP: Clinical research on the cicatrizing action of Madecassol in comparison of oropharyngeal mucosa. *Minerva Med* **56**, 2683–2686, 1965.
60. Riu R, *et al.*: Clinical study of Madecassol in otorhinology. *J Med Lyon* **47**, 693–706, 1966.
61. Sevin P: Some observations on the use of asiaticoside (Madecassol) in general surgery. *Prog Med (France)* **90**, 23–24, 1962.
62. King DS: Tuberculosis. *New Engl J Med* **243**, 530–536, 565–571, 1950.
63. Allegra C: Comparative capillaroscopic study of certain bioflavonoids and total triterpenic fractions of *Centella asiatica* in venous insufficiency. *Clin Terap* **110**, 555–559, 1984.
64. Allegra C, *et al.*: *Centella asiatica* extract in venous disorders of the lower limbs. Comparative clinico-instrumental studies with a placebo. *Clin Terap* **99**, 507–513, 1981.
65. Barletta S, Borgioli A, and Corsi C: Results with *Centella asiatica* in chronic venous insufficiency. *Gaz Med Ital* **140**, 33–35, 1981.
66. Basellini A, *et al.*: Varicose disease in pregnancy. *Ann Obstet Gyn Med Perinat* **106**, 337–341, 1985.
67. Boely C: Indications of titrated extract of *Centella asiatica* in phlebology. *Gaz Med Fr* **82**, 741–744, 1975.
68. Bolgert M and Gautron G: An extract from *Centella asiatica* in phlebology. *Prog Med (France)* **100**, 31–32, 1972.
69. Cappelli R: Clinical and pharmacological study on the effect of an extract of *Centella asiatica* in chronic venous insufficiency of lower limbs. *G Ital Angiol* **3**, 44–48, 1983.
70. Cospite M, *et al.*: Study about pharmacologic and clinical activity of *Centella asiatica* titrated extract in the chronic venous deficiency of the lower limbs: Valuation with strain gauge plethysmography. *G Ital Angiol* **4**, 200–205, 1984.
71. Frausini G, Rotatori T, and Oliva S: Controlled trial on clinical-dynamic effects of three treatments in chronic venous insufficiency. *G Ital Angiol* **5**, 147–151, 1985.
72. Marastoni F, *et al.*: *Centella asiatica* extract in venous pathology of the lower limbs and its evaluation as compared with tribenoside. *Minerva Cardioangiol* **30**, 201–207, 1982.
73. Mariani G and Patuzzo E: Treatment of venous insufficiency with extract of *Centella asiatica*. *Clin Eur (Italy)* **22**, 154–158, 1983.
74. Mazzola C and Gini MM: *Centella asiatica* extract in treatment of chronic venous insufficiency. *Clin Eur (Italy)* **21**, 160–166 1982.
75. Pointel JP, *et al.*: Titrated extract of *Centella asiatica* (TECA) in the treatment of venous insufficiency of the lower limbs. *Angiology* **38**, 46–50, 1987.
76. Ramaswamy AS, Periyasamy SM, and Basu N: Pharmacological studies on *Centella asiatica* L. (Brahma manduki) (N.O. Umbelliferae). *J Res Indian Med* **4**, 160–175, 1970.
77. Laerum OD and Iversen OH: Reticuloses and epidermal tumors in hairless mice after topical skin applications of cantharidin and asiaticoside. *Cancer Res* **32**, 1463–1469, 1972.

16

Grape seed extract and other sources of procyanidolic oligomers

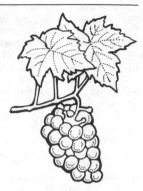

Key uses of grape seed extract:

- Antioxidant supplementation
- Atherosclerosis prevention
- Capillary fragility and easy bruising
- Diabetes
- Retinopathy (macular degeneration and diabetic retinopathy)
- Varicose veins
- Wound healing

General description

Grape seed extract is a rich source of one of the most beneficial groups of plant flavonoids—the proanthocyanidins (also referred to as procyanidins). These flavonoids exert many health-promoting effects. The most potent proanthocyanidins are those bound to other proanthocyanidins. Collectively, mixtures of proanthocyanidin dimers, trimers, tetramers, and larger molecules are referred to as procyanidolic oligomers, or PCOs for short.[1,2]

Although PCOs exist in many plants as well as red wine, commercially available sources of PCOs include extracts from grape seeds and the bark of the maritime (Landes) pine.[1,2] This chapter reviews these benefits of PCOs from grape seeds and pine bark.

History and folk use

In 1534, French explorer Jacques Cartier was leading an expedition up the Saint Lawrence river. Trapped by ice, Cartier and his crew were forced to survive on a ration of salted meat and biscuits. Cartier's crew began to exhibit signs and symptoms of scurvy—a severe deficiency of vitamin C. At the time, the cause of scurvy was unknown. Fortunately for Cartier and the surviving members of his crew, they came across a native American who told them to make a tea from the bark and needles of pine trees. As a result, Cartier and his men survived.

More than 400 years later, Professor Jacques Masquelier of the University of Bordeaux, France, read the book Cartier wrote detailing his expedition. Intrigued by Cartier's story, Masquelier and others concluded that pine bark must contain some vitamin C as well as being a good source of bioflavonoids, which can exert vitamin C-like effects.

Masquelier termed the active components of the pine bark "pycnogenols."[1,3] This term was used to describe an entire complex of proanthocyanidin complexes found in a variety of plants including pine bark, grape seed, lemon tree bark, peanuts, cranberries, and citrus peel. The term "pycnogenols" is now considered obsolete in the scientific community to describe these compounds giving way to the terms proanthocyanidins, oligomeric proanthocyanidin complexes (OPCs), and/or procyanidolic oligomers (PCO). In the United States, the term Pycnogenol® is a registered trademark of Horphag Research, Limited, Guernsey, UK and refers to the PCO extracted from the bark of the French maritime pine.

Masquelier patented the method of extracting PCO from pine bark in France in 1951 and from grape seeds in 1970. The PCO extract from grape seed emerged as the preferred source based on research between 1951 and 1971, as well as intensive research from 1972 to 1978.[1] The research in the 1970s was conducted with the goal of gaining the approval of PCOs as a medicinal agent by the French equivalent of the Food and Drug Administration (FDA). Detailed analytical, toxicity, pharmacological, and clinical studies were performed on the PCO derived from grape seeds.

PCOs from both grape seeds and pine bark have been marketed in France for decades. Sales for the grape seed extract in France are roughly 400 times greater than those for the pine bark. Owing to aggressive advertising and some misinformation, in the United States the pine bark extract currently outsells the grape seed extract.

Chemical composition

Grape seed and pine bark PCO extracts are well defined chemically. Available grape seed extracts contain 92 to 95 percent PCOs, while the pine bark extracts can vary from 80 to 85 percent.

Pharmacology

PCO extracts demonstrate a wide range of pharmacological activity. Their effects include an ability to increase intracellular vitamin C levels, decrease capillary permeability and fragility, scavenge oxidants and free radicals, and inhibit destruction of collagen.[1,2] Collagen, the most abundant protein of the body, is responsible for maintaining the integrity of "ground substance" as well as the integrity of tendons, ligaments, and cartilage. Collagen also is the support structure of the dermis and blood vessels. PCO extracts are remarkably effective in supporting collagen structures and preventing collagen destruction: (1) They cross-link collagen fibers, resulting in reinforcement of the natural cross-linking of collagen that forms the so-called collagen matrix of connective tissue[4,5]; they prevent free radical damage by their potent antioxidant and free radical scavenging action and inhibit cleavage of collagen by enzymes secreted by leukocytes during inflammation, by microbes during infection[6,7]; PCO extracts also prevent the release and synthesis of compounds that promote inflammation and allergies, such as histamine, serine proteases, prostaglandins, and leukotrienes.[1]

Perhaps the most celebrated effects of PCO in the United States are their potent antioxidant and free radical-scavenging effects. Antioxidants and free radical scavengers prevent free radical or oxidative damage. Free radical damage has been linked to the aging process and virtually every chronic degenerative disease including heart disease, arthritis, and cancer. Fats and cholesterol are particularly susceptible to free radical damage. When damaged, fats and cholesterol form toxic derivatives known as lipid peroxides and cholesterol epoxides, respectively. The antioxidant and free radical-scavenging effects of PCO were discovered by Masquelier in 1986.[1]

A recent study has shed more light on the antioxidant ativities and exact mechanisms underlying the primary clinical applications (e.g., varicose veins, capillary fragility, and easy bruising) of PCOs.[7] The study featured two primary goals: (1) to determine the free radical-scavenging activity of PCO and (2) to determine the inhibitory effects of PCO on xanthine oxidase (the primary generator of oxygen-derived free radicals) and the lysosomal enzyme system, which governs the release of enzymes that can damage the connective tissue framework surrounding capillary walls.

The results of some very sophisticated tests provide a detailed explanation of the vascular protective action of PCO and provide a strong rationale for their use in vascular disease. In these studies, PCOs demonstrated an ability to:

• Trap hydroxyl free radicals
• Trap lipid peroxides and free radicals

- Markedly delay the onset of lipid peroxidation
- Chelate to free iron molecules, thereby preventing iron-induced lipid peroxidation
- Inhibit production of free radicals by noncompetitively inhibiting xanthine oxidase
- Inhibit the damaging effects of the enzymes (e.g., hyaluronidase, elastase, and collagenase) that can degrade connective tissue structures

The activity of PCOs is approximately fifty times greater than that of vitamin C and vitamin E, in terms of antioxidant action. From a cellular perspective, one of the most advantageous features of PCO free radical-scavenging activity is that, because of its chemical structure, it is incorporated within cell membranes. This physical characteristic along with its ability to protect against both water- and fat-soluble free radicals provides incredible protection to the cells against free radical damage.

The researchers concluded their discussion with the following comment: "These findings, together [with] those of other investigators, provide a strong rationale for using these compounds in the therapeutic managements of microvascular disorders" (Facino et al., 1994).[7]

Uses of procyanidolic oligomer extracts

The primary uses of PCO extracts are in the treatment of venous and capillary disorders including venous insufficiency,[8-10] varicose veins, capillary fragility,[11] and disorders of the retina including diabetic retinopathy[12] and macular degeneration.[13] Clinical studies have shown positive results in the treatment of these conditions.

It appears that most individuals can benefit from an increased intake of PCOs. This suggestion is perhaps best illustrated by studies investigating the ability of grape seed PCO extract to improve visual function in healthy subjects.[14,15] In these studies, 100 normal volunteers with no retinal disorder received 200 milligrams per day of PCOs or placebo for 5 or 6 weeks and a control group received no treatment. The group receiving PCOs demonstrated significant improvement in visual performance in the dark and after glare tests compared to the placebo group. The improvement is related to improved retinal function.

On the basis of the relatively recent demonstration of potent antioxidant activity and vasculoprotective effects, the list of clinical uses of PCO extracts will surely increase. Perhaps the most significant use will eventually be in the prevention of atherosclerosis (hardening of the arteries) and its complications (heart attacks and strokes).

Numerous studies now demonstrate that the level of antioxidants may be a more significant factor than cholesterol levels in determining the risk of developing heart disease. Antioxidants prevent the oxidation of cholesterol and its carrier proteins as well as prevent the initial damage to the artery that ultimately leads to the process of atherosclerosis. Large-scale studies with vitamin E, vitamin C, and beta-carotene have shown that these antioxidants are capable of significantly reducing the risk of dying of a heart attack or a stroke. For example, one study of 87,245 nurses discovered that nurses who took 100 international units (IU) of vitamin E daily for more than 2 years had a 41 percent lower risk of heart disease compared to nonusers of vitamin E supplements.[16] In another study, 39,910 male health care professionals produced similar results: a 37 percent lower risk of heart disease with the intake of more than 30 IU of supplemental vitamin E daily.[17]

Since PCOs have a greater antioxidant effect compared to vitamins C and E, it is only natural to assume PCOs could offer greater protective effects. There is support for this contention. For example, several studies have shown the protective effects of red wine against heart disease and stroke by protecting against low-density lipoprotein (LDL) oxidation.[18] The active components in the wine are proanthocyanidins. A 7-year study, which began in 1985 and included 805 men, demonstrated an inverse correlation between flavonoid intake and death from a heart attack.[19] That is to say, when flavonoid intake was high the risk of having a heart attack was quite low. Conversely, if flavonoid intake was low, the risk of a heart attack was quite high.

In addition to preventing damage to cholesterol and the lining of arteries, PCO extracts have been shown in animal studies[1,20] to lower blood cholesterol levels and shrink the size of the cholesterol deposit in arteries. Additional ways in which PCOs prevent atherosclerosis include inhibition of platelet aggregation and inhibition of angiotensin I-converting enzyme.[21,22] Presumably PCO extracts may exert similar benefits in humans. PCO extracts, although in a supplement form, should be thought of as a necessary food in the prevention and treatment of atherosclerosis.

Grape seed versus pine bark

Grape seed and pine bark extracts are excellent sources of proanthocyanidins. Although both sources can be used interchangeably, for several valid reasons PCOs extracted from grape seeds have emerged as the preferred source.

- Most of the published clinical and experimental studies of the past 20 years have been performed on the grape seed extract, not the extract of pine bark.[23]
- Masquelier and others have demonstrated that grape seed extract may be more potent and effective than pine bark extract, in terms of free radical-scavenging activity. The reason? Only the grape seed extract contains the gallic esters of proanthocyanidins (in particular: proanthocyanidin B2-3'-0-gallate).[1,23] These compounds are the most active free radical-scavenging PCOs. They are found only in grape seed.
- It is far more economical to extract PCO from grape seeds than it is from pine bark. As a result, the grape seed extract provides greater value at a lower price.

Procyanidolic oligomers bound to phosphatidylcholine

The most beneficial PCO products may be those that utilize a special process to bind one part of the grape seed PCO extract with two parts of phosphatidylcholine. This process is referred to as the "Phytosome™ process." The result is a completely new molecule composed of a central molecule of PCO encased by two phosphatidylcholine molecules. The PCO–phosphatidylcholine complex offers significant advantages over unbound PCO.

The major advantage is improved absorption from the gastrointestinal tract. The phosphatidylcholine molecules envelope the PCO molecule, improving absorption and protecting the PCO molecules from degradation by digestion and gut bacteria. Absorption studies on unbound PCO indicate that only about 28 percent of an orally administered dose is retained in the body after 24 hours.[24] The majority (72 percent) is excreted in the feces (45 percent), urine (19 percent), or exhaled as carbon dioxide (6 percent). By binding the PCO to phosphatidylcholine, more PCO is absorbed.

Another advantage of the PCO–phosphatidylcholine complex is its improved utilization and incorporation into biological membranes: more PCOs are delivered to body tissue. Once delivered to the tissue, the bound PCOs exert much greater antioxidant effects compared to unbound PCOs.[25]

One 50-milligram capsule of phosphatidylcholine-bound PCO, in terms of absorption only, is equivalent to about 50 milligrams of unbound PCO whether they are derived from grape seed or pine bark. However, in terms of biological activity, one 50-milligram capsule of PCO-Phytosome may be as effective as 150 milligrams of unbound PCO.

Dosage

Regardless of the source, PCO extracts can be used to support good health. As a preventive measure and as antioxidant support, a daily dose of 50 milligrams of either the grape seed or pine bark extract is suitable. For comparison, it is now estimated that the average daily intake of total flavonoids in the United States is about 25 milligrams. An intake greater than 30 milligrams significantly reduces the risk of cardiovascular mortality.[19]

When used for therapeutic purposes, the daily dose should be increased to 150 to 300 milligrams. For PCO bound to phosphatidylcholine, the dose for general support is 50 milligrams; for therapeutic purposes, 150 milligrams.

Toxicity

PCO extracts exert no side effects.

References

1. Schwitters B and Masquelier J: *OPC in Practice: Biflavanols and Their Application.* Alfa Omega, Rome, 1993.
2. Masquelier J: Procyanidolic oligomers. *J Parfums Cosmet Arom* **95**, 89–97, 1990.
3. Masquelier J: Pycnogenols: Recent advances in the therapeutical activity of procyanidins. *Natural Prod Med Agents* **1**, 243–256, 1981.
4. Masquelier J, Dumon MC, and Dumas J: Stabilization of collagen by procyanidolic oligomers. *Acta Therap* **7**, 101–105, 1981.
5. Tixier JM, *et al.*: Evidence by in vivo and in vitro studies that binding of pycnogenols to elastin affects its rate of degradation by elastases. *Biochem Pharmacol* **33**, 3933–3939, 1984.
6. Meunier MT, Duroux E, and Bastide P: Free-radical scavenger activity of procyanidolic oligomers and anthocyanosides with respect to superoxide anion and lipid peroxidation. *Plant Med Phytother* **4**, 267–274, 1989.
7. Facino RM, *et al.*: Free radical scavenging action and anti-enzyme activities of procyanidines from *Vitis vinifera*. A mechanism for their capillary protective action. *Arzneimittel-Forsch* **44**, 592–601, 1994.
8. Henriet JP: Veno-lymphatic insufficiency: 4,729 patients undergoing hormonal and procyanidol oligomer therapy. *Phlebologie* **46**, 313–325, 1993.
9. Baruch J: Effect of Endotelon in postoperative edema. Results of a double-blind study versus placebo in 32 female patients. *Ann Chir Plast Esthet* **29**, 393–395, 1984.
10. Lagrue G, Oliver-Martin F, and Grillot A: A study of the effects of procyanidol oligomers on capillary resistance in hypertension and in certain nephropathies. *Semin Hosp Paris* **57**, 1399–1401, 1981.
11. Gomez Trillo JT: Varicose veins of the lower extremeties. Symptomatic treatment with a new vasculotrophic agent. *Prensa Med Mex* **38**, 293–296, 1973.
12. Soyeux A, *et al.*: Endotelon. Diabetic retinopathy and hemorrheology (preliminary study). *Bull Soc Ophtalmol Fr* **87**, 1441–1444, 1987.

13. Proto F, *et al.*: Electrophysical study of *Vitis vinifera* procyanoside oligomers effects on retinal function in myopic subjects. *Ann Ott Clin Ocul* **114**, 85–93, 1988.
14. Corbe C, Boisin JP, and Siou A: Light vision and chorioretinal circulation. Study of the effect of procyanidolic oligomers (Endotelon). *J Fr Ophtalmol* **11**, 453–460, 1988.
15. Boissin JP, Corbe C, and Siou A: Chorioretinal circulation and dazzling: Use of procyanidol oligomers. *Bull Soc Ophtalmol Fr* **88**, 173–174,177-9, 1988.
16. Stampfer MJ, *et al.*: Vitamin E consumption and the risk of coronary disease in women. *New Engl J Med* **328**, 1444–1448, 1993.
17. Rimm EB: Vitamin E consumption and the risk of coronary heart disease in men. *New Engl J Med* **328**, 1450–1455, 1993.
18. Frankel EN, *et al.*: Inhibition of oxidation of human low-density lipoprotein by phenolic substances in red wine. *Lancet* **341**, 454–457, 1993.
19. Hertog MG, *et al.*: Dietary antioxidant flavonoids and risk of coronary heart disease: The Zutphen Elderly Study. *Lancet* **342**, 1007–1011, 1993.
20. Wegrowski J, Robert AM, and Moczar M: The effect of procyanidolic oligomers on the composition of normal and hypercholesterolemic rabbit aortas. *Biochem Pharmacol* **33**, 3491–3497, 1984.
21. Chang WC and Hsu FL: Inhibition of platelet aggregation and arachidonate metabolism in platelets by procyanidins. *Prostaglandins Leukotrienes Essent Fatty Acids* **38**, 181–188, 1989.
22. Meunier MT, *et al.*: Inhibition of angiotensin I converting enzyme by flavanolic compounds: In vitro and in vivo studies. *Planta Medica* **54**, 12–15, 1987.
23. Masquelier J: *Historical Note on OPC*. Martillac, France, October 1991.
24. Harmand MF and Blanquet P: The fate of total flavanolic oligomers (OFT) extracted from "*Vitis vinifera* L." in the rat. *Eur J Drug Metab Pharmacokin* **1**, 15–30, 1978.
25. Bombardelli E, Cristoni A, and Morazzoni P: Botanical derivatives in functional cosmetics. *Drug Cosmet Ind* **155**, 44–51, 1994.

17
Green tea

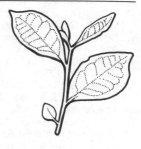

Key uses of green tea:

- Antioxidant supplementation
- Cancer prevention

General description

Both green tea and black tea are derived from the same plant, the tea plant (*Camellia sinensis*). The tea plant has long been cultivated in China. It is an evergreen shrub or tree that can grow to a height of 30 feet, but is usually maintained at a height of 2 to 3 feet by regular pruning. The shrub is heavily branched, with young hairy leaves. The parts used are the leaf bud and the two adjacent young leaves together with the stem, broken between the second and third leaf. Older leaves are considered inferior in quality.

Green tea is produced by lightly steaming the fresh-cut leaf, while to produce black tea the leaves are allowed to oxidize. During oxidation, enzymes present in the tea convert polyphenols, which possess outstanding therapeutic action, to compounds with much less activity. With green tea, oxidation is not allowed to take place because the steaming process inactivates these enzymes. Green tea is very high in polyphenols with potent antioxidant and anticancer properties. Oolong tea is partially oxidized.

Of the nearly 2.5 million tons of dried tea produced each year, only 20 percent is green tea (Table 17.1). In other words, nearly four times as much black tea is produced and consumed compared to green tea. India and Sri Lanka are the major producers of black tea. Green tea is produced and consumed primarily in China, Japan, and a few countries in North Africa and the Middle East.

Table 17.1 Yearly world tea production by type

Type of tea	Total dry weight[a]
Black	1940
Green	515
Oolong	60
Total	2515

[a]Measured in thousands of tons.

Chemical composition

The chemical composition of green tea varies with climate, season, horticultural practices, and age of the leaf (position of the leaf on the harvested shoot). The major components of interest are the polyphenols. The term *polyphenol* denotes the presence of multiple phenolic rings. The major polyphenols in green tea are flavonoids (e.g., catechin, epicatechin, epicatechin gallate, epigallocatechin gallate, and proanthocyanidins). Epigallocatechin gallate is viewed as the most significant active component. Not surprisingly, the leaf bud and the first leaves are richest in epigallocatechin gallate. The usual concentration of total polyphenols in dried green tea leaf is around 8 to 12 percent.[1,2]

Other compounds of interest in dried green tea leaf: caffeine (3.5 percent), an unusual amino acid known as theanine (one-half of the total amino acid content, which is usually 4 percent), lignin (6.5 percent), organic acids (1.5 percent), protein (15 percent), and chlorophyll (0.5 percent).

One cup of green tea usually contains about 300 to 400 milligrams of polyphenols and between 50 and 100 milligrams of caffeine.

Commercial preparations are available that have been decaffeinated and concentrated for polyphenols, anywhere from 60 to 80 percent total polyphenols.

Pharmacology

Most of the population and experimental studies on tea have focused on the cancer-causing and cancer-protective aspects. Green tea polyphenols are potent antioxidant compounds that have demonstrated greater antioxidant protection than vitamins C and E in experimental studies.[3]

In addition to exerting antioxidant activity on its own, green tea may increase the activity of antioxidant enzymes. In one study mice were fed green tea polyphenols via their drinking water for 30 days; researchers discovered a significant increase in the activity of antioxidant and detoxifying enzymes (glutathione peroxidase, glutathione reductase, glutathione S-transferase, catalase, and quinone reductase) in the small intestine, liver, and lungs.[4]

A number of experiments conducted *in vitro* and in animal cancer models have shown that green tea polyphenols may offer significant protection from cancer.[5–8] Specifically, green tea polyphenols inhibit cancer by blocking the formation of cancer-causing compounds such as nitrosamines, suppressing the activation of carcinogens, and detoxifying or trapping cancer-causing agents. In addition to these studies, human studies support the concept that green tea consumption can prevent some forms of cancer.[9]

The forms of cancer that appear to be best prevented by green tea are cancers of the gastrointestinal tract, including cancers of the stomach, small intestine, pancreas, and colon; lung cancer; and estrogen-related cancers including most breast cancers.[9]

Concerning breast cancer: *In vitro* studies show that green tea extracts inhibit the growth of mammary cancer cell lines.[8] Their primary mode of action is to inhibit the interaction of tumor promoters, hormones, and growth factors with their receptors: a kind of sealing-off effect. This effect would account for the reversible growth arrest noted in the *in vitro* studies.

Clinical applications

The primary clinical application for green tea is in the prevention of cancer. Population studies have demonstrated that green tea consumption may actually be one of the major reasons why the cancer rate is lower in Japan.[9] In contrast to green tea's protective effects, population studies seem to indicate that black tea consumption may increase the risk for certain cancers (e.g., cancer of the rectum, gallbladder, and endometrium).[10,11]

For example, in one study, the relationship between black tea consumption and cancer risk was analyzed using data from an integrated series of case-control studies conducted in northern Italy between 1983 and 1990.[10] The data set included 119 biopsy-confirmed cancers of the oral cavity and throat, 294 of the esophagus, 564 of the stomach, 673 of the colon, 406 of the rectum, 258 of the liver, 41 of the gallbladder, 303 of the pancreas, 149 of the larynx, 2,860 of the breast, 567 of the endometrium, 742 of the ovary, 107 of the prostate, 365 of the bladder, 147 of the kidney, 120 of the thyroid, and 6,147 controls admitted to hospital for acute noncancerous conditions. The risk of developing cancer due to tea consumption was derived after allowance for age, sex, area of residence, education, smoking, and coffee consumption. Results indicated an increased risk with tea consumption for cancers of the rectum, gallbladder, and endometrium. There was no association with cancers of the oral cavity, esophagus, stomach, bladder, kidney, prostate, or any other site considered.

In another study, men of Japanese ancestry were clinically examined from 1965 to 1968.[11] For 7,833 of these men, data on black tea consumption habits were recorded. Cancer cases identified among these men since 1965 include the following: 152 colon, 151 lung, 149 prostate, 136 stomach, 76 rectum, 57 bladder, 30 pancreas, 25 liver, 12 kidney, and 163 at other (miscellaneous) sites. Compared to almost-never drinkers, men who habitually drank black tea more than once a day had a four times greater chance of developing rectal cancer.

Anticancer properties of green tea

Green tea consumption with meals may inhibit the formation of nitrosamines.[12,13] Nitrosamines are formed when nitrites, such as those used in the curing of bacon and ham, bind to amino acids. Numerous studies have shown that green tea (including green tea polyphenols and extracts) exerts significant inhibitory effects on the formation of nitrosamines in various animal and human models. For example, when human volunteers ingested green tea along with 300 milligrams of sodium nitrate and 300 milligrams of proline, nitrosoproline formation was strongly inhibited.[12]

The popular custom of drinking green tea with meals in Japan is thought to be a major reason for the low cancer rate in this country. With the cancer rate in the United States rising, more Americans might want to start drinking green tea with their meals.

Dosage

The normal amount of green tea consumed by Japanese and other green tea-drinking cultures is about 3 cups daily or about 3 grams of soluble components, providing roughly 240 to 320 milligrams of polyphenols. To achieve some degree of protection, you should consume an amount of green tea or green tea polyphenols equivalent to the amount consumed in the positive population studies. For a green tea extract standardized for 80 percent total polyphenol and 55 percent epigallocatechin gallate content, this means a daily dose of 300 to 400 milligrams. (*Note*: When selecting commercial products, look for the level of epigallocatechin gallate, as well as total polyphenol content.)

Toxicity

Green tea is not associated with any significant side effects or toxicity. As with any caffeine-containing beverage, overconsumption may produce a stimulant effect (nervousness, anxiety, insomnia, irritability, etc.); however, for some reason green tea usually does not produce these symptoms even in those who are usually quite sensitive to caffeine (the author included).

References

1. Graham HN: Green tea composition, consumption, and polyphenol chemistry. *Prev Med* **21**, 334–350, 1992.
2. Min Z and Peigen X: Quantitative analysis of the active constituents in green tea. *Phytother Res* **5**, 239–240, 1991.
3. Ho C, *et al.*: Antioxidative effect of polyphenol extract prepared from various Chinese teas. *Prev Med* **21**, 520–525, 1992.
4. Khan SG, *et al.*: Enhancement of antioxidant and phase II enzymes by oral feeding of green tea polyphenols in drinking water to SKH-1 hairless mice: Possible role in cancer chemoprevention. *Cancer Res* **52**, 4050–4052, 1992.
5. Katiyar SK, Agarwal R, and Mukhtar H: Green tea in chemoprevention of cancer. *Compr Ther* **18**, 3–8, 1992.
6. Mukhtar H, *et al.*: Tea components: Antimutagenic and anticarcinogenic effects. *Prev Med* **21**, 351–360, 1992.
7. Wang ZY, *et al.*: Protection against polycyclic aromatic hydrocarbon-induced skin tumor initiation in mice by green tea polyphenols. *Carcinogenesis* **10**, 411–415, 1989.
8. Komori A, *et al.*: Anticarcinogenic activity of green tea polyphenols. *Jpn J Clin Oncol* **23**(3), 186–190, 1993.
9. Yang CS and Wang ZY: Tea and cancer. *J Natl Cancer Inst* **85**(13), 1038–1049, 1993.
10. La Vecchia C, *et al.*: Tea consumption and cancer risk. *Nutr Cancer* **17**, 27–31, 1992.
11. Heilbrun LK, Nomura A, and Stemmermann GN: Black tea consumption and cancer risk: A prospective study. *Br J Cancer* **54**, 677–683, 1986.
12. Stich HF: Teas and tea components as inhibitors of carcinogen formation in model systems and man. *Prev Med* **21**, 377–384, 1992.
13. Xu GP, Song PJ, and Reed PI. Effects of fruit juices, processed vegetable juice, orange peel and green tea on endogenous formation of *N*-nitrosoproline in subjects from a high-risk area for gastric cancer in Moping County, China. *Eur J Cancer Prev* **2**(4), 327–335, 1993.

18
Gugulipid

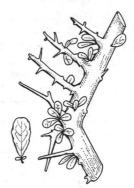

Key uses of gugulipid:

- High cholesterol levels
- High triglyceride levels

General description

Gugulipid is derived from the mukul myrrh tree (*Commiphora mukul*), a small thorny tree 4 to 6 feet tall that is native to Arabia and India. In its natural setting, the tree remains essentially free of foliage for most of the year. Its bark is ash-colored and comes off in rough flakes, exposing the underbark, which also peels off. On injury, the tree exudes a yellowish gum resin that has a balsamic odor. This oleoresin is referred to as "gum guggul" or "guggulu." This resin is used for medicinal purposes. When tapped during the winter, the average tree yields 700–900 grams of resin.[1]

Chemical composition

Guggulu contains a mixture of diverse chemical constituents that can be separated into several fractions.[1] The first step in the fractionation process (Figure 18.1) involves mixing guggulu with ethyl acetate, yielding a soluble and an insoluble fraction. The insoluble fraction, containing the carbohydrate constituents, is toxic and is the major reason why extracts of the soluble portion are preferred to crude gum guggul for medical use. The insoluble portion has no demonstrable pharmacological activity other than toxicity.[1]

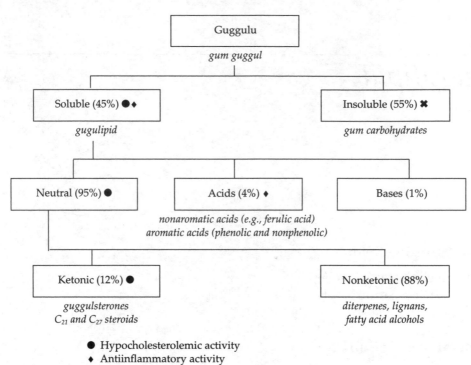

Figure 18.1 Chemical segregation of gum guggulu

In contrast, the soluble portion possesses significant cholesterol-lowering and antiinflammatory activity. The soluble portion can be further separated into base, acid, and neutral fractions. The neutral portion possesses almost all of the cholesterol-lowering activity, while the acid portion possesses the antiinflammatory components.[1]

On further purification of the neutral portion it was determined that the ketone fraction contains the most potent cholesterol-lowering components. The ketone fraction is composed of C_{21} or C_{27} steroids, with the major components being Z- and E-guggulsterone (Figure 18.2). These compounds are considered the major active components of gum guggul and its extracts.[1]

For medicinal purposes, a standardized extract known as gugulipid, which contains a minimum of 50 mg of guggulsterones per gram, is regarded as the most beneficial in terms of safety and effectiveness.[1,2] In addition to guggulsterones, gugulipid contains various diterpenes, sterols, esters, and fatty alcohols. These accessory components appear to exert a synergistic effect.[1,2]

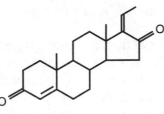

Figure 18.2 *E*-Guggulsterone

History and folk use

Guggulu is a highly valued botanical medicine in the Indian system of medicine, *Ayurveda*. It is included in formulas for a variety of health conditions including rheumatoid arthritis and lipid disorders. The classic Ayurvedic medical text, the *Sushrutasamhita*, describes in detail the usefulness of guggul in the treatment of obesity and other disorders of fats, including "coating and obstruction of channels."[1,2]

Inspired by this description, researchers began studying, in well-designed scientific studies, the clinical effectiveness of gum guggul and its extracts in disorders of lipid metabolism—specifically, its ability to lower cholesterol and triglyceride levels and promote weight loss. This research resulted in the development of a natural cholesterol-lowering substance that is safer and more effective than many cholesterol-lowering drugs, including niacin. Gugulipid was granted approval in India for marketing as a lipid-lowering drug in June 1986.[1,2]

Pharmacology

The pharmacology of gugulipid focuses primarily on its ability to lower cholesterol and triglyceride levels.

Cholesterol- and triglyceride-lowering effects

Numerous studies in humans and animals have shown that gum guggul (both crude and purified alcohol extract),[3-7] its petroleum ether extract (referred to as fraction A),[8-11] and gugulipid (standardized ethyl acetate extract)[12-13] all exert effective lipid-lowering activity. All three lower elevated cholesterol and triglyceride levels. The effect on cholesterol is particularly beneficial, as guggul lowers very low-density lipoprotein (VLDL) cholesterol and low-density lipoprotein (LDL) cholesterol while simultaneously elevating high-density lipoprotein (HDL) cholesterol, thus offering protection against heart disease due to atherosclerosis.

The primary mechanism of action for gum guggul and for gugulipid's cholesterol-lowering action is stimulation of liver metabolism of LDL cholesterol; that is, guggulsterones increase the uptake of LDL cholesterol from the blood by the liver.[14,15] However, another action of guggulsterone that also affects lipid levels is its ability to stimulate thyroid function.[16] This thyroid-stimulating effect may be responsible for some of gugulipid's weight loss activity.

Prevention and reversal of atherosclerosis

In addition to lowering lipid levels, gum guggul and its extracts, including gugulipid, prevent the development of atherosclerosis and aid in the regression of preexisting atherosclerotic plaques in animals. This implies that it may have a similar effect in humans.

Gum guggul and its extracts mildly inhibit platelet aggregation and promote fibrinolysis, implying that they may also prevent the development of a stroke or embolism.[2,14]

Cardioprotective activity

Gum guggul and gugulipid prevent the heart from being damaged by free radicals and improve the metabolism of the heart.[9,14]

Antiinflammatory effects

The guggulsterone fraction of gum guggul exhibits significant antiinflammatory action in experimental models of inflammation (e.g., raw paw edema and adjuvant arthritis method).[17-19] Its activity in models of acute inflammation is comparable to approximately one-fifth that of hydrocortisone, and equal to phenylbutazone and ibuprofen.[17] In models of chronic inflammation, it was shown to be more effective than hydrocortisone, phenylbutazone, and ibuprofen in reducing the severity of secondary lesions. The antiinflammatory action is thought to be due to inhibition of delayed hypersensitivity reactions.[18,19]

Clinical applications

The primary clinical application of gugulipid is in the treatment of elevated cholesterol and triglyceride levels. Research indicates that gugulipid offers

Table 18.1 Serum lipid effects of gugulipid compared to standard drugs

Agent	Total cholesterol (%)	HDL cholesterol (%)	Triglycerides (%)
Gugulipid	–24	+16	–23
Cholestyramine	–14	+8	+10
Gemfibrozil	–10	+11	–22
Lovastatin	–34	+8	–25

considerable benefit in preventing and treating atherosclerotic vascular disease, the leading cause of death in the United States.

Gugulipid appears most indicated in type IIb (increased LDL cholesterol, VLDL cholesterol, and triglycerides) and type IV (increased VLDL cholesterol and triglycerides) hyperlipidemias. In human clinical trials using gugulipid, cholesterol levels typically dropped 14 to 27 percent in a 4- to 12-week period while triglyceride levels dropped from 22 to 30 percent.[12–14] Table 18.1 compares the effects of gugulipid and standard drugs on serum lipids.

As seen in Table 18.1, the effect of gugulipid on serum cholesterol and triglycerides is comparable to that of other lipid-lowering drugs. However, while the drugs are associated with significant toxicity, appropriate extracts of gugulipid produce no side effects. In addition to the excellent safety demonstrated in human studies, safety studies in animals have demonstrated gugulipid to be virtually nontoxic (see Toxicity, below).

Dosage

While the crude oleoresin (gum guggul), alcohol extract, and petroleum ether extract all exert lipid-lowering and antiinflammatory action, they are associated with side effects (skin rashes, diarrhea, etc.) at the doses required to produce a clinical effect.

Gugulipid, the standardized extract of the gum guggul, not only has greater clinical efficacy, but patients tolerate it much better than they do crude or purified gum guggul. The dosage of gugulipid is based on its guggulsterone content. Clinical studies demonstrate that 25 milligrams of guggulsterone three times per day is an effective treatment for elevated cholesterol levels, elevated triglyceride levels, or both. For a 5 percent guggulsterone content extract this translates to an effective dose of 500 milligrams three times per day.

Toxicity

The side effects of crude gum guggul, and of alcoholic and petroleum ether extracts, are discussed above. In clinical studies, gugulipid has not displayed any untoward side effects, nor has it adversely affected liver function, blood sugar control, kidney function, or hematological parameters.[11–13]

Safety studies in rats, rabbits, and monkeys demonstrate gugulipid to be nontoxic.[14] It does not possess any embryotoxic/fetotoxic effects and is therefore considered safe to use in pregnancy. In mice the LD_{50} (50 percent lethal dose) is 1,600 milligrams per kilogram both orally and in injectible form.[1]

References

1. Satyavati GV: Gugulipid: A promising hypolipidaemic agent from gum guggul (*Commiphora wightii*). *Econ Med Plant Res* **5**, 47–82, 1991.
2. Satyavati GV: Gum guggul (*Commiphora mukul*)—the success story of an ancient insight leading to a modern discovery. *Indian J Med Res* **87**, 327–335, 1988.
3. Satyavati GV, Dwarakanath C, and Tripathi SN: Experimental studies of the hypocholesterolemic effect of *Commiphora mukul*. *Indian J Med Res* **57**, 1950–1962, 1969.
4. Khana DS, *et al.*: A biochemical approach to anti-atherosclerotic action of *Commiphora-mukul*: An Indian indigenous drug in Indian domestic pigs. *Indian J Med Res* **57**, 900–906, 1969.
5. Nityand S and Kapoor NK: Hypocholesterolemic effect of *Commiphora mukul* resin. *Indian J Exp Biol* **9**, 376–377, 1971.
6. Kuppurajan K, *et al.*: Effect of gugglu on serum lipids in obese hypercholesterolemic and hyperlipidemic cases. *J Assoc Physicians India* **26**, 367–371, 1978.
7. Baldwa VS, *et al.*: Effects of *Commiphora mukul* (Guggul) in experimentally induced hyperlipidemia and atherosclerosis. *J Assoc Physicians India* **29**, 13–17, 1981.
8. Malhotra SC and Ahuja MMS: Comparative hypolipidaemic effectiveness of gum guggulu (*Commiphora mukul*) fraction "A", ethyl-*p*-chlorophenoxyisobutyrate and Ciba-13437-Su. *Indian J Med Res* **10**, 1621–16232, 1971.
9. Arora RB, *et al.*: Effect of some fractions of *Commiphora mukul* on various serum lipid levels in hypercholesterolemic chicks and their effectiveness in myocardial infarction in rats. *Indian J Exp Biol* **11**, 166–168, 1973.
10. Malhotra SC, Ahuja MMS, and Sundaram KR: Long term clinical studies on the hypolipidaemic effect of *Commiphora mukul* (guggulu) and clofibrate. *Indian J Med Res* **65**, 390–395, 1977.
11. Verna SK and Bordia A: Effect of *Commiphora mukul* (gum guggulu) in patients of hyperlipidemia with special reference to HDL-cholesterol. *Indian J Med Res* **87**, 356–360, 1988.
12. Agarwal RC, *et al.*: Clinical trial of gugulipid a new hypolipidemic agent of plant origin in primary hyperlipidemia. *Indian J Med Res* **84**, 626–634, 1986.
13. Nityanand S, Srivastava JS, and Asthana OP: Clinical trials with gugulipid, a new hypolipidaemic agent. *J Assoc Physicians India* **37**, 321–328, 1989.
14. Gugulipid. *Drugs Future* **13**, 618–619, 1988.
15. Singh V, *et al.*: Stimulation of low density lipoprotein receptor activity in liver membrane of guggulsterone treated rats. *Pharmacol Res* **22**, 37–44, 1990.
16. Tripathi YB, *et al.*: Thyroid stimulatory action of (Z)-guggulsterone: Mechanism of action. *Planta Medica* **54**, 271–277, 1988.
17. Arora RB, *et al.*: Isolation of a crystalline steroidal compound from *Commiphora mukul* and its anti-inflammatory activity. *Indian J Exp Biol* **9**, 403–404, 1971.
18. Arora RB, *et al.*: Anti-inflammatory studies on a crystalline steroid isolated from *Commiphora mukul*. *Indian J Med Res* **60**, 929–931, 1972.
19. Sharma JN and Sharma JN: Comparison of the anti-inflammatory activity of *Commiphora mukul* (an indigenous drug) with those of phenylbutazone and ibuprofen in experimental arthritis induced by mycobacterial adjuvant. *Arzneimittel-Forsch* **27**, 1455–1457, 1977.

19
Hawthorn

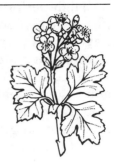

Key uses of hawthorn:

- Angina
- Atherosclerosis
- Congestive heart failure
- High blood pressure

General description

Hawthorn (*Crataegus oxyacantha*) is a spiny tree or shrub that is native to Europe. It may reach a height of 30 feet, but is often grown as a hedge plant. Its common name, hawthorn, is actually a corruption of "hedgethorn," as it was used in Germany to divide plots of land. Its botanical name, *Crataegus oxyacantha*, is from the Greek *kratos*, meaning hardness (of the wood), *oxus* meaning sharp, and *akantha* meaning a thorn. The fruit and blossoms are used medicinally.[1]

Other species of *Crataegus*, for example, *C. monogyna* and *C. pentagyna*, have pharmacological actions similar to that of *C. oxyacantha* and are suitable alternatives.[2,3]

Chemical composition

Hawthorn leaves, berries, and blossoms contain many biologically active flavonoid compounds, particularly anthocyanidins and proanthocyanidins.[4,5] These flavonoids are responsible for the red-to-blue colors not only of hawthorn berries, but also of blackberries, cherries, blueberries, grapes, and many flowers as well. These compounds are highly concentrated in haw-thorn berry and flower extracts.

High-performance liquid chromatography and thin-layer chromatogra-phy have demonstrated that extracts of the flowers are particularly rich in flavonoids (quercetin, quercetin-3-galactoside, vitexin, vitexin-4'-rhamno-side, etc.) and proanthocyanidins.[5,6]

In addition to flavonoids, hawthorn extracts also contain cardiotonic amines (e.g., phenylethylamine, o-methoxyphenylethylamine, tyramine, and isobutylamine), choline and acetylcholine, purine derivatives (e.g., adeno-sine, adenine, guanine, and caffeic acid), amygdalin, pectins, and triterpene acids (ursolic, oleanolic, and crataegolic acids).[7]

History and folk use

Hawthorn flowers and berries have been used primarily as heart tonics and mild diuretics in organic and functional heart disorders including conges-tive heart failure, angina, and high blood pressure. Hawthorn's astringent qualities were also utilized to relieve the discomfort of sore throats.[1]

Pharmacology

The pharmacology of hawthorn centers on its flavonoid components. The proanthocyanidins in hawthorn are largely responsible for its cardiovascu-lar activities.

Synergism with vitamin C

Hawthorn flavonoids have very strong "vitamin P" activity. Included in their effects are an ability to increase intracellular vitamin C levels, stabilize vita-min C (by protecting it from destruction or oxidation), and decrease capil-lary permeability and fragility.[4,8,9]

Collagen-stabilizing action

Hawthorn's flavonoid components possess significant collagen-stabilizing action. Collagen is the most abundant protein in the body and is responsible for maintaining the integrity of ground substance, tendons, ligaments, and cartilage. Collagen is destroyed during inflammatory processes that occur in rheumatoid arthritis, periodontal disease, and other inflammatory conditions involving bones, joints, cartilage, and other connective tissue. Anthocyanidins, proanthocyanidins, and other flavonoids are remarkable in their ability to prevent collagen destruction. They affect collagen metabolism in many ways, including:

- The unique ability to cross-link collagen fibers, resulting in reinforcement of the natural cross-linking of collagen that forms the collagen matrix of connective tissue (ground substance, cartilage, tendons, etc.)[4,8,9]
- The prevention of free radical damage, due to potent and free radical-scavenging action[4,8–10]
- The inhibition of enzymatic cleavage by enzymes secreted by white blood cells during inflammation[4,8,9]
- The prevention of the release and synthesis of compounds that promote inflammation, such as prostaglandins, serine proteases, histamine, and leukotrienes[9–12]

Cardiovascular effects

Hawthorn extracts are clinically effective in reducing blood pressure, angina attacks, and serum cholesterol levels and in preventing the deposition of cholesterol in arterial walls.[2,13,14] The beneficial pharmacological effects of hawthorn in the treatment of these conditions appear to be a result of the following actions:

- Improvement of the blood supply to the heart by dilating the coronary vessels[2,13,15–18]
- Improvement of the metabolic processes in the heart, which results in an increase in the force of contraction of the heart muscle and elimination of some types of rhythm disturbances[2,13,19–22]
- Inhibition of angiotensin-converting enzyme[23]

Hawthorn's ability to dilate coronary blood vessels, the vessels supplying the heart with vital oxygen and nutrients, has been repeatedly demonstrated in experimental studies.[2,13,15–18] This effect appears to be due to relaxation of the smooth muscle components of the vessel. Various flavonoid components in hawthorn have been shown to inhibit constriction of vessels by a variety of substances.[2,8,9] When blood vessels constrict, blood pressure goes up. In addition, procyanidins have been shown to inhibit angiotensin-converting enzyme.[23] This enzyme is responsible for converting angiotensin I to angiotensin II, which is a potent constrictor of blood vessels.

Recently, several proanthocyanidins have demonstrated a specific inhibition of angiotensin-converting enzyme similar to that of captopril.[23] Captopril is a synthetic angiotensin-converting enzyme inhibitor widely used in the treatment of high blood pressure. The proanthocyanidins that appear to have the highest activity are found in relatively high concentrations in hawthorn berries, flowers, and their extracts.[4,5]

Improvement in energy production within the heart has been demonstrated in humans and animals to whom hawthorn extracts have been administered.[2,13,19-21] The improvement is a result not only of increased blood and oxygen supply to the myocardium (muscle of the heart), but also a result of flavonoid–enzyme interactions. In particular, hawthorn extracts and various flavonoid components in hawthorn have been shown to inhibit several key enzymes within the myocardium (e.g., cyclic AMP phosphodiesterase).[22] The net result is an increase in the force of contraction. This is particularly beneficial in cases of congestive heart failure (discussed below).

A recent study has shed additional light on how hawthorn extracts enhance heart function.[19] A hawthorn extract standardized for proanthocyanidin content (3.3 percent) was studied utilizing an experimental model to determine the effects of a substance on heart function during ischemia. Although its effectiveness in this model was less than that of beta-blockers and calcium channel blockers, two classes of drugs often used in treating angina, there are two distinctions to be made: (1) the mechanism by which the drugs work in this model is by improving coronary blood flow and actually reducing the heart's need for oxygen by reducing its mechanical function. In contrast, hawthorn actually improves the mechanical function of the heart without increasing coronary blood flow.

Evidence that hawthorn improves energy metabolism and the utilization of oxygen by the heart was demonstrated by a decrease in accumulated lactic acid. Without oxygen, the heart muscle will shift to the breakdown of sugar for energy, but this can only go so far without oxygen. As a result, pyruvic acid is shunted to lactic acid. Recovery of heart function is inversely related to the level of lactic acid in the heart. The beneficial effects of hawthorn in angina appear to be related more to its ability to improve oxygen utilization, as noted by the reduction in heart tissue lactic acid levels, rather than to its ability to dilate coronary vessels. In fact, in this most recent study, hawthorn did not improve coronary blood flow.

Clinical applications

Hawthorn berries and hawthorn extracts are useful as food supplements in conditions affecting collagen structures, such as arthritis, periodontal disease, atherosclerosis, and inflammation. The clinical use of hawthorn revolves around its cardiovascular effects. Its use in atherosclerosis, hypertension, congestive heart failure, and arrhythmias is discussed below.

Atherosclerosis

Hawthorn extract, like other extracts containing proanthocyanidins (see Chapter 18—Grape Seed Extract, although in a supplement form, should be thought of as a necessary food in the prevention and treatment of athero-sclerosis. Increasing the intake of flavonoid compounds by taking hawthorn extracts has numerous health-promoting effects, including reducing choles-terol levels and decreasing the size of existing atherosclerotic plaques.[14] This again is probably a result of collagen stabilization.

A decrease in the integrity of the collagen matrix of the artery results in cholesterol being deposited within the artery. Many researchers feel that if the collagen matrix of the artery remains strong, the atherosclerotic plaque will never develop. Hawthorn flavonoids, by increasing the integrity of collagen structures, may offer significant protection against atherosclerosis. In addi-tion, feeding proanthocyanidin extracts to animals has resulted in the rever-sal of atherosclerotic lesions, as well as decreases in serum cholesterol levels.[14]

Flavonoids contained in hawthorn extracts appear to offer significant pre-vention, as well as potential reversing effects, in the treatment of atheroscle-rotic processes, which are still the major causes of death in the United States.

High blood pressure

Hawthorn exerts a mild blood pressure-lowering effect that has been demon-strated in many experimental and clinical studies.[2,13] Its action in lowering blood pressure is unique, in that it does so through a number of diverse phar-macological effects. Specifically, it dilates the coronary vessels, inhibits angiotensin-converting enzyme, increases the functional capacity of the heart, and possesses mild diuretic activity.

Hawthorn's effects generally require prolonged administration, and in many instances it may take up to 2 weeks before adequate tissue concentra-tions are achieved.

Congestive heart failure

Hawthorn has a long history of use in the treatment of congestive heart fail-ure, particularly in combination with digitalis or other herbs containing car-diac glycosides (e.g., *Cereus grandifloris*, also known as *Cactus grandifloris*, and *Convallaria majalis*). It potentiates the action of the cardiac glycosides.

Because of this enhancing effect, lower doses of cardiac glycosides can be used. In addition, magnesium has also been shown to augment digitalis action. For mild to moderate cases of congestive heart failure, hawthorn extract used alone may be sufficient, but for moderate to severe congestive heart failure, it should be used in combination with other cardiac glycosides as prescribed by a health care professional.

Hawthorn preparations are very effective in early stages of congestive heart failure and minor arrhythmias for which digitalis is not yet indicated. This has been repeatedly demonstrated in double-blind studies.[24–26] In the most recent study, thirty patients with congestive heart failure were assessed in a randomized double-blind study. Treatment consisted of a hawthorn extract standardized to contain 15 milligrams of procyanidin oligomers per 80-milligram capsule. Treatment duration was 8 weeks, and the substance was administered at a dose of one capsule taken twice a day. The group receiving the hawthorn extract showed a statistically significant advantage over placebo in terms of changes in heart function as determined by standard testing procedures. Systolic and diastolic blood pressure was also mildly reduced. Like all other studies with hawthorn extracts, no adverse reactions occurred.

Dosage

The dosage depends on the type of preparation and source material. Standardized extracts, similar to those used in Europe and Asia as prescription medications, are available commercially in the United States and are the preferred forms to use for clinical purposes. The doses listed below for the various forms of hawthorn are for use three times a day.

- Hawthorn berries or flowers (dried): 3–5 grams or as an infusion
- Hawthorn tincture (1:5): 4–5 milliliters (alcohol may elicit pressor response in some individuals)
- Hawthorn fluid extract (1:1): 1–2 milliliters
- Hawthorn freeze-dried berries: 1–1.5 grams
- Hawthorn flower extract (standardized to contain 1.8 percent vitexin-4'-rhamnoside or 20 percent procyanidins): 100–250 milligrams

Toxicity

Hawthorn has been shown to have low toxicity. In rats, the typical acute LD_{50} (50 percent lethal dose) of the tincture is about 25 milliliters per kilogram for oral administration; toxicity for chronic administration is found at about 5 milliliter per kilogram.[13] Similar results, adjusted for concentration, are found with other forms of hawthorn.

Although some studies have shown that proanthocyanidins may be carcinogenic, more careful evaluation has indicated that the carcinogenicity was probably due to contamination. Purified proanthocyanidins have been found to be nonmutagenic, according to the *Salmonella* mutagenicity assay system (Ames test).[27]

References

1. Grieve M: *A Modern Herbal*, Vol. 1. Dover Publications, New York, 1971, pp. 385–386.
2. Petkov V: Plants with hypotensive, antiatheromatous and coronarodilating action. *Am J Chin Med* **7**, 197–236, 1979.
3. Thompson EB, *et al.*: Preliminary study of potential antiarrhythmic effects of *Crataegus monogyna*. *J Pharm Sci* **63**, 1936–1937, 1974.
4. Kuhnau J: The flavonoids: A class of semi-essential food components: Their role in human nutrition. *World Rev Nutr Diet* **24**, 117–191, 1976.
5. Ficarra P, *et al.*: High-performance liquid chromatography of flavonoids in *Crataegus oxyacantha*. *Il Farmaco Ed Pr* **39**, 148–157, 1983.
6. Wagner H, Bladt S, and Zgainski EM: *Plant Drug Analysis*. Springer-Verlag, New York, 1984. pp. 166, 178, 179.
7. Wagner H and Grevel J: Cardiotonic drugs IV, cardiotonic amines from *Crataegus oxyacantha*. *Planta Medica* **45**, 98–101, 1982.
8. Gabor M: Pharmacologic effects of flavonoids on blood vessels. *Angiologica* **9**, 355–374, 1972.
9. Havsteen B: Flavonoids, a class of natural products of high pharmacological potency. *Biochem Pharm* **32**, 1141–1148, 1983.
10. Middleton E: The flavonoids. *Trends Pharm Sci* **5**, 335–338, 1984.
11. Amella M, *et al.*: Inhibition of mast cell histamine release by flavonoids and bioflavonoids. *Planta Medica* **51**, 16–20, 1985.
12. Busse WW, Kopp DE, and Middleton E: Flavonoid modulation of human neutrophil function. *J Allergy Clin Immunol* **73**, 801–809, 1984.
13. Ammon HPT and Handel M: Crataegus, toxicology and pharmacology. I. Toxicity. *Planta Medica* **43**, 105–120, 1981; II. Pharmacodynamics. *Planta Medica* **43**, 209–239, 1981; III. Pharmacodynamics and pharmacokinetics. *Planta Medica* **43**(4), 313–322, 1981.
14. Wegrowski J, Robert AM, and Moczar M: The effect of procyanidolic oligomers on the composition of normal and hypercholesterolemic rabbit aortas. *Biochem Pharm* **33**, 3491–3497, 1984.
15. Mavers VWH and Hensel H: Changes in local myocardial blood flow following oral administration of a crataegus extract to non-anesthetized dogs. *Arzneimittel-Forsch* **24**, 783–785, 1974.
16. Roddewig VC and Hensel H: Reaction of local myocardial blood flow in non-anesthetized dogs and anesthetized cats to oral and parenteral application of a crataegus fraction (oligomer procyanidins). *Arzneimittel-Forsch* **27**, 1407–1410, 1977.
17. Rewerski VW, *et al.*: Some pharmacological properties of oligomeric procyanidin isolated from hawthorn (*Crataegus oxyacantha*). *Arzneimittel-Forsch* **17**, 490–491, 1967.
18. Hammerl H, *et al.*: Klinixch-experimentelle toffwechseluntersuchungen mit einem crataegus-extrakt. *Arzneimittel-Forsch* **21**, 261–263, 1971.
19. Nasa Y, *et al.*: Protective effect of *Crataegus* extract on the cardiac mechanical dysfunction in isolated perfused working rat heart. *Arzneimittel-Forsch* **43**, 945–949, 1993.
20. Vogel VG: Predictability of the activity of drug combinations—yes or no? *Arzneimittel-Forsch* **25**, 1356–1365, 1975.
21. O'Conolly VM, *et al.*: Treatment of cardiac performance (NYHA stages I to II) in advanced age with standardized crataegus extract. *Forschr Med* **104**, 805–808, 1986.
22. Petkov E, Nikolov N, and Uzunov P: Inhibitory effect of some flavonoids and flavonoid mixtures on cyclic AMP phosphodiesterase activity of rat heart. *Planta Medica* **43**, 183–186, 1981.
23. Uchida S, *et al.*: Inhibitory effects of condensed tannins on angiotensin converting enzyme. *Jpn J Pharmacol* **43**, 242–245, 1987.
24. Blesken R: Crataegus in cardiology. *Forschr Med* **110**, 290–292, 1992.
25. O'Conolly VM, *et al.*: Treatment of cardiac performance (NYHA stages I to II) in advanced age with standardized crataegus extract. *Forschr Med* **104**, 805–808, 1986.
26. Leuchtgens H: Crataegus Special Extract WS 1442 in NYIIA II heart failure. A placebo controlled randomized double-blind study. *Forschr Med* **111**, 352–354, 1993.
27. Yu CL and Swaminathan B: Mutagenicity of proanthocyanidins. *Food Chem Toxicol* **25**, 135–139, 1987.

20
Kava

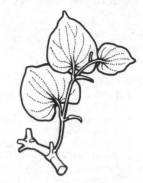

Key uses of kava:

- Anxiety
- Depression
- Insomnia

General description

Kava (*Piper methysticum*) is a member of the pepper family. It is a hardy, slow-growing perennial that generally resembles other members of the family Piperaceae. This attractive shrub can attain heights of more than 3 meters. The plant does not have many leaves, and those are thin, single, heart-shaped, alternate, petiolate, and 4 to 10 inches long and sometimes wider than they are long. Although *Piper methysticum* does flower, it is incapable of self-reproduction; its propagation is vegetative and solely due to human effort.[1,2]

The rootstock is used for medicinal purposes. The rootstock is knotty, thick, and sometimes tuberous, with holes or cracks created by partial destruction of the inner tissue. In other words, the rootstock is often somewhat pithy. Lateral roots up to 3 meters long extend from the main rootstock.[1,2]

Chemical composition

Analysis of the composition of the dried kava rootstock indicates that it contains approximately 43 percent starch, 12 percent water, 3.2 percent simple sugars, 3.6 percent proteins, 3.2 percent minerals (primarily potassium), and 15 percent kavalactones.[1,2]

On the basis of detailed analyses of kava's active ingredients (a laborious process spanning the past 110 years), many experts now believe the pharmacological activities of kava are due mostly, if not entirely, to the presence of the kavalactones (also referred to as kava alphapyrones). These compounds are found in the fat-soluble resin of the root. Although the kavalactones are the primary active components, it must be pointed out that other components appear to contribute to the sedative and anxiolytic activities of kava, as in one study the sedative activity of a crude preparation was more effective than that of the isolated kavalactones.[3] The kavalactone content of the root can vary between 3 and 20 percent. Therefore, for clinical use, preparations standardized for kavalactone content are preferred to crude preparations.

History and folk use

Oceania, that is, the island communities of the Pacific including Micronesia, Melanesia, and Polynesia, is one of the few areas of the world that did not have alcoholic beverages before European contact in the eighteenth century. However, these islanders did possess a "magical" drink used in ceremonies and celebrations because of its calming effect and ability to promote sociability. The drink, also called kava, is still used today in this region, where the people are often referred to as the happiest and friendliest in the world.

The origins of kava usage are not known, as it predates written history in Oceania.[1,2] It was first described for the western world by Captain James Cook in the account of his voyage to the South Seas in 1768. Many myths and legends surround the early use of kava. The plant itself probably originated in the New Guinea–Indonesia area and was spread, along with other plants, from island to island by early Polynesian explorers in canoes. Each culture has its own story on the origins of kava. For example, in Samoa a story is told about the origins of kava and sugar cane. The story goes that a Samoan girl went to Fiji, where she married a great chief. After some time, she returned to Samoa, but before doing so she noticed two plants growing on a hill. A rat was chewing on one of the plants, and it seemed to fall asleep. She concluded that the plant was a comforting food, and decided to take this plant (sugar cane) back to Samoa. Then she noticed that the rat awoke and began to chew the root of another plant—kava. The animal, which had been weak and shy, became bold, strong, and more energetic. She decided that she would take both plants back to Samoa. The plants grew very well in Samoa, and soon a chief from a neighboring island exchanged two laying hens for roots of the two plants. Hence, the Samoans take credit for the spread of both the sugar cane and kava.

In Tonga, the legend is told of a great chief named Loau, who lived on the island of Eua Iki and was visited by his servant Fevá anga. Fevá anga wanted to give a feast in honor of his chief, but it was a time of great famine. In desperation he and his wife killed and cooked their only daughter to be served to the chief. However, Loau recognized the human flesh in the food when it was served and would not eat it. He instructed Fevá anga to bury his daughter, and to bring him the plant that would spring forth. On receiving the mature plant, Loau instructed that a drink be prepared from it and consumed with due ceremony.

The kava ceremony

Regardless of exactly how kava originated, it has been used in ceremonies by the Oceanic people for thousands of years. There are three basic kava ceremonies: the full ceremonial as enacted on every formal occasion; that performed at the meeting of village elders, chiefs, and nobles and for visiting chiefs and dignitaries; and the less formal kava circle common to social occasions.[1,2]

The first step in any kava ceremony was the preparation of the beverage. A description of the classic process was given in 1777 by Georg Forster, a young naturalist on James Cook's second Pacific voyage:[1]

> [Kava] is made in the most disgustful manner that can be imagined, from the juice contained in the roots of a species of pepper-tree. This root is cut small, and the pieces chewed by several people, who spit the macerated mass into a bowl, where some water (milk) of coconuts is poured upon it. They then strain it through a quantity of fibres of coconuts, squeezing the chips, till all their juices mix with the coconut-milk; and the whole liquor is decanted into another bowl. They swallow this naseous stuff as fast as possible; and some old topers value themselves on being able to empty a great number of bowls.

This traditional method of preparation was frowned on or outlawed by colonial governments and missionaries, and more "sanitary" methods of preparation, involving grinding or grating, took its place in many parts of Oceania.

The full kava ceremony reserved for very highly honored guests involves leading all of the guests to a platform. The ceremony begins with the arrival of a group of young men dressed in ceremonial attire and carrying a bowl of the kava drink and necessary utensils. The bowl is placed between the kava preparers and the visitors. The kava is placed in a cup by a specially selected individual, the cup bearer, who then turns and faces the visitor and delivers the beverage to the chief guest. The guest is instructed to hold the cup with both hands and drink from it. If the whole cup is drained without stopping, everyone says *a maca* (pronounced "a matha," meaning "it is empty") and claps three times with cupped hands. The cup bearer then refills the kava bowl and proceeds to serve the person next in rank or importance.

Important people visiting Fiji and other islands of Oceania still participate in kava ceremonies. For example, during a 1992 presidential campaign visit to Hawaii, Hillary Clinton participated in a kava ceremony conducted by the Samoan community on Oahu.

The effects of drinking kava

Kava drinkers relate a pleasant sense of tranquillity and sociability on consumption. Subjective reports given by scientists who have sampled kava themselves are relatively abundant. One of the first scientific studies on kava was performed by the noted pharmacologist Louis Lewin in 1886. A later description, written in 1927, is as follows:[1]

> When the mixture is not too strong, the subject attains a state of happy unconcern, well-being and contentment, free of physical or psychological excitement. At the beginning conversation comes in a gentle, easy flow and hearing and sight are honed, becoming able to perceive subtle shades of sound and vision. Kava soothes temperaments. The drinker never becomes angry, unpleasant, quarrelsome or noisy, as happens with alcohol. Both natives and whites consider kava as a means of easing moral discomfort. The drinker remains master of his conscious and his reason. When consumption is excessive, however, the limbs become tired, the muscles seem no longer to respond to the orders and control of the mind, walking becomes slow and unsteady and the drinker looks partially inebriated. He feels the need to lie down. . . . He is overcome by somnolence and finally drifts off to sleep.

A more recent description is provided by researcher R. J. Gregory, who writes from his own experience:[1]

> Kava seizes one's mind. This is not a literal seizure, but something does change in the processes by which information enters, is retrieved, or leads to actions as a result. Thinking is certainly affected by the kava experience, but not in the same ways as are found from caffeine, nicotine, alcohol, or marijuana. I would personally characterize the changes I experienced as going from lineal processing of information to a greater sense of "being" and contentment with being. Memory seemed to be enhanced, whereas

restriction of data inputs was strongly desired, especially with regard to disturbances of light, movements, noise and so on. Peace and quiet were very important to maintain the inner sense of serenity. My senses seemed to be unusually sharpened, so that even whispers seemed to be loud while loud noises were extremely unpleasant.

Drinking about half a coconut shell (approximately 100 to 150 milliliters) of certain varieties of kava is enough to put most people into a deep, dreamless sleep within 30 minutes. Unlike alcohol and other sedatives, kava does not produce any morning hangover. The kava drinker awakens having fully recovered normal physical and mental capacities.

Standardized preparations of kava are now gaining greater popularity in Europe and the United States as mild sedatives and anxiolytics.

Pharmacology

Many of the the first comprehensive studies on the activities of kavalactones were conducted by a team of scientists from the Freiburg University Institute of Pharmacology in Germany, led by Hans J. Meyer, during the 1950s and 1960s.[3] Altogether, this research has determined that kavalactones exhibit sedative, analgesic, anticonvulsant, and muscle relaxant effects in laboratory animals. These studies seemed to confirm earlier empirical and subjective observations.

More recent studies, including those conducted by Dana D. Jamieson and colleagues at the University of New South Wales, have confirmed and/or elaborated on these effects. Most notable are the studies demonstrating that kavalactones exert many of their effects by nontraditional mechanisms. For example, most sedative drugs, including the benzodiazepines (e.g., Valium, Halcion, and Tranxene), work by binding to specific receptors (benzodiazepam or GABA [gamma-aminobutyric acid] receptors) in the brain, which then leads to the neurochemical changes (potentiation of GABA effects) that promote sedation. Studies in animals have shown that the kavalactones do not bind to benzodiazepam or GABA receptors.[4] Instead, the kavalactones somehow modify receptor domains rather than interact specifically with receptor-binding sites. In addition, other studies have indicated that the kavalactones appear to act primarily on the limbic system—an ancient part of the brain that affects all other brain activities and is the principal seat of the emotions.[5] It is thought that kava may also promote sleep by altering the way in which the limbic system modulates emotional processes. It appears that many of the laboratory models used to identify how a substance promotes a calming effect are simply not sophisticated enough to evaluate the kavalactones.

In another example of the uncharacteristic pharmacological qualities of kava, a study designed to evaluate its pain-relieving effects could not demonstrate any binding to opioid receptors.[6] The significance of this finding is that the study used models in which nonopiate analgesics such as aspirin and other nonsteroidal antiinflammatory drugs are ineffective. In addition, it was determined that the sedative or muscle-relaxing effects were not responsible for the pain-relieving effects. What all of these findings mean is that kava reduces pain in a manner unlike morphine, aspirin, or any other pain reliever.

An interesting effect of kava compared to many anxiolytic drugs is that, unlike the drugs, kava does not lose effectiveness with time. Loss of effectiveness of a drug is known as "tolerance." Kavalactones, even when administered in huge amounts, demonstrated absolutely no loss of effectiveness in animal studies.[7] Again, this is another example of the uncharacteristic qualities of kava.

Another pharmacological activity of kava worth mentioning is its ability to protect against brain damage due to ischemia.[8] This effect has been demonstrated in two animal models of focal cerebral ischemia. The effectiveness of the kavalactones was due to their ability to limit the infarct area as well to a mild anticonvulsant effect. Kava extract may prove useful in recovery from a stroke.

Clinical applications

Several European countries have approved kava preparations in the treatment of nervous anxiety, insomnia, and restlessness on the basis of detailed pharmacological data and favorable clinical studies.

Earlier clinical trials used D,L-kavain, a purified kavalactone, at a dose of 400 milligrams per day. For example, in one double-blind placebo-controlled study of eighty-four patients with anxiety symptoms, kavain was shown to improve vigilance, memory, and reaction time.[9] In another double-blind study, kavain was compared to the drug oxazepam (a drug similar to diazepam or Valium) in thirty-eight patients.[10] Both substances caused progressive improvements in two different anxiety scores (Anxiety Status Inventory and the Self-Rating Anxiety Scale) over a 4-week period. However, while oxazepam and similar drugs are addictive and produce side effects, kavain appeared to be free of these complications.

More recent studies have featured well-defined kava extracts. As mentioned earlier, evidence suggests that the whole complex of kavalactones together with other compounds naturally found in kava produce greater pharmacological activity. In addition, studies have shown that kavalactones are more rapidly absorbed when given orally as an extract of the root rather than as isolated kavalactones. The bioavailability of lactones, as measured by peak plasma concentrations, is up to three to five times higher from the extract than when given as isolated substances.[3] Further evidence that kava root extracts are superior to isolated kavalactones is offered by an animal study[11]; in this study isolated kavalactones were taken up well by brain tissue, but when a crude kava preparation was given the concentration of lactones was two to twenty times higher.[11] From this evidence it appears that crude extracts standardized for kavalactone content may offer the greatest therapeutic benefit.

Several clinical trials have featured a special kava extract standardized to contain 70 percent kavalactones; however, this high percentage of kavalactones may be sacrificing some of the other constituents that may contribute to the pharmacology of kava. More important than the actual percentage of kavalactones is the total dose of kavalactones and the assurance that the full range of kavalactones is present.

In perhaps the most significant study, a 70 percent kavalactone extract was shown to exhibit significant therapeutic benefit in patients suffering from anxiety.[12] In this double-blind study, twenty-nine patients were assigned to receive 100 milligrams of the kava extract three times daily while another twenty-nine patients received a placebo. Therapeutic effectiveness was assessed using several standard psychological assessments including the Hamilton Anxiety Scale. The result of this 4-week study indicated that individuals taking the kava extract had a statistically significant reduction in symptoms of anxiety, including feelings of nervousness and somatic complaints such as heart palpitations, chest pains, headache, dizziness, and feelings of gastric irritation. No side effects were reported with the kava extract.

In another double-blind study, two groups of twenty women with menopause-related symptoms were treated for a period of 8 weeks with a 70 percent kavalactone extract (100 milligrams three times daily) or placebo.[13] The target variable was once again the Hamilton Anxiety Scale. The group receiving the kava extract demonstrated significant improvement at the end of the very first week of treatment. Scores continued to improve over the course of the 8-week study. In addition to improvement in symptoms of stress and anxiety, a number of other symptoms also improved. Most notably, there was an overall improvement in subjective well-being, mood, and general symptoms of menopause including hot flashes. Again, no side effects were noted.

Two additional studies have shown that unlike benzodiazepines, alcohol, and other drugs, kava extract is not associated with depressed mental function or impairment in driving or the operation of heavy equipment.[14,15] In one of these studies twelve healthy volunteers were tested in a double-blind, cross-over manner to assess the effects of oxazepam (placebo on days 1–3, 15 milligrams on the day before testing, 75 milligrams on the morning of the experiment), an extract of kava standardized at 70 percent kavalactones (200 milligrams three times daily for 5 days), and a placebo on behavior and event-related potentials in electroencephalograph readings in a recognition memory task. The subjects' task was to identify, within a list of visually presented words, those that were shown for the first time and those that were being repeated. Consistent with other benzodiazepines, oxazepam inhibited the recognition of both new and old words, as noted by event-related potential. In contrast, kava showed a slightly increased recognition rate and a larger event-related potential difference between old and new words. The results of this study once again demonstrate the uncharacteristic effects of kava; in this case it reduced anxiety, but unlike standard anxiolytics, kava actually improves mental function and at the recommended levels does not promote sedation.

Dosage

The appropriate dose of a kava preparation depends on the level of kavalactones. On the basis of clinical studies using pure kavalactones or kava extracts standardized for kavalactones, the dosage recommendation for anxiolytic effects is 45 to 70 milligrams of kavalactones three times daily. For sedative effects, a dose providing 180 to 210 milligrams of kavalactones can be taken 1 hour before retiring.

To put the therapeutic dosage in perspective, remember that a standard bowl of traditionally prepared kava drink contains approximately 250 milligrams of kavalactones and several bowls may be consumed at one sitting.

Toxicity

Although no side effects have been reported when using standardized kava extracts at recommended levels, it is possible that side effects may present themselves at high doses. High doses of kava beverage consumed daily over a prolonged period (a few months to a year or more) is associated with "kava dermopathy"—a condition of the skin characterized by a peculiar, generalized scaly eruption known as kani.[16] The skin becomes dry and covered with scales, especially the palms of the hand, soles of the feet, forearms, the back, and shins. It was thought at one time that kava dermopathy may be due to interference with niacin. However, in one double-blind, placebo-controlled study no therapeutic effect with niacinamide (100 milligrams daily) could be demonstrated.[17] It appears that the only effective treatment for kava dermopathy is reduction or cessation of kava consumption. Again, no reported cases of kava dermopathy have been noted in individuals taking standardized kava extracts at recommended levels.

Other adverse effects following the consumption of extremely high doses of kava (e.g., more than 310 grams per week) for prolonged periods include biochemical abnormalities (low levels of serum albumin, protein, urea, and bilirubin), the presence of blood in the urine, increased red blood cell volume, decreased platelet and lymphocyte counts, and shortness of breath.[18] The attribution of these adverse effects to kava is questionable, because the subjects also reported heavy alcohol and cigarette usage. Nonetheless, high doses of kava are unnecessary and should not be encouraged.

References

1. Lebot V, Merlin M, and Lindstrom L: *Kava: The Pacific Drug.* Yale University Press, New Haven, CT, 1992.
2. Singh Y: Kava: An overview. *J Ethnopharmacol* **37**, 13–45, 1992.
3. Meyer HJ: Pharmacology of kava. In: *Ethnopharmacological Search for Psychoactive Drugs* (Holmstedt B and Kline NS, eds.). Raven Press, New York, 1979, pp. 133–140.
4. Davies LP, *et al.*: Kava pyrones and resin: Studies on $GABA_a$, $GABA_b$ and benzodiazepine binding sites in rodent brain. *Pharm Toxicol* **71**, 120–126, 1992.
5. Holm E, *et al.*: Studies on the profile of the neurophysiological effects of D,L-kavain: Cerebral sites of action and sleep-wakefulness-rhythm in animals. *Arzneimittel-Forsch* **41**, 673–683, 1991.
6. Jamieson DD and Duffield PH: The antinociceptive action of kava components in mice. *Clin Exp Pharmacol Physiol* **17**, 495–508, 1990.
7. Duffield PH and Jamieson D: Development of tolerance to kava in mice. *Clin Exp Pharmacol Physiol* **18**, 571–578, 1991.
8. Backhauss and Krieglstein J: Extract of kava (*Piper methysticum*) and its methysticum constituents protect brain tissue against ischemic damage in rodents. *Eur J Pharmacol* **215**, 265–269, 1992.
9. Scholing WE and Clausen HD: On the effect of d,l-kavain: Experience with neuronika. *Med Klin* **72**, 1301–1306, 1977.
10. Lindenberg D and Pitule-Schodel H: D,L-Kavain in comparison with oxazepam in anxiety disorders. A double-blind study of clinical effectiveness. *Forschr Med* **108**, 49–50, 53–54, 1990.
11. Keledjian J, *et al.*: Uptake into mouse brain of four compounds present in the psychoactive beverage kava. *J Pharm Sci* **77**, 1003–1006, 1988.
12. Kinzler E, Kromer J, and Lehmann E: Clinical efficacy of a kava extract in patients with anxiety syndrome: Double-blind placebo controlled study over 4 weeks. *Arzneimittel-Forsch* **41**, 584–588, 1991.
13. Warnecke G: Neurovegetative dystonia in the female climacteric. Studies on the clinical efficacy and tolerance of kava extract WS 1490. *Forschr Med* **109**, 120–122, 1991.

14. Herberg KW: The influence of kava-special extract WS 1490 on safety-relevant performance alone and in combination with ethyl alcohol. *Blutalkohol* **30**, 96–105, 1993.
15. Munte TF, *et al.*: Effects of oxazepam and an extract of kava roots (*Piper methysticum*) on event-related potentials in a word recognition task. *Neuropyschobiology* **27**, 46–53, 1993.
16. Norton SA and Ruze P: Kava dermopathy. *J Am Acad Dermatol* **31**, 89–97, 1994.
17. Ruze P: Kava-induced dermopathy: A niacin deficiency. *Lancet* **335**, 1442–1445, 1990.
18. Mathews JD, *et al.*: Effects of the heavy usage of kava on physical health: Summary of a pilot survey in an aboriginal community. *Med J Aust* **148**, 548–555, 1988.

21
LaPacho

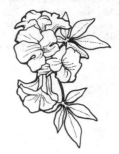

Key uses of LaPacho:

- Infections
- Cancer
- *Candida albicans*

General description

Although there are about 100 *Tabebuia* species native to tropical America, *Tabebuia avellanedae* or *Tabebuia ipe* is regarded as the true "LaPacho." This tree, native to Brazil, can rise to a height of 125 feet and has rose to violet-colored flowers that bloom in profusion just before the new leaves appear. The bark is the portion of the tree that is used medicinally.[1]

Chemical composition

Many of the studies and chemical analyses of *Tabebuia* species have been done on the heartwood, but it's the bark that is sold in the market place and used utilized in folk medicine. The major components of *Tabebuia avellanedae* are sixteen quinones (mostly with C_{15} skeletons) containing both naphtho-quinones (seven kinds, with carbon skeletons ranging in length from C_{10} to C_5) and anthraquinones (nine types, C_{14}–C_1); it is considered very rare to find both of these groups of quinones occurring in the same plant. The lapa-chol content is usually 2–7 percent. The quinones are listed in Table 21.1.

Other compounds found in the heartwood are lapachenole, quercetin, and *o*- and *p*-hydroxybenzoic acids.[2]

Table 21.1 Quinones in *Tabebuia avellanedae*

Naphthoquinones	Anthraquinones
Lapachol	2-Methylanthraquinone
Menaquinone-l	2-Hydroxymethylanthraquinone
Deoxylapachol	2-Acetoxymethylanthraquinone
beta-Lapachone	Anthraquinone-2-aldehyde
alpha-Lapachone	1-Hydroxyanthraquinone
Dehydro-alpha-lapachone	1-Methoxyanthraquinone
	2-Hydroxy-3-methylquinone
	Tabebuin (a newly discovered compound)

A recent analysis of twelve products found in the Canadian market place showed that only one contained lapachol (trace amounts) and the other eleven had none. This suggests that many of the products now present on the market are not truly from *Tabebuia* species, or the wrong part of the plant is being marketed, or processing and transportation have damaged the product. This might explain the variation in results practitioners have experienced. Standardization of LaPacho products for lapachol or naphthoquinone content would obviously solve this problem.

History and folk use

The native Indians of Brazil also refer to the tree as Pau d'Arco or Ipe Roxo. They use the inner bark as a folk remedy for a wide variety of afflictions, including boils; colitis; dysentery; bedwetting; fever; sore throat; snake bite; wounds; cancers of the esophagus, head, intestine, lung, prostate, and tongue; ulcers; respiratory problems; arthritis; cystitis; constipation; prostatitis; and poor circulation.[1-7]

Pharmacology

During the past century, LaPacho has come under scientific scrutiny. The first active constituent to be studied was lapachol; however, it is interesting to note that many of the studies show significantly better results with the whole extract and diminishing effectiveness as the extracts are refined or individual chemicals are tested.[8]

Antibacterial activity

In 1956, a research team at the Universidade do Recife in Brazil isolated lapachol from the *Tabebuia avellanedae* tree. de Lima and colleagues reported that it exhibited antimicrobial activity against gram-positive and acid-fast bacteria, and showed strong activity against *Brucella* species.[9]

It is important to note that de Lima *et al.* found that with progressive purification of LaPacho the antimicrobial activity of the extract decreased. This led to the conclusion that there was more than one active substance present in the original extract.

Later that year this team published a paper proclaiming a new antibiotic substance from *Tabebuia avellanedae* that demonstrated "strong anti-*Brucella* activity and fungistatic behavior."[10] de Lima's team eventually found that, along with lapachol, the extract of the *Tabebuia* tree contained alpha-lapachone, beta-lapachone, and a newly discovered quinone they named xyloidone.

In 1967, at the University of Aberdeen, Burnett and Thomson discovered the presence of seven naphthoquinones, nine anthraquinones, lapachenole, quercetin, and *o*- and *p*-hydroxy benzoic acids in the heartwood of the tree.[11] Several of these have strong microbicidal and fungicidal activities (see Table 21.2). Naphthoquinones are highly effective against *Candida albicans* and *Trichophyton mentagrophytes*.[12,13]

Lapachol has been shown to have antimicrobial[9] and antiviral[14] action. Beta-lapachone shows diversified antiparasitic activity[16] as well as antiviral action.[17] Alpha-lapachone is also active against certain parasites,[18] and xyloidone is active against numerous bacteria and fungi.[19] Another LaPacho component, the flavonoid quercetin, is cytotoxic for certain parasites.[20]

Table 21.2[21-32] lists some of the organisms against which xyloidone is effective. Several of the microorganisms listed are pathogenic, such as *Staphylococcus aureus* and the *Brucella* species. The causative agents of tuberculosis, dysentery, and anthrax are also inhibited by xyloidone. In addition to its activity against a variety of bacteria, this quinone inhibits several species of fungus, (including *Candida albicans*, *Candida kruzei*, and *Candida neoformans*).

Lapachol, like many naphthoquinones, acts as a respiratory poison by interfering with energy production in the microorganism.

Antiviral activity

Lapachol, beta-lapachone, hydroxynapthoquinone, and other LaPacho components are active against a number of viruses, including herpes virus types I and II, influenza virus, poliovirus, and vesicular stomatitis virus.[14,15,33]

Table 21.2 Antimicrobial activity of *Tabebuia avellanedae*[a]

Microorganism	Lapachol	Chorohidro-lapachol	Alpha-Lapachone	Beta-Lapachone	Xiloidona
Bac. sutilus	60.0–80.0	8.0–10.0	40.0–50.0	1.0–2.0	4.0–6.0
B. mycoides	40.0–60.0	10.0–15.0	40.0–50.0	5.0–8.0	20.0–30.0
B. anthracis	40.0–60.0	20.0–30.0	40.0–50.0	4.0–6.0	20.0–30.0
Staph. aureus	60.0–80.0	30.0–40.0	30.0–40.0	2.0–4.0	15.0–20.0
Sar. lutea	40.0–60.0	15.0–20.0	30.0–40.0	4.0–6.0	20.0–30.0
Strep. hemolyticus	>100.0	60.0–80.0	60.0–80.0	10.0–15.0	>50
M. tub. hom	80.0–100.0	40.0–60.0	30.0–50.0	10.0–15.0	10.0–15.0
M. smegmatis	80.0–100.0	60.0–80.0	30.0–50.0	15.0–20.0	15.0–20.0
M. phisi	60.0–80.0	40.0–60.0	20.0–30.0	10.0–15.0	8.0–10.0
N. asteroides	>100	40.0–60.0	60.0–80.0	10.0–15.0	20.0–30.0
N. catarrhalis	40.0–60.0	30.0–50.0	80.0–100.0	10.0–15.0	<20.0
E. coli	>100.0	>100.0	>100.0	>100.0	>100.0
K. pneumonia	>100.0	>100.0	>100.0	>100.0	>100.0
S. typhosa	>100.0	>100.0	>100.0	>100.0	>100.0
Br. suis	15.0–20.0	2.0–4.0	20.0–30.0	0.6–1.0	0.8–1.0
Br. abortus	15.0–20.0	2.0–4.0	30.0–40.0	1.0–2.0	1.5–2.0
Br. melirensis	10.0–15.0	2.0–4.0	30.0–40.0	1.0–2.0	1.5–2.0
C. albicans	>100.0	40.0–60.0	80.0–100.0	80.0–100.0	30.0–50.0
C. kruzei	>100.0	40.0–60.0	80.0–100.0	80.0–100.0	50.0–60.0
C. neoformans	>100.0	40.0–60.0	50.0–80.0	30.0–50.0	40.0–60.0

[a]Minimum concentration of inhibition (mcg/ml)

Studies of beta-lapachone's antiviral activity have offered insights into the mechanism of this powerful quinone. In experiments with viruses, beta-lapachone demonstrated its ability to inhibit certain key viral enzymes, such as DNA and RNA polymerases, and retrovirus reverse transcriptase.[17] These actions have great significance in the possible treatment of acquired immuno-deficiency syndrome (AIDS), Epstein–Barr virus, and other viral infections.

Antiparasitic activity

The parasite *Schistosoma mansoni* is the causative agent of the common tropical disease schistosomiasis. The larvae (cercariae) of this blood fluke live in water and enter the host by penetrating the skin. This debilitating disease, a serious problem in many tropical areas, causes weakening of the host and increases susceptibility to a variety of other pathogens, some of which may be fatal.

Lapachol has been tested as a topical barrier to the cercariae of schistosomes and found to be highly effective at preventing their penetration.[34,35] Oral lapachol was also tested and found to reduce penetration significantly. After consumption, the lapachol was secreted onto the skin, apparently by the sebaceous glands, where it again acted as a topical barrier. The cercariae seek to penetrate the host through or near the sebaceous glands, which suggests that dietary administration of lapachol would be an efficient means of protecting against infection.

Alpha-lapachone and beta-lapachone, both components of LaPacho, both exhibited activity against *Schistosoma mansoni*.[14]

Beta-lapachone is particularly effective against *Trypanosoma cruzi*, the parasite responsible for trypanosomiasis, or Chagas' disease. This disease occurs in both acute and chronic forms and is characterized in the acute form by swelling of the skin and enlargement of lymph nodes. In its chronic form it may affect the heart or nervous system.

Anticancer effects

After hearing about LaPacho's tumor-reducing qualities, the National Cancer Institute (NCI, Bethesda, MD) subjected it to extensive study. After initial positive results, it was determined that lapachol was the most active anticancer agent.

Lapachol entered phase I clinical trials at the NCI in 1968, on the basis of its activity against Walker 256 tumors (with a confidence rate greater than 90 percent). During these trials it was difficult to obtain therapeutic blood levels of lapachol without some mild toxic side effects such as nausea, vomiting, and anti-vitamin K activity. This is difficult to understand, as later studies found the toxicity to be very low, with an LD_{50} (50 percent lethal dose) of 487 milligrams per kilogram body weight—about the same as caffeine.[4] The Investigative New Drug status (IND) for the drug was withdrawn in 1970.[36]

It has been shown, however, that some of the anthraquinones in LaPacho have vitamin K activity, and therefore use of the whole herb would compensate for lapachol's effect on vitamin K.[37]

The approach described above indicates a flaw in the underlying philosophy of the pharmaceutical sciences and the NCI program. Since the initial studies involved the whole plant, the detailed studies should have been undertaken with the whole plant: some of the other quinones have also been shown to have anticancer activities. Was it too complex to consider the chemical reactions of the more than twenty components found in LaPacho? Or was the standard economic/political incentive for patenting an analog an impediment to the investigation of a plant species?

Lapachol is rapidly absorbed through the gastrointestinal tract after oral administration to rats bearing Walker 256 tumors. It is taken up by all tissues except the brain and blood cells. A significant amount appears in the tumor after 6 hours, with most of the drug disappearing from the other body tissues. The half-life of intravenous lapachol in mice is 33 minutes (75 minutes in dogs). Lapachol is extensively metabolized and excreted mostly in the feces.[1] Most other analogs had little effect on cancer.[38]

Antiinflammatory activity

Extracts of the bark from *Tabebuia avellanedae* demonstrate clear antiinflammatory activity with low toxicity.[21] Tampons soaked in an alcoholic extract of LaPacho have been shown to be very successful against a wide range of inflammations, such as cervicitis and cervicovaginitis.[2,13]

Clinical applications

Current use has focused on LaPacho's anticancer and antimicrobial activity. Its use is extremely popular in the treatment of intestinal candidiasis and vaginal candidiasis (topically and internally). There are also many anecdotal reports of remission of different forms of cancer following the use of this herb.[39]

Unfortunately, owing to lack of quality control and confusion about the portion of the plant to use (many of the studies and chemical analyses have been done on the heartwood, while the bark is the product available in the market place and discussed in folklore), it is highly likely that most consumers and practitioners are not using effective materials. This could explain varying clinical results.

Dosage

The usual form of administration of LaPacho is as a decoction, with the standard dose being 1 cup of decocted bark two to eight times per day. The decoction is made by boiling 1 teaspoon of LaPacho for each cup of water for 5 to 15 minutes.

A more precise dosage based on a lapachol content of 2–4 percent would be 15–20 grams of bark boiled in 500 milliliters or 1 pint of water for 5 to 15 minutes three to four times daily.

The dosage of other forms (aqueous extract, fluid extract, and solid extract) should be based on lapachol content, providing a daily lapachol intake of 1.5–2.0 grams per day.

A tampon that has been soaked in a decoction or fluid extract is used to treat vaginitis and cervicitis. The tampon is inserted vaginally and changed every 24 hours until resolution.

Toxicity

Although anti-vitamin K activity has been reported for lapachol, the presence of several vitamin K-like substances in the whole plant suggests this is not a problem. Lapachol has been reported to have an oral LD_{50} of 1.2–2.4 grams per kilogram in albino rats and 487–621 milligrams per kilogram in mice.[5,8] In comparison, the oral LD_{50} of caffeine is 192 milligrams per kilogram in rats and 620 milligrams per kilogram in mice.[5]

Chronic administration of lapachol at a dose of 0.0625–0.25 gram per kilogram per day to monkeys produces moderate to severe anemia. The anemia was most pronounced during the first 2 weeks of treatment. Death occurred in monkeys after six doses of lapachol at 0.5 grams per kilogram per day and after five doses of 1.0 grams per kilogram per day.[8]

There have been no reports in the literature of human toxicity when a whole-bark decoction is used.

References

1. Willard T: *Tabebuia* species. In: *A Textbook of Natural Medicine* (Pizzorno JE and Murray MT, eds.). JBC Publications, Seattle, WA, 1987, Chapter V.
2. Burnett AR and Thomson RH: Naturally occurring quinones. X. The quinonoid constituents of *Tabebuia avellanedae* (Bignoniaceae). *J Chem Soc (C)*, 2100–2104, 1967.
3. Pfizer C: Antitumor composition from lapachol and its salts. *Chemical Abstracts* 70, 9075B, 1956.
4. Canadian Health Protection Branch: Herbs and botanical preparations. *Inf Lett* Aug 13, 726, 1987.
5. Duke JA: *CRC Handbook of Medicinal Herbs*. CRC Press, Boca Raton, FL, 1985, pp. 470–473.
6. Bernarde A: *A Pocket Book of Brazilian Herbs (Folklore — History — Uses)*. Shogun Editora, Rio de Janeiro, Brazil, 1984, pp. 22–23.
7. Hartwell JL: *Plants Used against Cancer. A Survey*. Quarterman Publications, Lawrence, MA, 1982.
8. Morrison RK, *et al.*: Oral toxicology studies with lapachol. *Toxicol Appl Pharmacol* 17, 1–11, 1970.
9. de Lima OG, *et al.*: Primeiras observacoes sobre a acao antimicrobiana do lapachol. *Anais da Sociedade de Biologica de Pernambuco* XIV, 129–135, 1956.
10. de Lima OG, *et al.*: Uma nova substancia antibiotica isolada do "Pau d'Arco," *Tabebuia* sp. *Anais da Sociedade de Biologica de Pernambuco* XIV, 136–140, 1956.
11. Burnett AR and Thomson RH: Naturally occurring quinones. X. The quinonoid constituents of *Tabebuia avellanedae* (Bignoniaceae). *J Chem Soc (C)*, 2100–2104, 1967.
12. Gershon H and Shanks L: Fungitoxicity of 1,4-naphthoquinones to *Candida albicans* and *Trichophyton mentagrophytes*. *Can J Microbiol* 21, 1317–1321, 1975.
13. Wanick MC, *et al.*: Acao antiinflamatoria e cicatrizante do extrato hidroalcoolico do liber do Pau d'Arco roxo (*Tabebuia avellanedae*), em pacientes portadoras de cervicites e cervico-vaginites. *Separata da Revista do Instituto de Antibioticos* 10, 41–46, 1970.

14. Linhares MIS and De Santana CF: Estudo sobre of efeito de substancias antibioticas obtidas de *Streptomyces* e vegetais superiores sobre o herpesvirus hominis. *Revista Instituto Antibioticos, Recife* **15**, 25–32, 1975.

15. Lagrota M, *et al.*: Antiviral activity of lapachol, *Rev Microbiol* **14**, 21–26, 1983.

16. Lopes JN, *et al.*: In vitro and in vivo evaluation of the toxicity of 1,4-naphthoquinone and 1,2-naphthoquinone derivatives against *Trypanosoma cruzi*. *Ann Trop Med Parasit* **72**, 523–531, 1978.

17. Schuerch AR and Wehrli W: b-Lapachone, an inhibitor of oncornavirus reverse transcriptase and eukaryotic DNA polymerase-a: Inhibitory effect, thiol dependency and specificity. *Eur J Biochem* **84**, 197–205, 1978.

18. Pinto AV, Pinto MDR, and Gilbert B: *Schistosomiasis mansoni*: Blockage of cercarial skin penetration by chemical agents. I. Naphthoquinones and derivatives. *Trans R Soc Trop Med Hyg* **71**, 133–135, 1977.

19. de Lima OG, *et al.*: Comunicacao XX. Antividade antimicrobiana de alguns derivados do lapachol em comparacao com a xiloidona, nova ortonaftoquinona natural isolada de extractos do cerne do "Pau d'Arco" roxo, *Tabebuia avellanedae* Lor. ex. Griseb. Substancias antimicrobianas de plantas superiores. *Revista do Instituto de Antibioticos Recife* **4**, 1962.

20. Shapiro A, *et al.*: In vivo and in vitro activity by diverse chelators against *Trypanosoma brucei*. *J Protozool* **29**, 85–90, 1982.

21. Oga S and Sekino T: Toxicidade e atividade anti-inflamatoria de *Tabebuia avellanedae* Lorentz e Griesbach ("Ipe Roxo"). *Rev Fac Farm Bioquim S Paulo* **7**, 47–53, 1969.

22. Howland JL: Uncoupling and inhibition of oxidative phosphorylation by 2-hydroxy-3-alkyl-1,4-naphthoquinones. *Biochim Biophys Acta* **77**, 659–662, 1963.

23. Wendel WB: The influence of naphthoquinones upon the respiratory and carbohydrate metabolism of malarial parasites. *Fed Proc* **5**, 406–407, 1946.

24. Ball EG, Anfinsen CB, and Cooper O: The inhibitory action of naphthoquinones on respiratory processes. *J Biol Chem* **168**, 257–270, 1947.

25. Fieser LF and Richardson AP: Naphthoquinone antimalarials. II. Correlation of structure and activity against *Plasmodium lophurae* in ducks. *J Am Chem Soc* **70**, 3156–3165, 1948.

26. Gosalvez M, *et al.*: Effects and specificity of anticancer agents on the respiration and energy metabolism of tumor cells. *Canc Treat Rep* **60**, 1–8, 1976.

27. Crawford DR and Schneider DL: Identification of ubiquinone-50 in human neutrophils and its role in microbicidal events. *J Biol Chem* **257**, 6662–6668, 1982.

28. Wendel WB: The influence of naphthoquinones upon the respiratory and carbohydrate metabolism of malarial parasites. *Fed Proc* **5**, 406–407, 1946.

29. Howland JL: Influence of alkylhydroxynaphthoquinones on the mitochondrial oxidation of tetramethyl-*p*-phenylenediamine. *Biochim Biophys Acta* **131**, 247–254, 1967.

30. Hadler HI and Moreau TL: The induction of ATP energized mitochondrial volume changes by the combination of the two antitumour agents showdomycin and lapachol. *J Antibiot*, 513–520, 1969.

31. Douglas KT, *et al.*: Lapachol inhibition of alpha-ketoaldehyde metabolism. *IRCS Med Sci: Libr Compend* **10**, 683, 1982.

32. Koide SS: Inhibition of 3α-hydroxysteroid-mediated transhydrogenase of rat liver by various quinones and flavonoids. *Biochim Biophys Acta* **59**, 708–710, 1962.

33. Selway JWT: Antiviral activity of flavones and flavins. In: *Plant Flavonoids in Biology and Medicine: Biochemical, Pharmacological, and Structure–Activity Relationships*. Alan R. Liss, New York, 1986, pp. 521–536.

34. Austin FG: *Schistosoma mansoni* chemoprophylaxis with dietary lapachol. *Am J Trop Med Hyg* **23**, 412–419, 1974.

35. Gilbert B, *et al.*: Schistosomiasis. Protection against infection by terpenoids. *An Acad Brasil Cienc* **42**(Suppl), 397–400, 1970.

36. Block JB, *et al.*: Early clinical studies with lapachol (NSC-11905). *Cancer Chemo Rep* **4**, 27–28, 1974.

37. Preusch PC and Suttie J W: Lapachol inhibition of vitamin K epoxide reductase and vitamin K quinone reductase. *Arch Biochem Biophys* **234**, 405–412, 1984.

38. Rao KV: Quinone natural products: Streptonigrin (NSC-45383) and lapachol (NSC-11905) structure-activity relationships. *Cancer Chemo Rep* **4**, 11–17, 1974.

39. Weed B: Second opinion: Lapacho fight against cancer. Rostrum Communication, Vancouver, Canada, 1984.

22
Licorice

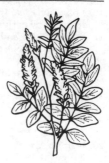

Key uses of licorice:

Oral:

- Viral infections including, the common cold, viral hepatitis, AIDS
- Inflammation
- Menstrual and menopausal disorders

As deglycyrrhizinated licorice (DGL):

- Peptic ulcers
- Canker sores

Topical glycyrrhetinic acid:

- Herpes
- Eczema
- Psoriasis

General description

Licorice (*Glycyrrhiza glabra*) is a perennial, temperate zone herb or subshrub, 3 to 7 feet high, with a long, cylindrical, branched, flexible, and burrowing rootstock with runners. The parts used are the dried runners and roots, which are collected in the fall. Licorice root is one of the most extensively used and scientifically investigated herbal medicines.

Chemical composition

The major active component of licorice root is glycyrrhizin (also known as glycyrrhizic acid or glycyrrhizinic acid), which is usually found in concentrations ranging from 6 to 10 percent. The intestinal flora are believed to hydrolyze glycyrrhizin, yielding the backbone molecule (glycyrrhetinic acid) and a sugar molecule, resulting in absorption of both.[2]

A special licorice extract, deglycyrrhizinated licorice (DGL), which is used in the treatment of peptic and mouth ulcers, is made by removing the glycyrrhizin molecule. The active components of DGL are flavonoids. These compounds have demonstrated impressive protection against chemically induced ulcer formation in animal studies.[3]

Other active constituents of licorice include isoflavonoids (isoflavonol, kumatakenin, licoricone, glabrol, etc.), chalcones, coumarins (umbelliferone, herniarin, etc.), triterpenoids and sterols, lignins, amino acids, amines, gums, and volatile oils.[1]

History and folk use

The medicinal use of licorice in both Western and Eastern cultures dates back several thousand years. It was used primarily as a demulcent, expectorant, antitussive, and mild laxative. Licorice is one of the most popular components of Chinese medicines. Its traditional uses include the treatment of peptic ulcers, asthma, pharyngitis, malaria, abdominal pain, insomnia, and infections.[1]

Pharmacology

Licorice is known to exhibit many pharmacological actions, including estrogenic; aldosterone-like; antiinflammatory (cortisol-like); antiallergic; antibacterial, antiviral, and anti-*Trichomonas*; antihepatotoxic; anticonvulsive; choleretic; anticancer; expectorant; and antitussive activities.[1] The majority of these actions are discussed individually below.

Although much of the pharmacology focuses on glycyrrhizin and glycyrrhetinic acid, remember that licorice has many other components, such as flavonoids, that may have significant pharmacological effect.

Estrogenic activity

Licorice is believed to exert an alterative action on estrogen metabolism—that is, when estrogen levels are too high, it will inhibit estrogen action, and when estrogens are too low, it will potentiate estrogen action when used in greater amounts.[4] Glycyrrhetinic acid antagonizes many of the effects of estrogens, particularly estrogens from outside sources.[5] The estrogenic action of licorice is due to its isoflavone content, as many isoflavone structures are known to possess estrogenic effects.[6] This effect has been demonstrated in experimental animal studies using the crude extract, suggesting that the estrogenic activity of the isoflavones is more significant than the estrogen antagonism of glycyrrhetinic acid.

Pseudoaldosterone activity

The chronic ingestion of licorice in large doses leads to a well-documented "aldosterone-like" syndrome, that is, high blood pressure, loss of potassium, and sodium and water retention.[7–12] These effects are due to glycyrrhetinic acid enhancing the activity of aldosterone largely by inhibiting its breakdown by the liver.[13] Glycyrrhizin and glycyrrhetinic acid suppress 5-beta-reductase, the main enzyme in humans responsible for inactivating cortisol, aldosterone, and progesterone. These effects are put to good use in the treatment of Addison's disease, a severe disease of adrenal insufficiency.[12]

Antiinflammatory and antiallergic activity

Licorice has significant antiinflammatory and antiallergic activity.[14,15] Although both glycyrrhizin and glycyrrhetinic acid bind to glucocorticoid receptors, and much of licorice's antiinflammatory activity has been explained by its "cortisol-like effects," many of the effects of licorice actually antagonize or counteract the negative effects of cortisol.[16] For example, licorice counteracts cortisol's stimulation of hepatic cholesterol synthesis, thymus atrophy, and adrenal atrophy.[17] Glycyrrhizin does, however, reinforce cortisol's inhibition of antibody formation, stress reaction, and inflammation. Like its mineralocorticoid effect, the major influence of licorice on glucocorticoid metabolism is probably related to its suppression of the breakdown of cortisol by the liver, thus increasing the half-life of cortisol.[14]

Licorice's major cortisol-like effect relates to its ability to inhibit phospholipase A_2.[18] This enzyme cleaves lipids from cellular membranes, thus beginning the manufacture of inflammatory prostaglandins and leukotrienes. In addition to this effect, glycyrrhizin also inhibits prostaglandin formation.[19]

Glycyrrhizin administered to animals has been shown to inhibit experimentally induced allergenic reactions and to be an antidote against many toxins, including diphtheria, tetanus, and tetrodotoxin.[17,19]

Immunostimulatory and antiviral effects

Glycyrrhizin and glycyrrhetinic acid induce interferon—the body's natural antiviral compound.[20] The induction of interferon leads to significant antiviral activity, because interferons bind to cell surfaces, stimulating synthesis of intracellular proteins that block viral DNA. The induction of interferon is also followed by activation of macrophages and augmentation of natural killer cell activity.

Glycyrrhizin inhibits the growth of several DNA and RNA viruses (vaccinia, herpes simplex, Newcastle disease, and vesicular stomatitis viruses) in cell cultures and inactivates herpes simplex virus type 1 irreversibly.[21]

Recent clinical research has focused on its ability to inhibit the human immunodeficiency virus (HIV) and acquired immunodeficiency virus (AIDS).

Antibacterial activity

Alcohol extracts of licorice have displayed antimicrobial activity *in vitro* against *Staphylococcus aureus*, *Streptococcus mutans*, *Mycobacterium smegmatis*, and *Candida albicans*.[22] The majority of the antimicrobial effects are due to isoflavonoid components, with glycyrrhetinic acid and derivatives having a lesser antibacterial effect.

Antihepatotoxic activity

Glycyrrhetinic acid inhibits chemical-induced liver damage in animal studies. It acts by preventing free radical damage as well as by inhibiting the formation of free radicals.[23]

Clinical applications

The clinical applications of licorice can be divided into three main categories: use of oral licorice preparations containing glycyrrhetinic acid; use of deglycyrrhizinated licorice (DGL); and use of topical prepations containing glycyrrhetinic acid.

Key uses of oral licorice preparations containing glycyrrhetinic acid include the treatment of viral infections (e.g., the common cold, HIV and AIDS, viral hepatitis), premenstrual syndrome (PMS), Addison's disease, and inflammation; and as a sweetening agent.

The key use of DGL is in ulcerative conditions of the gastrointestinal tract (e.g., peptic ulcers, canker sores, and inflammatory bowel disease).

Topical preparations containing glycyrrhetinic acid can be used in eczema, psoriasis, and herpes.

All of these uses are discussed in order below.

The common cold

Licorice has long been used to treat common cold symptoms. This historical use is justified by its immune-enhancing and antiviral effects.

HIV and AIDS

Glycyrrhizin-containing preparations are showing great promise in the treatment of HIV-related diseases, including AIDS. Much of the research features intravenous administration, but this route of administration may not be necessary because glycyrrhizin and glycyrrhetinic acid are easily absorbed orally and are well tolerated. This is most evident in a recent double-blind study on the clinical effectiveness of glycyrrhizin orally administered to sixteen hemophiliac patients with evidence of HIV infection.[24] Patients received daily doses of 150–225 milligrams of glycyrrhizin for 3 to 7 years. Helper and total T lymphocyte numbers, other immune system parameters, and glycyrrhizin and glycyrrhetinic acid levels in the blood were monitored. The results indicated that orally administered glycyrrhizin was converted into glycyrrhetinic acid, which was detected in sera without manifesting any side effect. None of the patients given the glycyrrhizin progressed in terms of immunological abnormalities or developed AIDS. In contrast, control group members not receiving glycyrrhetinic acid showed decreases in helper and total T cell counts and antibody levels. Two of the sixteen patients in the control group developed AIDS.

In another study, ten HIV-positive patients without AIDS took 150–225 milligrams of glycyrrhizin daily.[25] After 1–2 years, none developed symptoms associated with AIDS or AIDS-related complex (ARC), whereas one of ten patients in a matched control group developed ARC and two progressed to AIDS and subsequently died.

HIV-positive and AIDS patients given glycyrrhizin showed almost immediate improvement in immune function. In one study, nine symptom-free

HIV-positive patients received a daily dose of 200–800 milligrams of gly-cyrrhizin intravenously. After 8 weeks, the groups presented increased helper T cell counts, improved helper-to-suppressor T cell ratios, and improved liver function.[26]

In another study, six AIDS patients received a daily dose of 400–1600 milligrams of glycyrrhizin intravenously. After 30 days, five of the six showed a reduction or disappearance of the "p24 antigen," which indicates active disease.[27]

The results of these studies and others involving HIV-positive and AIDS patients are extremely encouraging.

Hepatitis

Some of the studies in HIV patients used an intravenous glycyrrhizin-containing product, Stronger Neominophagen C (SNMC), consisting of 0.2 percent glycyrrhizin, 0.1 percent cysteine and 2.0 percent glycine in a physiological saline solution. This product is used in Japan primarily for the treatment of hepatitis (discussed below). The other components, glycine and cysteine, appear to modulate glycyrrhizin's actions. Glycine prevents the aldosterone-like effects of glycyrrhizin, while cysteine assists the liver in detoxification reactions.

In addition to AIDS, SNMC has demonstrated impressive results in treating chronic hepatitis B, one of the most difficult infections for the body to throw off.[17,28–30] SNMC improves liver function and reduces blood levels of liver enzymes that signify liver damage. Approximately 40 percent of patients will experience complete resolution.

Premenstrual syndrome

The symptoms of the premenstrual syndrome (depression, craving for sweets, weight gain due to water retention, breast tenderness, etc.) have been largely attributed to an increase in the estrogen-to-progesterone ratio. Because licorice exerts alterative action on estrogen metabolism, and because both glycyrrhizin and glycyrrhetinic acid possess antiestrogenic properties and suppress the breakdown of progesterone, administration of licorice 2 weeks prior to the onset of menstruation (the midluteal phase) may help reduce the symptoms of PMS.

Addison's disease

As described above, licorice exerts an "aldosterone-like" effect that is useful in treating Addison's disease.

Inflammation

Virtually any inflammatory or allergic condition may be reduced by licorice by the mechanisms discussed above (see Pharmacology). Historically, licorice has been used successfully to treat asthma and other atopic conditions.[1,14]

Licorice enhances the action of corticosteroids such as prednisone and prednisolone, as well as the levels of the body's own corticosteroids.[31,32] In one study, six subjects received an intravenous dose of prednisolone with or without 200 milligrams of glycyrrhizin. Glycyrrhizin was found to increase significantly the concentration of total and free prednisolone by inhibiting its breakdown of prednisolone (PSL). Furthermore, the effects of prednisolone appeared to be potentiated by glycyrrhizin.[32]

Sweetening agent

As glycyrrhizin is 50 to 100 times sweeter than sucrose, licorice can be used as a sweetening or flavoring agent to mask the bitter taste of other medications.[1]

Peptic ulcer

By far, the most popular medicinal use of licorice in the United States is in the treatment of ulcers of the stomach or duodenum—collectively known as peptic ulcer. Original research focused on glycyrrhetinic acid. In fact, glycyrrhetinic acid was the first drug proven to promote healing of gastric and duodenal ulcers.[33] Most researchers and most physicians administering licorice in the treatment of peptic ulcers now use DGL. Deglycyrrhizinated licorice was actually shown to be more effective than glycyrrhetinic acid and is without side effects.[34]

The mode of action of DGL differs from that of current drugs such as antacids, Tagamet, and Zantac, which focus on reducing gastric acidity. Although effective, these treatments can be expensive, carry some risk of toxicity, disrupt normal digestive processes, and alter the structure and function of the cells that line the digestive tract. The latter factor is just one of the reasons why peptic ulcers will develop again if antacids, Tagamet, Zantac, and similar drugs are used.

Rather than inhibit the release of acid, DGL stimulates the normal defense mechanisms that prevent ulcer formation. Specifically, DGL improves both the quality and quantity of the protective substances that line the intestinal tract, increases the life span of the intestinal cell, and improves blood supply to the intestinal lining.[35,36]

Numerous clinical studies over the years have found DGL to be an effective antiulcer compound. In several head-to-head comparison studies, DGL has been shown to be more effective than either Tagamet, Zantac, or antacids in both short-term treatment and maintenance therapy of peptic ulcers.[14,37–40] However, while these drugs are associated with significant side effects (see above), DGL is extremely safe and inexpensive. For example, while Tagamet and Zantac typically cost well over $100 for a month's supply, DGL is available in health food stores at $15 for a month's supply.

Deglycyrrhizinated licorice in gastric ulcers

Deglycyrrhizinated licorice is extremely effective in the treatment of gastric ulcers.[38–42] In one study, thirty-three gastric ulcer patients were treated with either DGL (760 milligrams, three times a day) or a placebo for 1 month.[41] The reduction in ulcer size was significantly greater in the DGL group (78 percent), than in the placebo group (34 percent). Complete healing occurred in 44 percent of those receiving DGL, but in only 6 percent of the placebo group.

Subsequent studies show DGL to be as effective as Tagamet and Zantac for both short-term treatment and maintenance therapy of gastric ulcer.[38–40] For example, in a head-to-head comparison with Tagamet, 100 patients received either DGL (760 milligrams, three times a day between meals) or Tagamet (200 milligrams, three times a day and 400 milligrams at bedtime).[39] The percentage of ulcers healed after 6 and 12 weeks were similar in both groups. Yet, while Tagamet is associated with some toxicity, DGL is extremely safe to use.

Gastric ulcers are often a result of the use of alcohol, aspirin, nonsteroidal antiinflammatory drugs, caffeine, and other factors that decrease the integrity of the gastric lining. As DGL has been shown in human studies to reduce the gastric bleeding caused by aspirin, DGL is strongly indicated for the prevention of gastric ulcers in patients requiring long-term treatment with ulcerogenic drugs, such as aspirin, nonsteroidal antiinflammatory agents, and corticosteroids.[42]

Deglycyrrhizinated licorice in duodenal ulcers

Deglycyrrhizinated licorice is also effective in duodenal ulcers. This is perhaps best illustrated by one study in patients with severe duodenal ulcers. In the study, forty patients with chronic duodenal ulcers of 4 to 12 years' duration and more than six relapses during the previous year were treated with DGL.[43] All of the patients had been referred for surgery because of relentless pain, sometimes with frequent vomiting, despite treatment with bed rest, antacids, and anticholinergic drugs. Half of the patients received 3 grams of DGL daily for 8 weeks; the other half received 4.5 grams per day for 16 weeks. All forty patients showed substantial improvement, usually within 5 to 7 days, and none required surgery during the 1-year follow-up. Although both dosages were effective, the higher dose was significantly more effective than the lower dose.

In another, more recent study, the therapeutic effect of DGL was compared to that of antacids or cimetidine in 874 patients with confirmed chronic duodenal ulcers.[37] Ninety-one percent of all ulcers healed within 12 weeks; there was no significant difference in healing rate in the groups. However, there were fewer relapses in the DGL group (8.2 percent) than in those receiving cimetidine (12.9 percent), or antacids (16.4 percent). These results, coupled with DGL protective effects, suggest that DGL is a superior treatment of duodenal ulcers.

Deglycyrrhizinated licorice in canker sores

Recurrent canker sores are a common problem. Deglycyrrhizinated licorice may be effective in promoting healing. In one study, twenty patients were instructed to use a solution of DGL as a mouthwash (200 milligrams of powdered DGL dissolved in 200 milliliters warm water) four times daily. Fifteen of the twenty (75 percent) experienced 50–75 percent improvement within 1 day, followed by complete healing of the ulcers by the third day.[44] Deglycyrrhizinated licorice in tablet form may produce even better results.

Eczema and psoriasis

Glycyrrhetinic acid exerts an effect similar to that of topical hydrocortisone in the treatment of eczema, contact and allergic dermatitis, and psoriasis. In fact, in several studies, glycyrrhetinic acid was shown to be superior to topical cortisone, especially in chronic cases. For example, in one study in patients with eczema, 93 percent of the patients applying glycyrrhetinic acid demonstrated improvement compared to 83 percent using cortisone.[45]

Glycyrrhetinic acid can also be used to potentiate the effects of topically applied hydrocortisone by inhibiting 11-beta-hydroxysteroid dehydrogenase, which catalyzes the conversion of hydrocortisone to an inactive form.[46]

Herpes simplex

Topical glycyrrhetinic acid and derivatives have been shown, in clinical studies, to be quite helpful in reducing the healing time and pain associated with cold sores and genital herpes.[47,48] As mentioned earlier, glycyrrhizin inactivates herpes simplex virus type 1 irreversibly and stimulates the synthesis and release of interferon.[21]

Dosage

The dosage of licorice for most clinical applications is based on the level of glycyrrhetinic acid. The exception is in the treatment of peptic ulcer. In this application, DGL is preferred because it produces equally effective results compared to glycyrrhetinic acid, but is free from any side effects.

For most purposes, the goal is to achieve a high level of glycyrrhetinic acid in the blood without producing side effects (discussed below). In general, the following doses, administered three times a day, are safe and effective in raising glycyrrhetinic acid levels:

- Powdered root: 1–2 grams
- Fluid extract (1:1): 2–4 milliliters
- Solid (dry powdered) extract (4:1): 250 to 500 milligrams

In the treatment of AIDS, pure glycyrrhetinic acid products or extracts standardized for glycyrrhetinic acid are recommended. Patients taking licorice for any period longer than 1 month need to read the toxicity section below.

Dosage instructions for deglycyrrhizinated licorice

To heal peptic ulcers, DGL must mix with the saliva: DGL may promote the release of salivary compounds that stimulate the growth and regeneration of stomach and intestinal cells. Deglycyrrhizinated licorice in capsule form has not been shown to be effective.[49,50]

The standard dosage for DGL is two to four 380 milligram chewable tablets between or 20 minutes before meals. Taking DGL after meals is associated with poor results.[51] Deglycyrrhizinated licorice should be continued for 8 to 16 weeks, depending on the response.

Toxicity

The main hazard of licorice lies in its aldosterone-like effects. If ingested regularly, licorice root (more than 3 grams per day for more than 6 weeks) or glycyrrhizin (more than 100 milligrams per day) may cause sodium and water retention, hypertension, hypokalemia, and suppression of the renin–aldosterone system. Monitoring of blood pressure and electrolytes and increasing dietary potassium intake are suggested.[7,8]

People vary in their susceptibility to the symptom-producing effects of glycyrrhizin. Adverse effects are rarely observed at levels below 100 milligrams per day, while they are quite common at levels above 400 milligrams per day.[8]

Prevention of the side effects of glycyrrhizin may be possible by following a high-potassium, low-sodium diet. Although no formal trial has been performed, patients who normally consume high-potassium foods and restrict sodium intake, even those with high blood pressure and angina, have been reported to be free from the aldosterone-like side effects of glycyrrhizin.[52]

Licorice should probably not be used in patients with a history of hypertension, renal failure, or current use of digitalis preparations.

References

1. Chandler RF: Licorice, more than just a flavour. *Can Pharmacy J* September, 421–424, 1985.
2. Hattori M, *et al.*: Metabolism of glycyrrhizin by human intestinal flora. *Planta Medica* **48**, 38–42, 1983.
3. Yamamoto K, *et al.*: Gastric cytoprotective anti-ulcerogenic actions of hydroxychalcone in rats. *Planta Medica* **58**, 389–393, 1992.
4. Kumagai A, *et al.*: Effect of glycyrrhizin on estrogen action. *Endocrinol Jpn* **14**, 34–38, 1967.
5. Kraus S: The anti-estrogenic action of beta-glycyrrhetinic acid. *Exp Med Surg* **27**, 411–420, 1969.
6. Sharaf A and Goma N: Phytoestrogens and their antagonism to progesterone and testosterone. *J Endocrinol* **31**, 289–290, 1965.
7. Farese RV, *et al.*: Licorice-induced hypermineralocorticoidism. *N Engl J Med* **325**, 1223–1227, 1991.
8. Stormer FC, Reistad R, and Alexander J: Glycyrrhizic acid in liquorice—evaluation of health hazard. *Fd Chem Toxicol* **31**, 303–312, 1993.
9. Takeda R, *et al.*: Prolonged pseudoaldosteronism induced by glycyrrhizin. *Endocrinol Jpn* **26**, 541–547, 1979.
10. Baron J: Side-effects of carbonoxolone. *Acta Gastro-Enterol Belgica* **46**, 469–484, 1983.
11. Epstein M, *et al.*: Effect of eating liquorice on the renin-angiotensin aldosterone axis in normal subjects. *Br Med J* **1**, 488–490, 1977.
12. Armanini D, Karbowiak I, and Funder J: Affinity of liquorice derivatives for mineralocorticoid and glucocorticoid receptors. *Clin Endocrinol* **19**, 609–612, 1983.
13. Tamura Y, Nishikawa T, and Yamada K: Effects of glycyrrhetinic acid and its derivatives on delta4-5-alpha- and 5-beta-reductase in rat liver. *Arzneimittel-Forsch* **29**, 647–649, 1979.
14. Kuroyanagi T and Sato M: Effect of prednisolone and glycyrrhizin on passive transfer of experimental allergic encephalomyelitis. *Allergy* **15**, 67–75, 1966.
15. Cyong J: A pharmacological study of the anti-inflammatory activity of Chinese herbs. A review. *Acupunct Electro-Ther* **7**, 173–202, 1982.
16. Kumagai A, *et al.*: Effects of glycyrrhizin on thymolytic and immunosuppressive action of cortisone. *Endocrinol Jpn* **14**, 39–42, 1967.
17. Suzuki H, *et al.*: Effects of glycyrrhizin on biochemical tests in patients with chronic hepatitis—double blind trial. *Asian Med J* **26**, 423–438, 1984.
18. Okimasa E, *et al.*: Inhibition of phospholipase A2 by glycyrrhizin, an anti-inflammatory drug. *Acta Med Okayama* **37**, 385–391, 1983
19. Ohuchi K, *et al.*: Glycyrrhizin inhibits prostaglandin E2 formation by activated peritoneal macrophages from rats. *Prostaglandins Med* **7**, 457–463, 1981.
20. Abe N, Ebina T, and Ishida N: Interferon induction by glycyrrhizin and glycyrrhetinic acid in mice. *Microb Immunol* **26**, 535–539, 1982.

21. Pompei R, *et al.*: Antiviral activity of glycyrrhizic acid. *Experientia* **36**, 304–305, 1980.
22. Mitscher L, Park Y, and Clark D: Antimicrobial agents from higher plants. Antimicrobial isoflavonoids from *Glycyrrhiza glabra* L. var. typica. *J Nat Products* **43**, 259–269, 1980.
23. Kiso Y, *et al.*: Mechanism of antihepatotoxic activity of glycyrrhizin. I. Effect on free radical generation and lipid peroxidation. *Planta Medica* **50**, 298–302, 1984.
24. Ikegami N, *et al.*: Prophylactic effect of long-term oral administration of glycyrrhizin on AIDS development of asymptomatic patients. *Int Conf AIDS* **9**(1), 234, 1993. [Abstract No. PO-A25-0596]
25. Ikegami N, *et al.*: Clinical evaluation of glycyrrhizin in HIV-infected asymptomatic hemophiliac patients in Japan. Fifth International Conference on AIDS, June 1989. [Abstract W.B.P. 298]; cited in *AIDS Treatment News*, No. 103, May 18, 1990.
26. Mori K, *et al.*: The present status in prophylaxis and treatment of HIV infected patients with hemophilia in Japan. *Rinsho Byhori* **37**(11), 1200–1208, 1989.
27. Hattori T, *et al.*: Preliminary evidence for inhibitory effect of glycyrrhizin on HIV replication in patients with AIDS. *Antiviral Res* **11**, (5–6), 255–261, 1989.
28. Mori K, *et al.*: Effects of glycyrrhizin (SNMC: Stronger Neo-Minophagen C) in hemophilia patients with HIV-1 infection. *Tohoku J Exp Med* **162**(2), 183–193, 1990.
29. Eisenburg J: Treatment of chronic hepatitis B. 2. Effect of glycyrrhizinic acid on the course of illness. *Forschr Med* **110**, 395–398, 1992.
30. Acharya SK, *et al.*: A preliminary open trial on interferon stimulator (SNMC) derived from *Glycyrrhiza glabra* in the treatment of subacute hepatic failure. *Ind J Med Res* **98**, 75–78, 1993.
31. MacKenzie MA, *et al.*: The influence of glycyrrhetinic acid on plasma cortisol and cortisone in healthy young volunteers. *J Clin Endocrinol Metab* **70**, 1637–1643, 1990.
32. Chen MF, *et al.*: Effect of glycyrrhizin on the pharmacokinetics of prednisolone following low dosage of prednisolone hemisuccinate. *Endocrinol Jpn* **37**(3), 331–341, 1990.
33. Doll R, *et al.*: Clinical trial of a triterpenoid liquorice compound in gastric and duodenal ulcer. *Lancet* **ii**, 793–796, 1962.
34. Wilson JA: A comparison of carbenoxolone sodium and deglycyrrhizinated liquorice in the treatment of gastric ulcer in the ambulant patient. *Br J Clin Pract* **26**, 563–566, 1972.
35. van Marle J, *et al.*: Deglycyrrhizinised liquorice (DGL) and the renewal of rat stomach epithelium. *Eur J Pharmacol* **72**, 219–225, 1981.
36. Johnson B and McIssac R. Effect of some anti-ulcer agents on mucosal blood flow. *Br J Pharmacol* **1**, 308, 1981.
37. Kassir ZA: Endoscopic controlled trial of four drug regimens in the treatment of chronic duodenal ulceration. *Irish Med J* **78**, 153–156, 1985.
38. Morgan AG, *et al.*: Maintenance therapy: A two year comparison between Caved-S and cimetidine treatment in the prevention of symptomatic gastric ulcer. *Gut* **26**, 599–602, 1985.
39. Morgan AG, *et al.*: Comparison between cimetidine and Caved-S in the treatment of gastric ulceration, and subsequent maintenance therapy. *Gut* **23**, 545–551, 1982.
40. Glick L: Deglycyrrhizinated liquorice in peptic ulcer. *Lancet* **ii**, 817, 1982.
41. Turpie AG, Runcie J, and Thomson TJ: Clinical trial of deglycyrrhizinate liquorice in gastric ulcer. *Gut* **10**, 299–303, 1969.
42. Rees WDW, *et al.*: Effect of deglycyrrhizinated liquorice on gastric mucosal damage by aspirin. *Scand J Gastroenterol* **14**, 605–607, 1979.
43. Tewari SN and Wilson AK: Deglycyrrhizinated liquorice in duodenal ulcer. *Practitioner* **210**, 820–825, 1972.
44. Das SK, Gulati AK, and Singh VP: Deglycyrrhizinated liquorice in aphthous ulcers. *J Assoc Physicians India* **37**, 647, 1989.
45. Evans FQ: The rational use of glycyrrhetinic acid in dermatology. *Br J Clin Pract* **12**, 269–279, 1958.
46. Teelucksingh S, *et al.*: Potentiation of hydrocortisone activity in skin by glycyrrhetinic acid. *Lancet* **335**, 1060–1063, 1990.
47. Partridge M and Poswillo D: Topical carbonoxolone sodium in the management of herpes simplex infection. *Br J Oral Maxillofac Surg* **22**, 138–145, 1984.
48. Csonka G and Tyrrell D: Treatment of herpes genitalis with carbonoxolone and cicloxolone creams: A double blind placebo controlled trial. *Br J Ven Dis* **60**, 178–181, 1984.
49. Bardhan, *et al.*: Clinical trial of deglycyrrhizinised liquorice in gastric ulcer. *Gut* **19**, 779–782, 1978.
50. Multicentre Trial: Treatment of duodenal ulcers with glycyrrhinizin acid-reduced liquorice. *Br Med J* **3**(773), 501–503,1973.
51. Feldman H and Gilat T: A trial of deglycyrrhizinated liquorice in the treatment of duodenal ulcer. *Gut* **12**, 449–451, 1971.
52. Baron J, *et al.*: Metabolic studies, aldosterone secretion rate and plasma renin after carbonoxolone sodium as biogastrone. *Br Med J* **2**, 793–795, 1969.

23
Lobelia

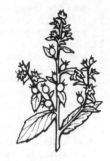

Key uses of lobelia:

- Smoking deterrent
- Asthma
- Bronchitis
- Pneumonia

General description

Lobelia or Indian tobacco is an indigenous North American annual or biennial plant with an erect, angular, hairy stem that contains a milky sap and grows from 6 inches to 3 feet in height. Numerous small, two-lipped, blue flowers grow in spikelike racemes from July to November.

Chemical composition

Lobelia contains about 0.48 percent pyridine (piperidine) alkaloids composed mainly of lobeline, with lesser amounts of lobelanine, lobelanidine, and other alkaloids. Other constituents include resin, gum, lipids, and chelidonic acid.[1-3]

History and folk use

Lobelia was used extensively by Thomsonians (see *The History of Herbal Medicine*) as an emetic (inducer of vomiting), diaphoretic, expectorant, sedative, antispasmodic, and antiasthmatic. Conditions for which it has been used include the treatment of asthma, whooping cough, bruises, sprains, ringworm, insect bites, poison ivy symptoms, and many others. Thomson stated, "there is no vegetable which the earth produces more harmless in its effect on the human system, and none more powerful in removing disease and promoting health than lobelia."[4] Lobelia has also been used as a stop-smoking aid.

Pharmacology

The pharmacology of lobelia centers around its lobeline content. Lobeline has many of the same pharmacological actions as nicotine, but is generally regarded as being less potent.[5,6] Lobeline was at one time approved for use by the Food and Drug Administration (FDA) as a smoking deterrent to lessen the difficulty of nicotine withdrawal.[1,2]

Gastrointestinal effects

The emetic action of lobeline is a result of its stimulation of the vomiting center at the base of the brain, the area postrema of the medulla oblongata, which is outside the blood–brain barrier.[7]

Respiratory effects

Lobelia is a very effective expectorant. Expectorants modify the quality and quantity of the secretions of the respiratory tract, resulting in the expulsion of secretions and improvement in respiratory tract function.

Lobelia is primarily used as an expectorant in such conditions as pneumonia, asthma, and bronchitis. It appears that its major action is a result of stimulating the adrenal gland to release hormones that cause the bronchial muscles to relax.[8]

Although often effective when used alone in the treatment of asthma, it has traditionally been used in combination with other herbs. Typically it is combined with cayenne pepper (*Capsicum frutescens*), licorice (*Glycyrrhiza glabra*), or Ma Huang (*Ephedra sinica*).

Dosage

Many of lobelia's effects are related to its lobeline content. Lobelia is particularly useful as an expectorant in respiratory tract conditions such as asthma, pneumonia, and bronchitis.[9] Lobelia can be used as a smoking deterrent.

Administer the following doses three times a day:

- Dried herb or as infusion (tea): 0.5–1 gram
- Tincture (1:5): 3–5 milliliters
- Fluid extract (1:1): 0.5–1 milliliter
- Solid (dried powdered) extract (1 percent lobeline content): 200 milligrams

Toxicity

Ingestion of toxic levels of lobelia usually results in vomiting, thereby lessening the likelihood of a fatal outcome.[4] Like nicotine poisoning, toxic symptoms include nausea, salivation, diarrhea, disturbed hearing and vision, mental confusion, and marked weakness. Faintness and prostration ensue; blood pressure falls; the pulse becomes weak, rapid, and irregular; breathing is difficult; and collapse occurs followed by convulsions. Death may result from respiratory failure.[5] The antidote in acute poisoning is 2 milligrams of atropine, given subcutaneously.[10]

References

1. Leung A: *Encyclopedia of Common Natural Ingredients Used in Food, Drugs, and Cosmetics.* John Wiley & Sons, New York, 1980, pp. 220–223.
2. Tyler V, Brady L, and Robbers J: *Pharmacognosy*, 8th Ed. Lea & Febiger, Philadelphia, 1981, pp. 68–70.
3. *Merck Index*, 10th Ed. Merck & Co, Rahway, NJ, 1983, p. 4374.
4. Christopher J: *School of Natural Healing.* BiWorld Publishers, Provo, UT, 1976, pp. 358–367.
5. Gilman A, Goodman L, and Gilman A: *The Pharmacological Basis of Therapeutics.* Macmillan, New York, 1980, pp. 212–214.
6. Mansuri S, Kelkar V, and Jindal M: Some pharmacological characteristics of ganglionic activity of lobeline. *Arzneimittel-Forsch* **23**, 1271–1275, 1973.
7. Laffan R and Borison H: Emetic action of nicotine and lobeline. *J Pharmacol Exp Ther* **121**, 468–476, 1957.
8. Halmagyi D, Kovacs A, and Neumann P: Adrenocortical pathway of lobeline protection in some forms of experimental lung edema of the rat. *Dis Chest* **33**, 285–296, 1958.
9. Cambar P, Shore S, and Aviado D: Bronchopulmonary and gastrointestinal effects of lobeline. *Arch Int Pharmacodyn* **177**, 1–27, 1969.
10. Dreisbach RH: *Handbook of Poisoning.* Lange Medical Publishing, Los Altos, CA, 1983, p. 553.

24
Milk thistle

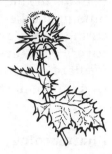

Key uses of milk thistle:

- Liver disorders
- Hepatitis
- Cirrhosis of the liver
- Gallstones
- Psoriasis

General description

Milk thistle (*Silybum marianum*) is a stout, annual or biennial plant, found in dry rocky soils in southern and western Europe and some parts of the United States. The branched stem grows 1 to 3 feet high and bears alternate, dark green, shiny leaves with spiny, scalloped edges that are markedly streaked with white along the veins. The solitary flower heads are reddish-purple with bracts ending in sharp spines. Flowering season is from June to August. The seeds, fruit, and leaves are used for medicinal purposes.[1]

Milk thistle has also been referred to as Mary thistle, Marian thistle, Lady's thistle, Holy thistle, and the wild artichoke.

Chemical composition

Milk thistle contains silymarin, a mixture of flavonolignans consisting chiefly of silibin, silidianin, and silichristine.[1-5] The concentration of silymarin is highest in the fruit, but it is also found in the seeds and leaves. Silibin is the silymarin component that yields the greatest degree of biological activity.

History and folk use

Perhaps the most widespread folk use of this plant has been in assisting the nursing mother in the production of milk. It was also used in Germany for curing jaundice and biliary derangements. It is interesting to note that the discovery of the liver-protecting compound silymarin in milk thistle was not the result of extensive pharmacological screening, but rather of investigation of silybum's empirical effects in liver disorders.[1]

Pharmacology

Milk thistle extracts (usually standardized to contain 70 to 80 percent silymarin) are currently widely used in European pharmaceutical preparations for hepatic disorders. Silymarin is one of the most potent liver-protecting substances known.[1-9]

Actions relating to the liver

Milk thistle's ability to prevent liver destruction and enhance liver function is due largely to silymarin's inhibition of the factors that are responsible for liver damage, coupled with its ability to stimulate the growth of new liver cells to replace old damaged cells.

One of the ways the liver can be damaged is a result of certain toxins producing or acting as free radicals. Free radicals are highly reactive molecules that can damage other molecules, including those in cells. Silymarin prevents free radical damage by acting as an antioxidant.[1-5] Silymarin is at least ten times more potent in antioxidant activity than vitamin E.[1-4]

Silymarin also increases the glutathione (GSH) content of the liver by over 35 percent in healthy subjects and by over 50 percent in rats, and increases considerably the level of the important antioxidant enzyme superoxide dismutase in cell cultures.[10,11] Glutathione is responsible for detoxifying a wide range of hormones, drugs, and chemicals. Increasing the glutathione content of the liver means the liver has an increased capacity for detoxification reactions.

Another way in which the liver can be damaged is by the action of leukotrienes. These compounds are produced by the transfer of an oxygen molecule to polyunsaturated fatty acids, a reaction catalyzed by the enzyme lipoxygenase. Silymarin has been shown to be a potent inhibitor of this enzyme, thereby inhibiting the formation of damaging leukotrienes.[12]

Free radical damage to membrane structures due to organic disease or toxic chemicals results in increased release of fatty acids. This leads, among other things, to increased leukotriene synthesis and inflammation. Silymarin counteracts this deleterious process by suppressing the pathological decomposition of membrane lipids and inhibiting leukotriene formation and inflammation.[13]

The protective effect of silymarin against liver damage has been demonstrated in a number of experimental and clinical studies.[1-36] Experimental liver damage in animals can be produced by such diverse toxic chemicals as carbon tetrachloride, galactosamine, ethanol, and praseodymium nitrate. Silymarin has been shown to protect the liver from all of these toxins.[1-6,8,14]

Perhaps the most impressive of silymarin's protective effects is against the severe poisoning of *Amanita phalloides* (the deathcap or toadstool mushroom), an effect that has long been recognized in folk medicine.[6-8] Ingestion of *Amanita phalloides* or its toxins causes severe poisoning and, in approximately 30 percent of victims, death.

Among the experimental models for measuring protection against liver damage, those based on amanitin or phalloidin toxicity are the most important, because these two peptides from *Amanita phalloides* are the most powerful liver-damaging substances known. Silymarin has demonstrated impressive results in these experimental models. When silymarin was administered before amanita toxin poisoning, it was 100 percent effective in preventing toxicity.[6,8] Even if given 10 minutes after the amanita toxin, it completely counteracted the toxic effects. If given within 24 hours, silymarin would still prevent death and greatly reduce the amount of liver damage.[7]

Perhaps the most interesting effect of milk thistle components on the liver is their ability to stimulate protein synthesis.[5,15,16] This stimulation results in an increase in the production of new liver cells to replace the damaged old ones. Interestingly enough, silymarin does not have a stimulatory effect on malignant liver tissue.[15]

From the above-described actions, it is apparent that milk thistle, and more specifically silymarin, exerts both a protective and restorative effect on the liver.

Clinical applications

Obviously, silymarin is useful as an aid to the liver. It can be used to support detoxification reactions or in the treatment of more severe liver disease.

In numerous clinical studies, silymarin has been shown to have positive effects in treating several types of liver disease, including cirrhosis, chronic hepatitis, fatty infiltration of the liver (chemical- and alcohol-induced fatty liver), subclinical cholestasis of pregnancy, and cholangitis and pericholangitis.[17-35] The therapeutic effect of silymarin in these disorders has been confirmed by histological, clinical, and laboratory data. Silymarin may also be useful in improving the solubility of the bile in the treatment of gallstones and in psoriasis.

The therapeutic effect of silymarin in these disorders is described below, along with a discussion on a new form of silymarin (phosphatidylcholine-bound silymarin) and its clinical effects.

Chemical-induced liver damage

In one of the first extensive double-blind clinical trials investigating silymarin's therapeutic effect in liver disorders, silymarin demonstrated impressive results in 129 patients with toxic metabolic liver damage, fatty degeneration of the liver of various origins, or chronic hepatitis, as compared with a control group composed of fifty-six patients. The results might have been even more impressive if the study had lasted longer than 35 days.[17]

A follow-up study of patients with liver damage due to alcohol, diabetes viruses, or toxic exposure demonstrated even more striking results. Patients were followed for a long period of time (e.g., 7 weeks). Not only were clinical findings markedly improved in the silymarin-treated groups, but laboratory and liver biopsy data improved as well. Highly significant results were obtained in bromsulfophthalein retention, SGPT, iron, and cholesterol levels. There were remarkable tissue restorative effects as evidenced by biopsy. On completion of silymarin therapy, the liver showed restitution of normal cell structure, even in severely damaged livers. These effects on the tissue level correlated well with improvements in blood chemistry.[18]

A more recent study highlights the benefit of silymarin in individuals exposed to toxic chemicals. In the study, abnormal results of liver function tests (elevated levels of two liver enzymes, AST and ALT activity) and/or abnormal hematological values (low platelet counts, increased white blood cell counts, and a relative increase in lymphocytes compared to other white blood cells) were observed in 49 of 200 workers exposed to toxic toluene and/or xylene vapors for 5–20 years. Thirty of the affected workers were treated with silymarin, the remaining nineteen were left without treatment. Under the influence of silymarin the liver function tests and the platelet counts significantly improved. The white blood counts also showed a non-significant tendency toward improvement.

Cirrhosis

As described above, silymarin is quite effective in treating alcohol-related liver disease. There is a tremendous range in severity of alcohol-related liver disease, from relatively mild to serious damage. Serious damage to the liver results in cirrhosis—severe scarring (fibrosis). Even in this severe state, silymarin has shown benefit. Perhaps the most significant benefit is to extend the life span of these patients.

In one study, eighty-seven cirrhotics (forty-six with alcoholic cirrhosis) received silymarin, while eighty-three cirrhotics (forty-five with alcoholic cirrhosis) received a placebo. The mean observation period was 41 months. In the treatment group, there were twenty-four deaths with eighteen related to liver disease; among the controls, there were thirty-seven deaths with thirty-one related to liver disease. The 4-year survival rate was 58 percent in the treatment group compared to 39 percent in the controls.

Silymarin can also improve immune function in patients with cirrhosis.[32] Whether this effect is involved in the hepatoprotective action or a result of improved liver function has yet to be determined.

Viral hepatitis

Silymarin is also useful in treating viral-induced liver damage. It is effective in both acute and chronic viral hepatitis.

In a study of acute viral hepatitis, silymarin administered to twenty-nine patients showed a definite therapeutic influence on the characteristic increased serum levels of bilirubin and liver enzymes compared with a placebo group. The laboratory parameters in the silymarin group regressed more than in the placebo group after the fifth day of treatment. The number of patients having attained normal liver values after 3 weeks' treatment was significantly higher in the silymarin group than in the placebo group.

In a study in chronic viral hepatitis, silymarin was shown to result in dramatic improvement. Used at a high dose (420 milligrams of silymarin) for periods of 3 to 12 months, silymarin resulted in a reversal of liver cell damage (as noted by biopsy), an increase in protein level in the blood, and a lowering of liver enzymes. Common symptoms of hepatitis (e.g., abdominal discomfort, decreased appetite, and fatigue) were all improved.[34]

Gallstones

Silymarin may help prevent or treat gallstones via its ability to increase the solubility of the bile, according to the results of a recent study.[35] In the study, the composition of the bile was assayed in nineteen patients with a history of gallstones (four) or removal of the gallbladder due to gallstones (fifteen) before and after silymarin (420 milligrams per day for 30 days) or placebo.

Silymarin treatment led to significant reduction in the biliary cholesterol concentration and bile saturation index.

Silymarin in psoriasis

Correction of abnormal liver function is indicated in the treatment of psoriasis. Silymarin has been reported to be of value in the treatment of psoriasis, and this may be due to its ability to inhibit the synthesis of leukotrienes, and improve liver function.[36,37]

The connection between the liver and psoriasis relates to one of the liver's basic tasks—filtering the blood. Psoriasis has been shown to be linked to high levels of circulating endotoxins, such as those found in the cell walls of gut bacteria. If the liver is overwhelmed by an increased number of endotoxins or chemical toxins, or if the liver's functional ability to filter and detoxify is decreased, the psoriasis gets much worse.

Another factor in psoriasis is excessive production of leukotrienes. Silymarin has been shown to reduce leukotriene formation by inhibiting lipoxygenase.[12] Therefore, silymarin would inhibit one of the causes of the excessive cellular replication.

Silymarin has other effects that would be of value in patients with psoriasis. Most of these effects revolve around correcting the abnormal cAMP-to-cGMP ratio observed in the skin of patients with psoriasis. The ratio of these two cellular control agents controls cellular replication. In psoriasis, cGMP levels are high in ratio to cAMP levels. Silymarin works to lower cGMP levels while raising cAMP levels.[36]

Silymarin bound to phosphatidylcholine

Recently, a new form of silymarin has emerged that may provide the greatest benefit. The new form binds silymarin to phosphatidylcholine, the key component of cellular membranes throughout our bodies. Preliminary research indicates that bound silymarin is absorbed better and produces better clinical results.

Absorption studies with phosphatidylcholine-bound silymarin

Several human and animal studies have shown that phosphatidylcholine-bound silymarin is better absorbed. In one study, the excretion of silibin, the major component of silymarin, in the bile was evaluated in patients undergoing gallbladder removal (cholecystectomy). A special drainage tube, the T-tube, was used to obtain the samples of bile necessary. Patients were given either a single oral dose of the silymarin–phosphatidylcholine complex or silymarin. The amount of silibin recovered in the bile in free and conjugated form within 48 hours was 11 percent for the silymarin–phosphatidylcholine group and 3 percent for the silymarin group.[38]

One of the significant features of this study is the fact that silymarin has been shown to improve the solubility of the bile. Since more silymarin is being delivered to the liver and gallbladder when the phosphatidylcholine-bound silymarin is used, this form is ideal for individuals with gallstones or fatty infiltration of the liver—two conditions characterized by decreased bile solubility.

In another study designed to assess the absorption of silymarin bound to phosphatidylcholine, plasma silibin levels were determined after administration of single oral doses of silymarin–phosphatidylcholine complex and a similar amount of silymarin to nine healthy volunteers. Although absorption was rapid with both preparations, the bioavailability of the silymarin–phosphatidylcholine complex was much greater than that of silymarin, as indicated by higher plasma silibin levels at all sampling times after intake of the complex. The authors concluded that complexation with phosphatidylcholine greatly increases the oral bioavailability of silymarin, probably by facilitating its passage across the gastrointestinal mucosa.[39]

Clinical studies with phosphatidylcholine-bound silymarin

Several clinical studies have also shown phosphatidylcholine-bound silymarin to be more effective. In one study, eight patients with chronic viral hepatitis (three with hepatitis B, three with both hepatitis B and hepatitis C, and two with hepatitis C) were given one capsule of phosphatidylcholine-bound silymarin (equivalent to 140 milligrams of silymarin) between meals for 2 months.[40] After treatment, serum malondialdehyde levels (an indicator of lipid peroxidation) decreased by 36 percent, and the quantitative liver function evaluation, as expressed by galactose elimination capacity, increased by 15 percent. A statistically significant reduction of liver enzymes was also seen: AST decreased by 17 percent and ALT decreased by 16 percent.

In another study designed primarily to evaluate the dose–response relationship of phosphatidylcholine-bound silymarin, positive effects were again displayed.[41] In the study, patients with chronic hepatitis due to either a virus or alcohol were given different doses: twenty patients received 80 milligrams twice daily, twenty patients received 120 milligrams twice daily, and twenty patients received 120 milligrams three times daily for 2 weeks. At all tested doses, phosphatidylcholine-bound silymarin produced a remarkable and statistically significant decrease of mean serum and total bilirubin levels. When used at the dosage of 240 or 360 milligrams per day, it also resulted in a remarkable and statistically significant decrease in ALT and GGTP liver enzymes. These results indicate that even short-term treatment of viral or alcohol-induced hepatitis with relative low doses of phosphatidylcholine-bound silymarin can be effective, but for the best results higher doses are indicated.

Dosage

The standard dose of milk thistle is based on its silymarin content (70–210 milligrams three times daily). For this reason, standardized extracts are preferred. The best results are achieved at higher dosages, that is, 140 milligrams of silymarin three times daily.

The dosage for silymarin bound to phosphatidylcholine is 100 milligrams to 200 milligrams twice daily.

Alcohol-based extracts are virtually always contraindicated, due to the need to administer relatively high amounts of alcohol in order to obtain an adequate dose of silymarin.

Toxicity

Silymarin preparations are widely used medications in Europe, where a considerable body of evidence points to very low toxicity.[1]

When used at high doses for short periods of time, silymarin given by various routes to mice, rats, rabbits, and dogs has shown no toxic effects. Studies in rats receiving silymarin for protracted periods have also demonstrated a complete lack of toxicity.[1]

As silymarin possesses choleretic activity, it may produce a looser stool as a result of increased bile flow and secretion. If higher doses are used, it may be appropriate to use bile-sequestering fiber compounds (e.g., guar gum, pectin, psyllium, and oat bran) to prevent mucosal irritation and loose stools. Because of silymarin lack of toxicity, long-term use is feasible when necessary.

References

1. Awang D: Milk thistle. *Can Pharm J* **422**, 403–404, 1993.
2. Wagner H: Antihepatotoxic flavonoids. In: *Plant Flavonoids in Biology and Medicine: Biochemical, Pharmacological, and Structure–Activity Relationships* (Cody V, Middleton E, and Harbourne JB, eds.). Alan R. Liss, New York, 1986, pp. 545–558.
3. Adzet T: Polyphenolic compounds with biological and pharmacological activity. *Herbs Spices Med Plants* **1**, 167–184, 1986.

4. Hikino H, *et al.*: Antihepatotoxic actions of flavonolignans from *Silybum marianum* fruits. *Planta Medica* **50**, 248–250, 1984.

5. Wagner H: Plant constituents with antihepatotoxic activity. In: *Natural Products as Medicinal Agents* (Beal JL and Reinhard E, eds.). Hippokrates-Verlag, Stuttgart, Germany, 1981.

6. Vogel G, *et al.*: Protection against *Amanita phalloides* intoxication in beagles. *Toxicol Appl Pharm* **73**, 355–362, 1984.

7. Desplaces A, *et al.*: The effects of silymarin on experimental phalloidin poisoning. *Arzneimittel-Forsch* **25**, 89–96, 1975.

8. Vogel G, *et al.*: Studies on pharmacodynamics, site and mechanism of action of silymarin, the antihepatotoxic principle from *Silybum marianum* (L.) Gaert. *Arzneimittel-Forsch* **25**, 179–185, 1975.

9. Sarre H: Experience in the treatment of chronic hepatopathies with silymarin. *Arzneimittel-Forsch* **21**, 1209–1212, 1971.

10. Valenzuela A, *et al.*: Selectivity of silymarin on the increase of the glutathione content in different tissues of the rat. *Planta Medica* **55**, 420–422, 1989.

11. Muzes G, *et al.*: Effect of the bioflavonoid silymarin on the in vitro activity and expression of super oxide dismutase (SOD) enzyme. *Acta Physiol Hungarica* **78**, 3–9, 1991.

12. Fiebrich F and Koch H: Silymarin, an inhibitor of lipoxygenase. *Experientia* **35**, 148–150, 1979.

13. Fiebrich F and Koch H: Silymarin, an inhibitor of prostaglandin synthetase. *Experientia* **35**, 150–152, 1979.

14. Valenzuela A, *et al.*: Silymarin protection against hepatic lipid peroxidation induced by acute ethanol intoxication in the rat. *Biochem Pharm* **34**, 2209–2212, 1985.

15. Sonnenbichler J, *et al.*: Stimulatory effect of silibinin on the DNA synthesis in partially hepatectomized rat livers: Non-response in hepatoma and other malignant cell lines. *Biochem Pharm* **35**, 538–541, 1986.

16. Sonnenbichler J and Zetl I: Biochemical effects of the flavonolignan silibinin on RNA, protein and DNA synthesis in rat livers. In: *Plant Flavonoids in Biology and Medicine: Biochemical, Pharmacological, and Structure–Activity Relationships* (Cody V, Middleton E, and Harbourne JB, eds.). Alan R. Liss, New York, 1986, pp. 319–331.

17. Schopen RD, *et al.*: Searching for a new therapeutic principle. Experience with hepatic therapeutic agent legalon. *Med Welt* **20**, 888–893, 1969.

18. Schopen RD and Lange OK: Therapy of hepatoses. Therapeutic use of silymarin. *Med Welt* **21**, 691–698, 1970.

19. Sarre H: Experience in the treatment of chronic hepatopathies with silymarin. *Arzneimittel-Forsch* **21**, 1209–1212, 1971.

20. Canini F, *et al.*: Use of silymarin in the treatment of alcoholic hepatic steatosis. *Clin Ther* **114**, 307–314, 1985.

21. Salmi HA and Sarna S: Effect of silymarin on chemical, functional, and morphological alteration of the liver. A double-blind controlled study. *Scand J Gastroenterol* **17**, 417–421, 1982.

22. Scheiber V and Wohlzogen FX: Analysis of a certain type of 2×3 tables, exemplified by biopsy findings in a controlled clinical trial. *Int J Clin Pharm* **16**, 533–535, 1978.

23. Boari C, *et al.*: Occupational toxic liver diseases. Therapeutic effects of silymarin. *Min Med* **72**, 2679–2688, 1981.

24. Grossi F and Viola F: Protettori di membrana e silimarina nella terapia epatologica. *Cl Terap* **96**, 11–23, 1981.

25. Maneschi M, Tiberio C, and Cittadini E: Impegno metabolico dell'epatocita in gravidanza: Profilassi e terapia con un farmaco stabilizzante di membrana. *Clinica Terapeutica* **97**, 625–630, 1981.

26. Bulfoni A and Gobbato F: Evaluation of the therapeutic activity of silymarin in alcoholic hepatology. *Gaz Med Ital* **138**, 597–608, 1979.

27. Cavalieri S: A controlled clinical trial of Legalon in 40 patients. *Gaz Med Ital* **133**, 628–635, 1974.

28. Saba P, *et al.*: Therapeutic effects of silymarin in chronic liver diseases due to psychodrugs. *Gaz Med Ital* **135**, 236–251, 1976.

29. De Martis M, *et al.*: La silymaina, farmaco membranotropo: Ossevazioni cliniche e sperimentali. *Cl Terap* **81**, 333–362, 1977.

30. Szilard S, Szentgyorgyi D, and Demeter I: Protective effect of Legalon in workers exposed to organic solvents. *Acta Med Hung* **45**, 249–256, 1988.

31. Ferenci P, *et al.*: Randomized controlled trial of silymarin treatment in patients with cirrhosis of the liver. *J Hepatol* **9**, 105–113, 1989.

32. Deak G, *et al.*: Immunomodulator effect of silymarin therapy in chronic alcoholic liver diseases. *Orv Hetil* **131**, 1291–1292, 1295–1296, 1990.

33. Magliulo E, Gagliardi B, and Fiori GP: Results of a double blind study on the effect of silymarin in the treatment of acute viral hepatitis, carried out at two medical centres. *Med Klin* **73**, 1060–1065, 1978.

34. Berenguer J and Carrasco D: Double-blind trial of silymarin versus placebo in the treatment of chronic hepatitis. *Muench Med Wochenschr* **119**, 240–260, 1977.

35. Nassauto G, *et al.*: Effect of silibinin on biliary lipid composition. Experimental and clinical study. *J Hepatol* **12**, 290–295, 1991.

36. Kock HP, Bachner J, and Loffler E: Silymarin: Potent inhibitor of cyclic AMP phosphodiesterase. *Meth Find Exp Clin Pharm* **7**, 409–413, 1985.

37. Weber G and Galle K: The liver, a therapeutic target in dermatoses. *Med Welt* **34**, 108–111, 1983.

38. Schandalik R, Gatti G, and Perucca E: Pharmacokinetics of silybin in bile following administration of silipide and silymarin in cholecystectomy patients. *Arzneimittel-Forsch* **42**(7), 964–968, 1992.

39. Barzaghi N, *et al.*: Pharmacokinetic studies on IdB 1016, a silybin-phosphatidylcholine complex, in healthy human subjects. *Eur J Drug Metab Pharmacokinet* **15**(4), 333–338, 1990.

40. Mascarella S, *et al.*: Therapeutic and antilipoperoxidant effects of silybin-phosphatidylcholine complex in chronic liver disease: Preliminary results. *Curr Ther Res* **53**(1), 98–102, 1993.

41. Vailati A, *et al.*: Randomized open study of the dose-effect relationship of a short course of IdB 1016 in patients with viral or alcoholic hepatitis. *Fitoterapia* **44**(3), 219–228, 1993.

25
Mistletoe

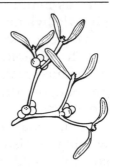

Key uses of European mistletoe:

- Cancer
- Impaired thymus gland activity
- Immune system enhancement
- High blood pressure

General description

Viscum album or European mistletoe is an evergreen, semiparasitic plant found on the branches of deciduous trees in Europe and northern Asia. The roots of the plant penetrate through the bark into the wood of the host tree. The green branches, 40–60 centimeters long, form pendent bushes with leaves that are opposite, leathery, yellow-green, and narrowly obovate. Pale yellow or green, inconspicuous flowers appear from March to May, the female developing into sticky white berries that ripen from September to November.[1,2]

Viscum is most commonly seen on old apple, ash, and hawthorn trees. Traditionally, mistletoe from oak has been the most widely used although it does not grow as well on oak as on the previously mentioned trees.[1,2]

Chemical composition

Viscum album contains a variety of pharmacologically active substances including alkaloids, polysaccharides, phenylpropanes, lignans, lectins, and "viscotoxins."[3–10] Other compounds found in viscum include a wide range of carbohydrates including simple sugars as well as polysaccharides;[5]

phenolic compounds such as flavonoids, caffeic acid, syringin, and eleuthero-sides;[6,10] sterols including beta-sitosterol, stigmasterol, and triterpenes; various amino acids as well as vasoactive amines including tyramine, phenylethylamine, and histamine; and fatty acids such as linoleic, palmitic, and oleic acids.[2]

The alkaloids isolated from viscum appear to be related to those found in the host plant.[3,4] For example, strychnine has been found in mistletoe growing on *Strychnos* species and caffeine in mistletoe growing on coffee plants.

Since pharmacologically active compounds appear to be concentrated within the mistletoe, different host trees providing different chemical constituents could be used for different therapeutic action.

In addition, the proteins/lectins are present only in aqueous (water) extracts, indicating therapeutic activity may differ from aqueous and alcoholic/aqueous (tincture) extracts. The alcoholic/aqueous extracts would also demonstrate considerably less toxicity.

History and folk use

Mistletoe was held in great reverence by the druids. Dressed in white robes, they would search for the sacred plant. When it was discovered, a great ceremony would ensue, with a druid finally separating the mistletoe from the oak with a golden knife. The druids believed that the mistletoe protected them from all evil, and the oaks on which it was seen growing were to be respected because of the wonderful cures that the priests were able to produce with it.[1]

Mistletoe's use was recorded in the Middle East, Africa, India, and Japan. Mistletoe was mentioned as an anticancer drug by Pliny, Dioscorides, and Galen.[3]

In 1720, an English physician, Sir John Colbatch, extolled the virtues of viscum in a pamphlet entitled "The Treatment of Epilepsy by Mistletoe." For many years mistletoe was used in the treatment of a variety of nervous system disorders including convulsions, delirium, hysteria, neuralgia, and nervous debility.[1,3]

Probably owing to toxicity, viscum use appeared to fall into some disrepute shortly after Colbatch's work. For many years it was used only in external preparations for the treatment of dermatitis. In 1906 a study demonstrating a blood pressure-lowering action in animals and humans was published. This appears to have restored viscum's medical prestige, initially in France and eventually throughout Europe.[3]

Pharmacology

Viscum album exhibits diverse pharmacological actions. The herb and various extracts have demonstrated blood pressure-lowering, vasodilating, cardiac depressant, sedative, antispasmodic, immune system stimulation, and anticancer activities.

Cardiovascular effects

Viscum has exhibited a variety of effects on components of the cardiovascular system.[3,11] Specifically, viscum has repeatedly demonstrated blood pressure-lowering action in animal studies.

The mechanism of action for its blood pressure-lowering effect is still not entirely clear, as no recent investigations exist. Viscum has been shown to affect blood pressure control centers in the brain.[11]

The blood pressure-lowering activity may depend on the form in which the mistletoe is administered and the host tree from which it was collected. Studies indicate aqueous extracts are more effective and the highest hypotensive activity was demonstrated by a macerate of leaves of mistletoe growing on willow, gathered in January.[11]

If nonprotein viscum components (e.g., flavonoids, phenol carboxylic acids, phenylpropanes, and lignans) were shown to possess blood pressure-lowering action, then alcoholic solutions (tinctures and fluid extracts) may be useful solutions. Alcoholic solutions would contain these compounds but no viscotoxins or lectins. However, as stated above, aqueous extracts appear to be more effective.

In Europe, several viscum preparations for hypertension exist. In fact, in Britain alone more than 150 different mistletoe preparations exist in the market place.[3] These preparations typically have small amounts of viscum in combination with other herbs thought to possess hypotensive action, for example, garlic, *Crataegus oxyacantha*, and *Tilia platyphyllos*.

Anticancer and immune system effects

Viscum preparations have been used clinically in Europe in the treatment of cancer since 1926, when a fermented product, Iscador, made from the crude, pressed-out juice of mistletoe was introduced as a therapeutic agent for cancer. Since that time numerous studies have been performed on this preparation as well as other viscum preparations and components.[12–29]

It must be pointed out that the standard route of administration of Iscador is by subdermal or intravenous injection. The effects of oral administration of Iscador, as well as other preparations and viscum compounds, have not been described.

Iscador and other fermented viscum preparations differ from nonfermented extracts in several ways that are thought to reduce toxicity and increase effectiveness.[12] Specifically, the major viscotoxin, mistletoe lectin I (ML I), is not found in Iscador.[13] Fermentation results in a rapid decrease in lectin concentration; it is thought that ML I breaks down during fermentation into its component A and B chains. These chains are less toxic than ML I, but retain important immunological properties.[14]

The pharmacological activity of Iscador is due to its viscum components rather than to other constituents. For example, Iscador contains lactobacilli (organisms assisting in the fermentation process), which possess immune-enhancing activity; but it has been clearly demonstrated that the viscum components—not the lactobacilli—are the components largely responsible for Iscador's activity, as unfermented plant juice has demonstrated comparable activity to Iscador.[15,16]

Iscador is most effective when administered near a tumor (i.e., locally), although systemic administration has also yielded positive results. On local administration, an inflammatory process ensues that promotes white blood cell infiltration and a "walling off" of the tumor.

The nonspecific host defense factors stimulated by *Viscum album* include enhanced macrophage phagocytic and cytotoxic activity;[12,16] neutrophilia;[12] increased thymic weight and enhanced cortical thymocyte activity and proliferation;[17,19] enhanced natural killer cell activity;[12,18,20] and increased antibody-dependent, cell-mediated cytotoxicity.[12,18] Iscador's effects on these immunological parameters have been confirmed in patients with cancer.[12,18]

Iscador stimulates the thymus gland, as demonstrated in several studies.[17,19] Its ability to stimulate the thymic cortex and accelerate the regeneration of hematopoietic cells following X-irradiation is much greater than anything else reported to date.[17] In addition, thymic lymphocytes became twenty-nine times more responsive to concanavalin A as a result of Iscador administration.

It is interesting to note that purified mistletoe lectins, in general, are not as active in experimental studies as crude preparations.[21,22] Presumably, a number of compounds in viscum act synergistically. It has also been proposed that alkaloid components are responsible for the maintenance of lectin structure and activity.[5] During isolation and purification procedures, alkaloid linkages are cleaved from the lectins, resulting in a loss of specifity for target molecules. Unfermented viscum preparations are typically toxic to tumor cells, owing to their higher concentrations of the viscotoxin ML I.[14,23,24]

Clinical applications

Early clinical investigations of viscum preparations (i.e., Iscador) were not very well documented. Owing to a lack of acceptable scientifically controlled clinical trials, the use of Iscador as a cancer treatment in Europe has remained controversial even though positive effects with Iscador in the postoperative treatment of lung, breast, colon, and cervical carcinomas have been shown in well-controlled studies to be of benefit.[25-27] At this time, mistletoe preparations appear most useful as adjuncts to standard therapy.

Recently, several clinical trials have been started that should provide greater information about mistletoe's effectiveness. In addition, new-generation mistletoe preparations standardized for mistletoe lectin I content (e.g., Eurixor) are emerging. This greater standardization offers significant advantages. Mistletoe lectin I is a potent inducer of cytokines such as interleukin 1, interleukin 6, and tumor necrosis factor (all of which enhance the immune system).

In one study the effect of Eurixor was examined in forty patients with advanced carcinoma of the breast. Along with standard chemotherapy [Vincristine Epirubicin Cyclophosphamide (VEC) regimen], twenty-one patients received mistletoe (treatment group) while nineteen patients were given a placebo (control group).[28] After the fourth cycle of chemotherapy, the treatment group had achieved higher (statistically significant) leukocyte levels ($p < 0.001$) compared to the control group. The treatment group had an average white blood cell count of 3,000 per cubic millimeter while the control group had an average count of 1,000 per cubic millimeter. Furthermore, patient responses concerning quality of life and anxiety revealed significantly better values in the treatment group than in the control group. These results show that adjuvant treatment with mistletoe extract, in this case Eurixor, is a valuable addition to standard chemotherapy for advanced breast cancer patients. The significance of these results is quite important, as advanced breast cancer carries with it a very poor prognosis.

Clearly, additional investigations on the pharmacology of *Viscum album* are needed. Specifically, it must be determined whether the effects noted in animals, and in patients receiving injectable viscum preparations, can be attained by oral administration.

In addition, greater clarification is needed in determining optimal viscum preparations. What host tree should be selected for which condition? What is the optimal harvesting time? In what form should the viscum be administered—crude herb? Aqueous or alcoholic extract? Fermented or nonfermented?

Viscum is undoubtedly one of the most complex medicinal herbs; yet, after examining currently available data, it can be said with much confidence that the future medicinal use of *Viscum album* is quite promising.

Dosage

The standard dose of *Viscum album*, based on the information given in the *British Herbal Pharmacopoeia*, is as follows (administer three times a day):[29]

- Dried leaves: 2–6 grams (or by infusion)
- Tincture (1:5) (45 percent alcohol): 1–3 milliliters
- Fluid extract (1:1) (25 percent alcohol): 0.5 milliliter
- Dried aqueous extract (4:1): 100–250 milligrams

Toxicity

Viscum album possesses significant toxicity. Historically, the berries have been regarded as significantly more toxic than the leaves and stems, despite the fact that they both contain similar toxic compounds. The reason the berries are considered more toxic probably stems from fatal poisonings in children that have occurred after ingestion of the berries.

Lethal doses of viscum lectins administered by various routes in mice produce two types of toxicity—a typical type characterized by death with globalized wasting away after 3 to 4 days and an atypical type characterized by immediate death caused by respiratory paralysis.[19]

The definitive toxicity of orally administered *Viscum album* or extracts of *Viscum album* has not yet been determined. As stated earlier, alcohol-based extracts contain virtually no viscum proteins. This implies that alcohol-based extracts are significantly less toxic. However, this also implies loss of activity, as much of the pharmacology of viscum relates to its protein content, especially its immune-enhancing activity.

It is interesting to note that the toxicity of Korean mistletoe, *Viscum album coloratum*, appears to be less than that of European mistletoe.[30,31] This species has also demonstrated anticancer effects, but the effects appear to be due to alkaloids rather than lectins.[5,30] Studies comparing Korean viscum extracts to European extracts, as well as their alkaloid components, have demonstrated that Korean mistletoe is more active in inhibiting cancer cells. In addition, fresh Korean mistletoe extracts exhibit greater activity compared to fermented extracts.[5,30] In future, Korean mistletoe may prove to be superior to European mistletoe.

References

1. Grieve M: *A Modern Herbal.* Dover Publications, New York, 1971, pp. 547–548.
2. Becker H: Botany of European mistletoe (*Viscum album* L.). *Oncology* **43**(Suppl. 1), 2–7, 1986.
3. Anderson LA and Phillippson JD: Mistletoe—the magic herb. From the Department of Pharmacognosy, School of Pharmacy, University of London, 1982.
4. Khwaja TA, Dias CB, and Pentecost S: Recent studies on the anticancer activities of mistletoe (*Viscum album*) and its alkaloids. *Oncology* **43**(Suppl. 1), 42–50, 1986.
5. Jordan E and Wagner H: Structure and properties of polysaccharides from *Viscum album* (L.). *Oncology* **43**(Suppl. 1), 8–15, 1986.
6. Wagner H, Jordan E, and Feil B: Studies on the standardization of mistletoe preparations. *Oncology* **43**(Suppl. 1), 16–22, 1986.
7. Franz H, Ziska P, and Kindt A: Isolation and properties of three lectins from mistletoe (*Viscum album* L.). *Biochem J* **195**, 481–484, 1981.
8. Olsnes S, *et al.*: Isolation and characterisation of viscumin, a toxic lectin from *Viscum album* L. (mistletoe). *J Biol Chem* **257**, 13263–13270, 1982.
9. Petricic J and Kalogjera Z: Isolation of glucosides from mistletoe leaves (*Viscum album* L.). *Acta Pharm Jugosl* **30**, 163, 1980.
10. Wagner H, *et al.*: Phenylpropanes and lignanes of *Viscum album*. *Planta Medica* **2**, 102, 1986.
11. Petkov V: Plants with hypotensive, antiatheromatous and coronary dilatating action. *Am J Chin Med* **7**, 197–236, 1979.
12. Hajto T: Immunomodulating effects of Iscador: A *Viscum album* preparation. *Oncology* **43**(Suppl. 1), 51–65, 1986.
13. Jordan E and Wagner H: Detection and quantitative determination of lectins and viscotoxins in mistletoe preparations. *Arzneimittel-Forsch* **36**, 428–433, 1986.
14. Ribereau-Gayon G, *et al.*: Comparison of the effects of fermented and unfermented mistletoe preparations on cultured tumor cells. *Oncology* **43**(Suppl. 1), 35–41, 1986.
15. Bloksma N, *et al.*: Cellular and humoral adjuvant activity of a mistletoe extract. *Immunobiology* **156**, 309–319, 1979.
16. Bloksma N, *et al.*: Stimulation of humoral and cellular immunity by viscum preparations. *Planta Medica* **46**, 221–227, 1982.
17. Rentea R, Lyon E, and Hunter R: Biological properties of Iscador: A *Viscum album* preparation. *Lab Invest* **44**, 43–48, 1981.
18. Hajto T and Lanzrein G: Natural killer and antibody-dependent cell-mediated cytotoxicity activities and large granular lymphocyte frequencies in *Viscum album*-treated breast cancer patients. *Oncology* **43**, 93–97, 1986.
19. Nienhaus J, Stoll M, and Vester F: Thymus stimulation and cancer prophylaxis by *Viscum* proteins. *Experientia* **26**, 523–525, 1970.
20. Hamprecht K, *et al.*: Mediation of human NK-activity by components in extracts of *Viscum album*. *Int J Immunopharm* **9**, 199–209, 1987.
21. Evans MR and Preece AW: *Viscum album*—a possible treatment for cancer? *Bristol Med Chir J* **88**, 17–20, 1973.
22. Klamerth O, Vester F, and Kellner G: Inhibitory effects of a protein complex from *Viscum album* on fibroblasts and HeLa cells. *Z Physiol Chem* **349**, 863–864, 1968.
23. Hulsen H, Doser C, and Mechelke F: Differences in the in vitro effectiveness of preparations produced from mistletoes of various host trees. *Arzneimittel-Forsch* **36**, 433–436, 1986.
24. Hulsen H and Mechelke F: The influence of a mistletoe preparation on suspension cell cultures of human leukemia and human myeloma cells. *Arzneimittel-Forsch* **32**, 1126–1127, 1982.
25. Leroi R: Nachbehandling des operierten Mammakarzinoms mit *Viscum album*. *Helv Chir Acta* **44**, 403–414, 1977.
26. Leroi R: Neuere resultate aus dem gebeit del malignombehandlung mit *Viscum album*. *Erfahrungsheilkunde* **25**, 41–54, 1977.

27. Salzer G and Havelec L: Rezidivprophyl bei operierten bronchuskarzinoompatiienten mit mistelpra-parat Iscador. *Onkologie* **1**, 264–267, 1978.
28. Heiny BM: Adjuvant treatment with standardized mistletoe extract reduces leukopenia and improves the quality of life of patients with advanced carcinoma of the breast getting palliative chemotherapy (VEC regimen). *Krebsmedizin* **12**, 3–14, 1991.
29. British Herbal Medicine Association, Scientific Committee: *British Herbal Pharmacopoeia.* British Herbal Medicine Association, Cowling, England, 1983, pp. 235–236.
30. Khwaja TA, *et al.*: Isolation of biologically active alkaloids from Korean mistletoe *Viscum album, coloratum. Experientia* **36**, 599–600, 1980.
31. Manjikian S, Pentecost S, and Khwaja TA: Isolation of cytotoxic proteins form *Viscum album, coloratum. Proc Am Assoc Cancer Res* **27**, 266, 1986.

26
Onion

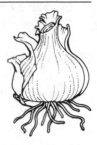

Key uses of onion:

- Infections
- Elevated cholesterol levels
- High blood pressure
- Diabetes

General description

Numerous forms and varieties of onion, a perennial or biennial herb, are cultivated worldwide. The part used is the fleshy bulb. Common varieties are White Globe, Yellow Globe, and Red Globe.

As onion is chiefly regarded as a food or seasoning, this raises questions about the medicinal effects of other common vegetables and/or seasonings. Many common vegetables may have significant pharmacological effects that have not yet been investigated. A diet rich in vegetables, spices, or seasonings may offer protection and possibly treatment for a wide variety of diseases, particularly the major chronic degenerative diseases such as heart disease, diabetes, and cancer.

Chemical composition

Onion, like garlic, contains a variety of organic sulfur compounds, including S-methylcysteine sulfoxide, trans-S-(1-propenyl)cysteine sulfoxide, S-propyl-cysteine sulfoxide, and dipropyl disulfide. Onion also contains the enzyme alliinase, which is released when the onion is cut or crushed, causing conversion of trans-S-(1-propenyl)cysteine sulfoxide to the so-called lacrimatory (crying) factor (propanethiol S-oxide). Other constituents include flavonoids (primarily quercetin), phenolic acids (e.g., caffeic, sinapic, and p-coumaric acids), sterols, saponins, pectin, and volatile oils.[1,2]

History and folk use

Although not as valued a medicinal agent as garlic, onion has been used almost as widely. Like garlic, onion is used as an antispasmodic, carminative, diuretic, expectorant, stomachic, anthelmintic, and antiinfective agent. It has been applied externally as a rubefacient and poultice, giving relief in skin diseases and insect bites.[1–3]

Pharmacology

Onion and garlic, owing to their similar chemical composition, have many of the same pharmacological effects. There are, however, some significant differences that make one more advantageous than the other under certain conditions.

Antimicrobial activity

Although onion does exhibit some antibacterial, antifungal, and anthelmintic (intestinal worm killing) activity, it is not nearly as potent as garlic.[2,4] Although this suggests that garlic may be better indicated in cases of infection, onions can usually be consumed in larger quantity than garlic, which may increase the concentration of antimicrobial compounds to approximate those of garlic.

Cardiovascular effects

Like garlic, onions and onion extracts have been shown to decrease blood lipid levels, prevent clot formation, and lower blood pressure in several clinical studies.[5–7] Garlic and onion consumption is associated with lower levels of cholesterol and triglycerides, and a lower incidence of heart disease.[8,9] As the quantity of onion consumed in the study by Sainani et al. was so much larger than that of garlic (600 grams of onion per week compared with 50 grams of garlic), it could be argued that onion consumption was the major determinant.

Diabetes

Onion's ability to lower blood sugar levels is comparable to that of the prescription drugs tolbutamide and phenformin, which are often given to diabetics.[10,11] The active blood sugar-lowering principle in onion is believed to be allyl propyl disulfide, although other constituents, such as flavonoids, may play a significant role as well. Experimental and clinical evidence suggests that allyl propyl disulfide lowers glucose by competing with insulin (also a disulfide molecule) for degradation sites in the liver, thereby increasing the life span of insulin. Other mechanisms, such as increased liver metabolism of glucose or increased insulin secretion, have also been proposed.

Antiasthmatic action

Onion has been used historically as an antiasthmatic agent.[2,3] Its action in asthma is due to its ability to inhibit the production of compounds that cause the bronchial muscle to spasm, along with its ability to relax the bronchial muscle.[12,13]

Antitumor effects

An onion extract was found to destroy tumor cells in test tubes and to arrest tumor growth when tumor cells were implanted in rats.[14] The onion extract was shown to be unusually nontoxic, since a dose as high as forty times that of the dose required to kill the tumor cells had no adverse effect on the host. Another species of *Allium*, *Allium ascalonicum* (shallots), exhibits significant activity against leukemia in mice.[15]

Dosage

Dosages of the various forms are typically equivalent to 2 to 5 ounces of fresh onion (roughly ¼ to 1 cup of chopped onions) per day.

Toxicity

There are no significant reports of toxicity caused by onions.

References

1. Leung A: *Encyclopedia of Common Natural Ingredients Used in Food, Drugs, and Cosmetics.* John Wiley & Sons, New York, 1980, pp. 246–247.
2. Raj KP and Patel NN: Onion—the vegetable drug. *Indian Drugs* **14**, 156–160, 1977.
3. Vahora SB, Rizwan M, and Khan JA: Medicinal uses of common Indian vegetables. *Planta Medica* **23**, 381–393, 1973.
4. Elnima EI, *et al.*: The antimicrobial activity of garlic and onion extracts. *Pharmazie* **38**, 747–748, 1983.
5. Louria DB, *et al.*: Onion extract in treatment of hypertension and hyperlipidemia: A preliminary communication. *Curr Ther Res* **37**, 127–131, 1985.
6. Mittal MM, *et al.*: Effects of feeding onion on fibrinolysis, serum cholesterol, platelet aggregation and adhesion. *Indian J Med Sci* **24**, 144–148, 1972.
7. Menon IS: Fresh onions and blood fibrinolysis. *Br Med J* **i**, 845, 1969.
8. Norwell DY and Tarr RS: Garlic, vampires, and CHD. *Osteopath Ann* **11**, 546–549, 1983.
9. Sainani GS, *et al.*: Effect of dietary garlic and onion on serum lipid profile in Jain community. *Indian J Med Res* **69**, 776–780, 1979.
10. Bever BO and Zahnd GR: Plants with oral hypoglycemic action. *Q J Crude Drug Res* **17**, 139–196, 1979.
11. Sharma KK, *et al.*: Antihyperglycemic effect of onion: Effect on fasting blood sugar and induced hyperglycemia in man. *Indian J Med Res* **65**, 422–429, 1977.
12. Dorsch W, *et al.*: Antiasthmatic effects of onion extracts—detection of benzyl- and other isothiocyanates in mustard oils as antiasthmatic compounds of plant origin. *Eur J Pharmacol* **107**, 17–24, 1985.
13. Dorsch W and Weber J: Prevention of allergen-induced bronchial constriction in sensitized guinea pigs by crude alcohol onion extract. *Agents Action* **14**, 626–630, 1984.
14. Nepkar DP, *et al.*: Cytotoxic effect of onion extract on mouse fibrosarcoma 180 A cells. *Indian J Exp Biol* **19**, 598–600, 1981.
15. Caldes G and Prescott B: A potential antileukemic substance present in *Allium ascalonicum. Planta Medica* **23**, 99–100, 1973.

27

Panax ginseng

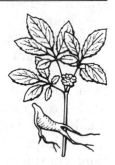

Key uses of *Panax ginseng*:

- Fatigue
- Recovery from illness
- Stress
- Diabetes

General description

Panax ginseng, also referred to as Korean or Chinese ginseng, is a small perennial plant that originally grew wild in the damp woodlands of northern
China, Manchuria, and Korea. Wild ginseng is now extremely rare. However,
ginseng is a widely cultivated plant, especially in Korea, but also in Russia,
China, and Japan. In addition to *Panax ginseng* C.A. Meyer, four other closely
related species are often used: *Panax quinquefolium* (American ginseng), *Panax
japonicum* C.A. Meyer (Japanese ginseng), *Panax pseudoginseng* (Himalayan
ginseng), and *Panax trifolium. Panax ginseng* C.A. Meyer is the most widely
used and most extensively studied species. Its pharmacology is the major
focus of this chapter.[1,2]

Fully mature, Korean ginseng is an herbaceous plant with a tap root,
five-lobed palmate leaves, and greenish-white flowers arranged in an
umbel. In its first year, ginseng bears only a single leaf with three leaflets.
In the second year, it bears a single leaf with five leaflets, and in its third
year it produces two leaves with five leaflets. It usually starts flowering in
its fourth year, while bearing three leaves. The roots of the cultivated plant
are 3–4 millimeters in diameter and 10 centimeters long, while the roots
of wild plants may attain 10 centimeters in diameter and a length of 50–
60 centimeters.

Ginseng is often processed in two forms: white and red ginseng. White ginseng is the dried root, whose peripheral skin is frequently peeled off. Red ginseng is the steamed root, which shows a caramel-like color.[2]

There are many types and grades of ginseng and ginseng extracts depending on the source, age, and parts of the root used, and on the methods of preparation. Old, wild, well-formed roots are the most valued, while rootlets of cultivated plants are considered the lowest grade. For largely economic purposes, most ginseng in the American market place is derived from the lowest grade root, diluted with excipients, blended with adulterants, or totally devoid of active constituents, that is, ginsenosides.[3]

High-quality roots and extracts are available, however. These preparations consist of the main root of plants between 4 and 6 years of age, or extracts that have been standardized for ginsenoside content and ratio to ensure optimum pharmacological effect.

Chemical composition

Ginseng contains at least thirteen different triterpenoid saponins, collectively known as ginsenosides, which are believed to be the most important active constituents. The usual concentration of ginsenosides is between 1 and 3 percent. The ginsenosides have been designated R0, Rb1, Rb2, Rb3, Rc, Rd, Re, Rf, 20-gluco-Rf, Rg1, and Rg2. The ginsenosides differ primarily in their sugar groups that are attached to the steroid molecule.

Ginsenosides Rb1, Rb2, Rc, Re, and Rg1 are present in significant concentrations in Korean ginseng. In contrast, American ginseng (*Panax quinquefolium*) contains primarily ginsenosides Rb1 and Re, and does not contain ginsenosides Rb2, Rf, or, in some instances, Rg1. This difference allows for easy detection of species, using high-pressure liquid chromatography.[1,2,4]

Other components include panacene, a volatile oil; free and glucoside-bound sterols (e.g., beta-sitosterol and its beta-glucoside); polyacetylene derivatives B-elemene and panaxinol; 8–32 percent starch; low molecular weight polysaccharides; pectin; vitamins (e.g., thiamin, riboflavin, B_{12}, nicotinic acid, pantothenic acid, and biotin); 0.1–0.2 percent choline; minerals; simple sugars (glucose, fructose, sucrose, maltose, trisaccharides, etc.); and various flavonoids.[1,2,4]

Although it had been reported that ginseng contains large amounts of germanium (i.e., 300 parts per million [ppm]), a follow-up study using highly sensitive (detection limit of 1 part per billion [ppb]), flameless atomic absorption spectrometry combined with solvent extraction demonstrated that the highest concentration of germanium measured in samples of ginseng purchased in the Osaka market was only 6 ppb.[5] More research is needed to determine accurately the germanium content of herbal medicines, as the reported concentrations vary widely. Such low levels suggest that a connection between the pharmacology of ginseng and its germanium content is unlikely.

History and folk use

Perhaps the most famous medicinal plant of China, ginseng is generally administered alone or in combination with other herbs to restore the *yang* quality. It is also used as a tonic for its revitalizing properties, especially after a long illness. Ginseng is utilized in folk medicine for amnesia, anemia, anorexia, asthma, atherosclerosis, boils, bruises, cachexia, cancer, convulsions, cough, debility, diabetes, diuretic, divination, dysentery, dysmenorrhea, dyspepsia, enterorrhagia, epilepsy, epistaxis, fatigue, fear, fever, forgetfulness, gastritis, hangover, headache, heart, hemoptysis, hemorrhage, hyperglycemia, hypertension, hypotension, impotence, insomnia, intestinal complaints, longevity promotion, malaria, menorrhagia, nausea, neurasthenia, palpitations, polyuria, pregnancy, puerperium, rectocele, rhinitis, rheumatism, shortness of breath, sores, spermatorrhea, splenitis, swelling, and vertigo. It has been used as an alterative, anodyne, aperitif, aphrodisiac, cardiotonic, carminative, emetic, estrogenic, expectorant, gonadotropic, nervine, sedative, sialagogue, stimulant, stomachic, and tranquilizer.[1,2]

As can be seen from this list, ginseng is used to treat most conditions, reflecting a broad range of nutritional and medicinal properties.

Pharmacology

Since the 1950s, a great amount of research has been conducted worldwide to determine whether the therapeutic properties attributed to ginseng belong in the realm of legend or fact. Unfortunately, inconsistent results (due mostly to different procedures in the preparation of extracts, use of nonmedicinal parts of the plant, use of adulterants, and lack of quality control in the ginseng used) have made determination of ginseng's true properties difficult. Nonetheless, enough good research does exist to indicate that ginseng possesses pharmacological activity consistent with its near-legendary status, especially when high-quality extracts, standardized for active constituents, are used.

Ginseng exerts numerous pharmacological effects in humans and laboratory animals, including a general stimulatory effects during stress; a decrease in sensitivity to stress; an increase in mental and physical capacity for work; improved endocrine system function; prevention of radiation sickness, neurosis, and cancer; enhanced protein synthesis and cell reproduction; improved glucose control in humans and diabetic (alloxan-induced) rats; modulation of various immune system parameters; and lowering of serum cholesterol; and protection of the liver from toxic substances.[1,2,4,5] Some of these actions are discussed in greater detail below.

Adaptogenic activity

Ginseng was originally investigated for its adaptogen qualities. An *adaptogen* as defined in 1957 by the Russian pharmacologist I. Brekhman, is a substance that (1) must be innocuous and cause minimal disorders in the physiological functions of an organism, (2) must have a nonspecific action (i.e., it should increase resistance to adverse influences by a wide range of physical, chemical, and biochemical factors), and (3) usually has a normalizing action irrespective of the direction of the pathological state.[2] According to tradition and scientific evidence, ginseng possesses this kind of equilibrating, tonic, antistress action, and so the term adaptogen is quite appropriate in describing its general effects.[1,2,6,7]

Antifatigue (mental and physical) activity

Some of the first studies of ginseng's adaptogenic activities were performed during the late 1950s and early 1960s by Brekhman and Dardymov in Russia, and by Petkov in Bulgaria.[6–10]

In one of Brekhman's experiments, Soviet soldiers given an extract of ginseng ran faster in a 3-kilometer race than those given a placebo. In another, radio operators tested after administration of ginseng extract transmitted text significantly faster and with fewer mistakes than those given placebo. These and similar results found by European researchers, who demonstrated improvement in human physical and mental performance after the administration of ginseng extracts, prompted researchers to confirm the results in experimental models using mice.[2,6–8]

In perhaps the best known of these experiments, mice were subjected to swimming in cold water or running up an apparently endless rope to determine if ginseng could increase the time to exhaustion. The results indicated that ginseng possessed significant antifatigue activity, as a clear dose-dependent increase in time to exhaustion was noted in mice receiving ginseng.[2,7,11–14] In one study, the time to exhaustion was increased up to 183 percent in the mice given ginseng 30 minutes prior to exercising, compared with controls.[7]

Experimental animal studies indicated that much of the antifatigue action of ginseng was due to the stimulant effect of ginseng on the central nervous system (i.e., the brain and spinal cord). Ginseng ingestion improves energy metabolism during prolonged exercise.[9–14]

Ginseng has been shown to increase muscle stimulation by nerve impulses,[15] modify brain-wave tracings,[9] improve metabolic activity in the brain,[16] and affect the hypothalamo–pituitary–adrenal axis (discussed below), all of which could be largely responsible for ginseng's antifatigue activity on mental and physical performance. The brain activity of ginseng is essentially different from that of the usual stimulants. While stimulants are active under most situations, ginseng reveals its stimulatory action only under the challenge of stress.[16] An analogy often used is that stimulants are like pushing on the gas pedal, whereas ginseng is like giving the engine a tune-up.

On the physical level, ginseng's antifatigue properties appear to be closely related to its ability to spare glycogen utilization in exercising muscle.[13] Glycogen is the storage form of glucose (a sugar) in muscle. Exercise physiologists have clearly established that during prolonged exercise, the development of fatigue is closely related to the depletion of glycogen stores and the build-up of lactic acid, both in skeletal muscle and the liver. If an adequate supply of oxygen is available to the working muscle, fatty acids are the preferred source for energy production, thus sparing utilization of muscle glycogen. The greater the ability to conserve body glycogen stores by using fatty acids as the energy source, the greater the amount of time to exhaustion. Ginseng enhances the transformation of fatty acids to energy during prolonged exercise, thereby sparing muscle glycogen stores.[13]

In summary, the mental and physical antifatigue effects of ginseng have been demonstrated in both animal studies and double-blind, clinical trials in humans.[1,2,17,18]

Antistress activity

Stress is a term widely used in our fast-paced society. The daily demands placed on us often build and accumulate to a point at which it is almost impossible to cope. Job pressures. Family arguments. Financial pressures. Deadlines. These are common examples of "stressors." Actually, a stressor may be almost anything that creates a disturbance, including exposure to heat or cold, environmental toxins, toxins produced by microorganisms, physical trauma, and, of course, strong emotional reactions.

Ginseng has been shown to enhance the ability to cope with various stressors, both physical and mental. Presumably, this is a result of delaying the alarm phase (fight or flight) response in Selye's classic model of stress. Ginseng's antistress effects are due largely to its effect on the adrenal glands.[4,13,19–22] The adrenal glands maintain the balance of many bodily functions during stress by secreting several important hormones.

Italian researchers have studied the effect of a standardized ginseng extract on rats exposed to cold.[4,19] The ginseng extract significantly counteracted body temperature decline without affecting blood glucose or cortisone levels. In a group of rats that had their adrenal glands surgically removed, the ginseng extract had no significant effects. This study demonstrated that ginseng's antistress effect depends on adrenal function.

It appears, on the basis of extensive research, that ginseng acts through nervous system control mechanisms to adjust metabolic and functional systems that maintain the body during the challenge of stresses.[11,12] This is very similar to how a thermostat maintains temperature.

Researchers have demonstrated that ginseng acts predominantly on the hypothalamus or pituitary to promote secretion of adrenocorticotropic hormone (ACTH), a hormone that promotes the manufacture and secretion of adrenal hormones. This release of ACTH and associated pituitary substances (e.g., endorphins, enkephalins, and beta-lipoprotein) is probably responsible for many of the antifatigue and antistress actions of ginseng, as ACTH and adrenal hormones have been shown to bind directly to brain tissue, thereby increasing mental activity during stress.

From a practical perspective, it is apparent that ginseng exerts a balancing effect on the hypothalamic–pituitary–adrenal axis by adjusting metabolic and functional systems governing hormonal control of homeostasis. This assists the body's response to the challenge of stress and therefore is indicated when disruption of this axis is apparent.

Ginseng may prove especially effective in restoring normal adrenal function and preventing adrenal atrophy associated with corticosteroid administration. In rats, ginseng has been found to inhibit cortisone-induced adrenal and thymic atrophy.[23] Ginseng, like Chinese thoroughwax,[24] curcumin,[25] licorice,[26] and Siberian ginseng,[27] appears to be very useful in restoring adrenal function in patients taking corticosteroids.

Diabetes

Ginseng, used either alone or in combination with other herbs, has long been used in the treatment of diabetes. Ginseng has confirmed hypoglycemic (i.e., blood sugar-lowering) activity. The ginseng components responsible for this effect include five types of substances: five glycans (polysaccharides designated panaxans A to E), adenosine, a carboxylic acid, a peptide, and a fraction designated DPG-3-2.[28-32] The ginsenosides are without hypoglycemic action. This fact highlights the importance of using crude, standardized extracts containing all active principles rather than isolated ginsenosides or pure ginsenoside extracts.

It is interesting to note that ginseng will increase serum cortisol levels in nondiabetic individuals, whereas in patients with diabetes serum cortisol levels will be reduced.[33] Because cortisol, an adrenal hormone, antagonizes insulin, this is presumably a beneficial effect in the diabetic. In addition, the ginseng compound DPG-3-2 exhibits hypoglycemic action or provokes insulin secretion only in diabetic and glucose-loaded normal mice; it has no effect on normal mice fed a standard diet.[28] This again demonstrates ginseng's nonspecific balancing effect, which is baffling to researchers accustomed to investigating compounds with consistent pharmacological effects.

Reproductive effects

Although ginseng is claimed to be a "sexual rejuvenator," human studies supporting this belief are scanty. Ginseng has, however, been shown to promote the growth of the testes and increase sperm formation in rabbits, accelerate the growth of the ovary and enhance ovulation in frogs, stimulate egg laying in hens, increase gonadal weight in both male and female rats, and increase sexual activity and mating behavior in male rats.[34] These animal study results seem to support ginseng's use as a fertility and virility aid.

In other experimental animal studies, ginseng has been shown to increase testosterone levels while decreasing prostate weight.[35] This suggests that ginseng should have favorable effects in the treatment of benign prostatic enlargement; however, no clinical trials have yet been reported.

Anticancer properties

Long-term oral administration of ginseng to newborn mice has been shown to reduce the incidence and also inhibit the proliferation of tumors induced by various chemical carcinogens, including DMBA, urethane, and aflatoxin B_1.[36-38] These results are consistent with more recent population studies (discussed in Clinical Applications, below).

Cell proliferating and antiaging effects

Ginseng has a dual effect on cell growth: it stimulates cell division in an adequate nutritional environment, but it acts to inhibit cell growth under adverse conditions.[39] Furthermore, ginseng has yielded impressive results in lengthening the life span of cells in culture.[40]

This enhancement of cellular proliferation and function occurs in a variety of cell types (epithelial, hepatic, lymphocyte, fibroblast, thymic, neural, etc.) and may be a result of potentiation of nerve growth factor by ginsenosides.[3,41] Nerve growth factor levels typically decline with age.

These results indicate a potential use of ginseng in healing virtually all tissue types as well as inhibiting the aging process.

Immunostimulating effects

Ginseng possesses immunostimulating activity as evidenced by its ability to enhance antibody responses, cell-mediated immunity, natural killer cell activity, the production of interferon, and lymphocyte and reticuloendothelial system proliferative and phagocytic functions.[42,43] The clinical significance of these effects is discussed below.

Ginseng has been shown to prevent viral infections in experimental animals,[44] presumably a result of the combination of effects listed above.

Perhaps the most important of ginseng's immune-enhancing effects is its ability to enhance the activity of the cells of the reticuloendothelial system. This system is composed of white blood cells known as macrophages, which filter the blood and lymph by engulfing and destroying bacteria, viruses, worn-out red blood cells, and other particulate waste matter. Macrophages are found in highest concentrations in the liver, spleen, and lymph nodes. Ginseng stimulates these cells, thus increasing host defense capacity immensely.

Note: Do not use large dosages of ginseng during an acute infection. Highly concentrated ginseng can inhibit some immune functions.[42,45,46]

Liver effects

Obviously, any adaptogenic substance must impact the liver, owing to the liver's central role in metabolic and detoxification reactions. Ginseng affects the liver in several ways. As previously mentioned, ginseng enhances the activity of macrophages. The liver contains specialized macrophages known as Kupffer cells.[4,19] As these cells are responsible for removing toxins and debris from the circulation, increasing their activity could have a profound effect.

Ginseng has also been shown to increase protein synthesis in the liver.[3,47-49] Because protein synthesis is often reduced in the elderly, enhancement of hepatic protein synthesis by ginseng would be extremely beneficial. However, these results have yet to be confirmed by clinical studies.

Ginseng has also been shown to reverse diet-induced fatty liver in animals and to protect the liver from damage by chemicals.[50,51]

The clinical indications of these hepatic actions of ginseng are quite broad and support its general tonic/adaptogen properties.

Clinical applications

The therapeutic applications of ginseng are varied, owing to its adaptogenic qualities. Ginseng can be applied as a general tonic, especially in debilitated and feeble individuals; whenever fatigue or lack of vigilance is apparent; to increase mental and physical performance; to prevent the negative effects of stress and enhance the body's response to stress; to offset the negative effects of cortisone; as a supportive therapy in the treatment of diabetes; in conditions involving the reproductive system, including decreased sperm counts, testicular atrophy or hypofunction, and other organic causes of male infertility, and ovarian atrophy or hypofunction, absence of menstruation, and other organic causes of female infertility; to enhance liver function; and to protect against radiation damage. The more pertinent clinical applications are discussed below.

Antifatigue and antistress

In addition to several Russian studies,[6] other studies showing the antifatigue and antistress effects of ginseng have been published.[1,2,17,18]

In one double-blind, clinical study, nurses who had switched from day to night duty rated themselves for competence, mood, and general well being, and were given a test for mental and physical performance; blood cell counts and blood chemistry evaluations were also performed. The group-administered ginseng demonstrated higher scores in competence, mood parameters, and mental and physical performance when compared with those receiving a placebo.[17]

In a double-blind, cross-over study on university students in Italy, ginseng extract was compared with placebo in various tests of mental performance. A favorable effect of ginseng relative to baseline performance was observed in attention, mental arithmetic, logical deduction, integrated brain–body function, and reaction time to sounds. It is interesting to note that in the course of the trial the students taking ginseng reported a greater sensation of well being.[18]

From a practical standpoint, ginseng's antifatigue and antistress properties may be useful whenever fatigue or the negative effects of stress are apparent. Athletes, in particular, may derive some benefit from ginseng use.

Diabetes

Ginseng is indicated as a supportive therapy in the treatment of diabetes, both for its hypoglycemic effect as well as for its ability to decrease atherosclerosis (see below).

Cardiovascular effects

Ginseng has paradoxical effects on blood pressure. It appears that at low doses it possesses a hypertensive (blood pressure-increasing) effect, but when administered at larger doses a hypotensive (blood pressure-lowering) effect is noted.[52] Accordingly, it has been reported useful in the treatment of high blood pressure in humans, but it has also been shown to have blood pressure-raising effects as well.[53] This latter effect must be kept in mind when administering ginseng to both normotensive and hypertensive individuals.

Ginseng administered to human subjects with hyperlipidemia (elevated lipids or fats in the blood) has been shown to reduce total serum cholesterol, triglyceride, and fatty acid levels, while raising serum high-density lipoprotein (HDL) cholesterol levels (HDL cholesterol has been shown to actually protect against atherosclerosis). Platelet adhesiveness was also decreased.[50]

These results in humans confirmed earlier studies on rats fed high-cholesterol diets.[54,55] The mechanism of action appears to be through accelerated degradation, conversion, and excretion of cholesterol and triglyceride.

From a clinical perspective, it appears that ginseng may offer some protection against atherosclerotic disease, further supporting its use as a general tonic. Ginseng may also regulate blood pressure.

Menopause

Ginsenosides exert an estrogen-like action on the vaginal epithelium. This effect is significant enough to prevent the atrophic vaginal changes associated with postmenopause and other menopausal symptoms.[36] It should be noted that breast tenderness has been reported by women taking ginseng (see Toxicity, below).

Reproductive system enhancement

Therapeutic indications of *Panax ginseng* involving the reproductive system (on the basis of historical use and experimental evidence) include decreased sperm counts, testicular atrophy or hypofunction, and other organic causes of male infertility; and ovarian atrophy or hypofunction, absence of menstruation, other organic causes of female infertility, and menopause.

Cancer prevention

Regular ginseng consumption may protect against cancer. In a large population study,[56] the risk of developing cancer was significantly lower among people who consumed ginseng on a regular basis. Interestingly, ginseng extract and powder were shown to be more effective than fresh sliced ginseng, ginseng juice, or ginseng tea in reducing the cancer risk. A statistically highly significant dose–response relationship between ginseng intake and cancer risk was observed—that is, the higher the intake of ginseng the lower the risk of cancer. These results support the preventive effects of ginseng suggested by earlier animal studies.

Immune system enhancement

The regular ingestion of ginseng by individuals with mild immune deficiency (frequent colds) may reduce the risk of viral infection. Use in this manner is consistent with the historical use of ginseng by debilitated individuals. *Panax ginseng* has been shown to enhance many immune functions, including natural killer cell activity, interferon production, and macrophage activity. In one clinical study, three groups (twenty healthy volunteers each) were treated with capsules containing either 100 milligrams of an aqueous extract of *Panax ginseng* (group A), 100 milligrams of lactose (group B), and with capsules containing 100 milligrams of a standardized extract (4 percent ginsenoside content) of *Panax ginseng* (group C).[57] All of the volunteers took one capsule every 12 hours for 8 weeks. Blood samples were drawn before the beginning of treatment and at weeks 4 and 8. Immune parameters examined included the following: the ability of neutrophils to move toward chemical toxins, the ability of neutrophils to engulf and destroy particulate matter (phagocytosis index, PHI), total lymphocytes (T3), helper T cell (T4) subset, suppressor T cell (T8) subset, and natural killer (NK) cells. Improvements noted: improved neutrophil function; increased PHI; increased total lymphocytes, increased helper T cells, increased T4/T8 subset, and increased NK cell activity. Although most of these effects were evident by 4 weeks, consistently greater effects were noted after 8 weeks, implying that ginseng's beneficial effects on the immune system are cumulative.

Radiation protection

In experimental studies, ginseng has been shown to offer some protection against harmful radiation and to hasten recovery from radiation damage.[58,59] In the wake of ever-increasing environmental radiation contamination, ginseng use may be an appropriate preventive measure.

Dosage

The appropriate dose of ginseng depends on the ginsenoside content; if an extract or ginseng preparation contains high concentrations of ginsenosides (and presumably other active components), a lower dose will suffice.

Currently, almost no quality control is imposed on ginseng products marketed in the United States. Independent research and published studies clearly document the tremendous variation in ginsenoside content of commercial preparations.[3,4] In fact, the majority of products on the market contain only trace amounts of ginsenosides, and many formulations contain no ginseng at all. This has led to several problems, ranging from toxicity reactions[60] (discussed below) to lack of medicinal effect. The widespread disregard for quality control in the health food industry has done much to tarnish the reputation of ginseng as well as other important herbal treatments.

The use of standardized ginseng preparations is recommended to ensure sufficient ginsenoside content, consistent therapeutic results, and reduced risk of toxicity. Products should be standardized by their ginsenoside content. The typical dose (taken one to three times daily) for general tonic effects should contain a saponin content of at least 10 milligrams of ginsenoside Rg1, with a ratio of Rg1 to Rb1 of 1:2. For example, for a high-quality ginseng root extract containing 5 percent ginsenosides, the dose would be 200 milligrams; for a standardized *Panax ginseng* extract containing an 10 percent saponin content calculated as ginsenoside Rg1, the standard dose would be 100 milligrams. The standard dose for high-quality ginseng root is in the range of 4 to 6 grams daily.

As each individual's response to ginseng is unique, care must be taken to observe possible ginseng toxicity (see below). It is best to begin at lower doses and increase gradually. The Russian approach for long-term administration is to use ginseng cyclically for a period of 15–20 days, followed by a 2-week interval without any ginseng.

Toxicity

The problem of quality control makes ginseng toxicology difficult to address. This is exemplified by an article entitled "Ginseng Abuse Syndrome" (published in 1979 in the *Journal of the American Medical Association [JAMA]*.[60] In this article, a number of side effects are reported, including hypertension, euphoria, nervousness, insomnia, skin eruptions, and morning diarrhea.

Given the extreme variation in quality of ginseng in the American market place and the use both of nonmedical parts of the plant and of adulterants, it is not surprising that side effects were noted. None of the commercial preparations used in the trial had been subjected to controlled analysis. Furthermore, the species of ginseng used included *Panax ginseng*, *Panax quinquefolium*, *Eleutherococcus senticosus*, and *Rumex hymenosepalus* in a variety of different forms, that is, roots, capsules, tablets, teas, extracts, cigarettes, chewing gum, and candies.

It is virtually impossible to derive any firm conclusions from the data presented in the *JAMA* article. The author's final words do, however, seem sensible and appropriate:

> An important caveat is that these GAS [ginseng abuse syndrome] effects are neither uniformly negative nor uniformly predictable. Nevertheless, long-term ingestion of large amounts of ginseng should be avoided, as even a panacea can cause problems if abused.

Studies performed on standardized extracts of ginseng have demonstrated the absence of side effects as well as the lack of mutagenic or teratogenic effects.[4,12,61,62]

Women taking *Panax ginseng* may experience breast tenderness. Reducing the dose, or stopping the treatment altogether, will cause the pain to cease.[63,64]

References

1. Hikino H: Traditional remedies and modern assessment: The case of ginseng. In: *The Medicinal Plant Industry* (Wijeskera ROB, ed.). CRC Press, Boca Raton, FL, 1991, pp. 149–166.
2. Shibata S, *et al.*: Chemistry and pharmacology of *Panax*. *Econ Med Plant Res* **1**, 217–284, 1985.
3. Liberti LE and Marderosian AD: Evaluation of commercial ginseng products. *J Pharm Sci* **67**, 1487–1489, 1978.
4. Bombardelli E: *Ginseng: Chemical, Pharmacological, and Clinical Profile.* Indena S.p.A., Milan, Italy, 1989.
5. Minmo Y, *et al.*: Determination of germanium in medicinal plants by atomic absorption spectrometry with electrothermal atomization. *Chem Pharm Bull* **28**, 2687–2691, 1980.
6. Brekhman II and Dardymov IV: New substances of plant origin which increase nonspecific resistance. *Annu Rev Pharmacol* **9**, 419–430, 1969.
7. Brekhman II and Dardymov IV: Pharmacological investigation of glycosides from ginseng and *Eleutherococcus*. *Lloydia* **32**, 46–51, 1969.
8. Petkov W: Pharmacological studies of the drug *P. ginseng* C.A. Meyer. *Arzniemittel-Forsch* **9**, 305–311, 1959.

9. Petkov W: The mechanism of action of *P. ginseng. Arzneimittel-Forsch* **11**, 288–295, 418–422, 1961.
10. Petkov W: Effect of ginseng on the brain biogenic monoamines and 3',5'-AMP system. Experiments in rats. *Arzneimittel-Forsch* **28**, 388–393, 1978.
11. Saito H, Yoshida Y, and Takagi K: Effect of *Panax ginseng* root on exhaustive exercise in mice. *Jpn J Pharmacol* **24**, 119–127, 1974.
12. Kaku T, *et al.*: Chemicopharmacological studies on saponins of *Panax ginseng* C.A. Meyer. *Arzneimittel-Forsch* **25**, 539–547, 1975.
13. Avakia EV and Evonuk E: Effects of *Panax ginseng* extract on tissue glycogen and adrenal cholesterol depletion during prolonged exercise. *Planta Medica* **36**, 43–48, 1979.
14. Sterner W and Kirchdorfer AM: Comparative work load tests on mice with standardized ginseng extract and a ginseng containing pharmaceutical preparation. *Z Gerontol* **3**, 307–312, 1970.
15. Hong SA, *et al.*: The effects of ginseng saponin on animal behavior. Proceedings of the 1st International Ginseng Symposium, 1975, Korean Ginseng Research Institute, pp. 33–44.
16. Samira MMH, *et al.*: Effect of the standardized ginseng extract G115 on the metabolism and electrical activity of the rabbit's brain. *J Int Med Res* **13**, 342–348, 1985.
17. Hallstrom C, Fulder S, and Carruthers M: Effect of ginseng on the performance of nurses on night duty. *Comp Med East West* **6**, 277–282, 1982.
18. D'Angelo L, *et al.*: A double-blind, placebo controlled clinical study on the effect of a standardized ginseng extract on psychomotor performance in healthy volunteers. *J Ethnopharmacol* **16**, 15–22, 1986.
19. Bombardelli E, Cirstoni A, and Lietti A: The effect of acute and chronic (*Panax*) ginseng saponins treatment on adrenal function; biochemical and pharmacological. Proceedings 3rd International Ginseng Symposium, 1980, Korean Ginseng Research Institute, pp. 9–16.
20. Fulder SJ: Ginseng and the hypothalamic-pituitary control of stress. *Am J Chin Med* **9**, 112–118, 1981.
21. Hiai S, Yokoyama H, and Oura H: Features of ginseng saponin-induced corticosterone secretion. *Endocrinol Jpn* **26**, 737–740, 1979.
22. Hiai S, *et al.*: Evaluation of corticosterone secretion-inducing effects of ginsenosides and their prosapogenins and sapogenins. *Chem Pharm Bull* **31**, 168–174, 1983.
23. Tanizawa H, *et al.*: Study of the saponin of *P. ginseng* C.A. Meyer. I. Inhibitory effect on adrenal atrophy, thymus atrophy and the decrease of serum potassium ion concentration induced by cortisone acetate in unilaterally adrenalectomized rats. *J Pharm Soc Jpn* **101**, 169–173, 1981.
24. Hiai S, *et al.*: Stimulation of the pituitary-adrenocortical axis by saikosaponin of *Bupleuri radix. Chem Pharm Bull* **29**, 495–499, 1981.
25. See Chapter 37—Turmeric.
26. See Chapter 24—Licorice.
27. Farnsworth NR, *et al.*: Siberian ginseng (*Eleutherococcus senticosus*): Current status as an adaptogen. *Econ Med Plant Res* **1**, 156–215, 1985.
28. Ng TB and Yeung HW: Hypoglycemic constituents of *Panax ginseng. Gen Pharmacol* **6**, 549–552, 1985.
29. Waki I, *et al.*: Effects of a hypoglycemic component of ginseng radix on insulin biosynthesis in normal and diabetic animals. *J Pharm Dyn* **5**, 547–554, 1982.
30. Konno C, *et al.*: Isolation and hypoglycaemic activity of panaxans A, B, C, D and E, glycans of *Panax ginseng* roots. *Planta Medica* **51**, 434–436, 1984.
31. Kimura M, *et al.*: Pharmacological sequential trials for the fractionation of components with hypoglycemic activity in alloxan diabetic mice from ginseng radix. *J Pharm Dyn* **4**, 402–409, 1981.
32. Kimura M, *et al.*: Effects of hypoglycemic components in ginseng radix on blood insulin level in alloxan diabetic mice and on insulin release from perfused rat pancreas. *J Pharm Dyn* **4**, 410–417, 1981.
33. Yamamoto M and Uemura T: Endocrinological and metabolic actions of *P. ginseng* principles. Proceeding 3rd International Ginseng Symposium, 1980, Korean Ginseng Research Institute, pp. 115–119.
34. Kim C, *et al.*: Influence of ginseng on mating behavior of male rats. *Am J Chin Med* **4**, 163–168, 1976.
35. Fahim WS, *et al.*: Effect of *Panax ginseng* on testosterone level and prostate in male rats. *Arch Androl* **8**, 261–263, 1982.
36. Punnonen R and Lukola A: Oestrogen-like effect of ginseng. *Br Med J* **281**, 1110, 1980.
37. Yun TK, Yun YS, and Han IW: Anticarcinogenic effect of long-term oral administration of newborn mice exposed to various chemical carcinogens. *Cancer Detect Prev* **6**, 515–525, 1983.
38. Lee KD and Huemer RP: Antitumoral activity of *Panax ginseng* extracts. *Jpn J Pharmacol* **21**, 299–302, 1971.
39. Fulder SJ: The growth of cultured human fibroblasts treated with hydrocortisone and extracts of the medicinal plant *Panax ginseng. Exp Gerontol* **12**, 125–131, 1977.
40. Saito H: Ginsenoside-Rb1 and nerve growth factor (*P. ginseng*). Proceeding 3rd International Ginseng Symposium, 1981, Korean Ginseng Research Institute, pp. 181–185.

41. Yamamoto M, *et al.*: Stimulatory effect of ginsenosides on DNA, protein and lipid synthesis in bone marrow. *Arzneimittel-Forsch* **28**, 2238–2241, 1978.
42. Jie YH, Cammisuli S, and Baggiolini M: Immunomodulatory effects of *Panax ginseng* C.A. Meyer in the mouse. *Agents Actions* **15**, 386–391, 1984.
43. Gupta S, *et al.*: *Panax*: A new mitogen and interferon producer. *Clin Res* **28**, 504A, 1980.
44. Singh VK, Agarwal SS, and Gupta BM: Immunomodulatory activity of *Panax ginseng* extract. *Planta Medica* **51**, 462–465, 1984.
45. Chong SKF, *et al.*: In vitro effect of *Panax ginseng* on phytohaemagglutinin-induced lymphocyte transformation. *Int Arch Allergy Appl Immun* **73**, 216–220, 1984.
46. Yeung HW, Cheung K, and Leung KN: Immunopharmacology of Chinese medicine. I. Ginseng induced immunosuppression in virus infected mice. *Am J Chin Med* **10**, 44–54, 1982.
47. Oura H, Hiai S, and Seno H: Synthesis and characterization of nuclear RNA induced by *Radix ginseng* extract in rat liver. *Chem Pharm Bull* **19**, 1598–1605, 1971.
48. Oura H, *et al.*: Effect on ginseng on endoplasmic reticulum and ribosome. *Planta Medica* **28**, 76–88, 1975.
49. Oura H, *et al.*: Effect of radix ginseng on serum protein synthesis. *Chem Pharm Bull* **20**, 980–986, 1972.
50. Hikino H, *et al.*: Antihepatotoxic actions of ginsenosides from *Panax ginseng* roots. *Planta Medica* **52**, 62–64, 1985.
51. Oh JS, *et al.*: The effect of ginseng on experimental hypertension. *Korean J Pharmacol* **4**, 27–31, 1968.
52. Siegel RK: Ginseng and high blood pressure. *JAMA* **243**, 32, 1980. [Letter]
53. Yamamoto M, *et al.*: Serum HDL-cholesterol-increasing and fatty liver-improving action of *Panax ginseng* in high cholesterol diet-fed rats with clinical effect on hyperlipidemia in man. *Am J Chin Med* **11**, 96–101, 1983.
54. Yamamoto M and Kumagai S: Plasma lipid lowering actions of ginseng saponins and mechanisms of the action. *Am J Chin Med* **11**, 84–87, 1983.
55. Joo CN: The preventative effect of Korean (*P. ginseng*) saponins on aortic atheroma formation in prolonged cholesterol-fed rabbits. Proceeding 3rd International Ginseng Symposium, 1980, Korean Ginseng Research Institute, pp. 27–36.
56. Yun TK, *et al.*: A case-control study of ginseng intake and cancer. *Int J Epidemiol* **19**, 871–876, 1990.
57. Scaglione F, *et al.*: Immunomodulatory effects of two extracts of *Panax ginseng* C.A. Meyer. *Drugs Exp Clin Res* **16**, 537–542, 1990.
58. Ben-Hur E and Fulder S: Effect of *P. ginseng* saponins and *Eleutherococcus* S. on survival of cultured mammalian cells after ionizing radiation. *Am J Chin Med* **9**, 48–56, 1981.
59. Yonezawa M: Restoration of radiation injury by intraperitoneal injection of ginseng extract in mice. *J Radiat Res* **17**, 111–113, 1976.
60. Siegel RK: Ginseng abuse syndrome. *JAMA* **241**, 1614–1615, 1979.
61. Hess FG, *et al.*: Effects of subchronic feeding of ginsenoside extract G115 in beagle dogs. *Food Chem Toxicol* **21**, 95–97, 1983.
62. Hess FG, *et al.*: Reproduction study in rats of ginseng extract G115. *Food Chem Toxicol* **20**, 189, 1982.
63. Palmer BV, Montgomery ACV, and Monteiro JCMP: Ginseng and mastalgia. *Br Med J* **i**, 1284, 1978. [Letter]
64. Koriech OM: Ginseng and mastalgia. *Br Med J* **i**, 1556, 1978. [Letter]

28
Peppermint and other mints

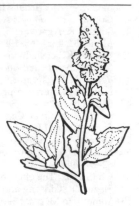

Key uses of peppermint and other mints:

Oral:

- Gallstones
- Irritable bowel syndrome
- Common cold

Topical:

- Musculoskeletal pain

General description

Peppermint is a natural hybrid of garden spearmint (*Mentha spicata*) and water mint (*Mentha aquatica*). First described in England in 1696, peppermint and other members of the mint family grow almost everywhere.[1] The two most popular varieties are white peppermint (*Mentha piperita* var. *officinalis*) and black peppermint (*Mentha piperita* var. *vulgaris*). Both are typical members of the mint family, that is, herbs with square stems, horizontal rhizomes, and lanceolated leaves with a serrated edge. Black peppermint has deep red stems with purplish-tinged dark green leaves, while the white has green stems with lighter green leaves. Both varieties produce purple flowers during the summer months. For medicinal effects, the aerial portion of the plant is the most widely used.

Chemical composition

The major medicinal component of peppermint is its volatile oil, which can be found in concentrations of up to 1.5 percent in the herb, but is usually present in the 0.3 to 0.4 percent range. The principal components of the oil

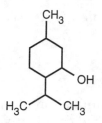

Figure 28.1 Menthol

are menthol (29–28 percent; Figure 28.1), menthone (20–31 percent), and menthyl acetate (3–10 percent), although analysis of peppermint oil will typically show more than forty different compounds. Most of the volatile oil components are terpenoids.[1]

The proportion of menthol relative to other components in peppermint oil depends on climate and latitude, as well as on the maturity of the plant. Pharmaceutical-grade peppermint oil is produced by distilling the fresh aerial parts of the plant harvested at the very beginning of the flowering cycle. The oil is standardized to contain not less than 44 percent free menthol and a minimum of 5 percent esters calculated as menthyl acetate. The ketone component (calculated as menthone) usually ranges from 15 to 30 percent, with the remainder of the oil being composed of various terpenoids.[1] Menthol is also synthesized by hydrogenation of thymol.

Other components of peppermint herb that may contribute to its medicinal effects include polymerized polyphenols (19 percent of dry weight), flavonoids (12 percent), tocopherols, carotenes, betaine, and choline.[2]

History and folk use

Although peppermint was not officially recognized until the seventeenth century, mints have been used for their medicinal effects for thousands of years. Records from the ancient Egyptian, Greek, and Roman eras show that other members of the mint family, particularly spearmint (*Mentha spicata*), were used.[1]

Peppermint is used medicinally to treat indigestion and intestinal colic, as well as colds, fever, and headache.

Pharmacology

The pharmacology of peppermint focuses almost entirely on its menthol components. Peppermint and menthol possess carminative, antispasmodic, and choleretic properties, and are also used as an external analgesic and nasal decongestant.

Carminative effects

Carminatives promote the elimination of intestinal gas. Peppermint and peppermint oil are well-accepted carminatives. Although the exact mechanism of action has not been determined, one proposed mechanism is by relaxation of the esophageal sphincter, leading to released gas pressure in the stomach.[3]

Antispasmodic effects

The mechanism behind peppermint oil's antispasmodic effects has recently been determined. Researchers believe that peppermint oil's inhibition of isolated smooth muscle contractions occurs via blockage of calcium influx into the muscle cells.[4,5] Researchers hypothesize that the clinical effectiveness of peppermint oil in the treatment of irritable bowel syndrome results from inhibition of the hypercontractility of intestinal smooth muscle, thereby returning the muscle to its proper tone.

Choleretic effects

Choleretics stimulate the flow of bile. Menthol and related terpenes exert a choleretic effect as well as improve the solubility of the bile.[6–10]

External analgesic effects

The external analgesic and counterirritant effects of menthol are well accepted. When applied to the skin, peppermint oil or menthol stimulates the nerves that perceive cold, while simultaneously depressing those for pain. The initial cooling effect is followed by a period of warmth.

Clinical applications

Peppermint oil is the most extensively used of all the volatile oils. Pharmaceutical preparations often utilize peppermint oil or menthol for its therapeutic and flavoring properties. For example, it is used extensively in antacid products and irritant laxatives both for its flavor and its therapeutic effects. The same is true for its inclusion in mouthwash preparations and after-dinner mints.

The pharmacological effects of peppermint and peppermint oil are useful in a number of clinical situations; the most notable include irritable bowel syndrome, intestinal colic, gallstones, musculoskeletal pain, and the common cold.

Irritable bowel syndrome

Peppermint oil has been used to treat irritable bowel syndrome for many years. Irritable bowel syndrome can include a combination of any of the following symptoms: abdominal pain and distension; more frequent bowel movements with pain, or relief of pain with bowel movements; constipation or diarrhea; excessive production of mucus in the colon; symptoms of indigestion such as flatulence, nausea, or anorexia; and varying degrees of anxiety or depression. Hypercontractility of intestinal smooth muscle is one of the central findings in irritable bowel syndrome. As described above, peppermint oil inhibits the hypercontractility of intestinal smooth muscle, making it useful in cases of irritable bowel syndrome as well as intestinal colic.

The preferred delivery of peppermint oil in the treatment of irritable bowel syndrome is via enteric-coated preparations, which prevent the oil from being released in the stomach. Without enteric coating, peppermint oil tends to produce heartburn. With the coating, the peppermint oil travels to the small and large intestines, where it relaxes intestinal muscles. Several clinical studies have demonstrated that enteric-coated peppermint oil is quite effective in reducing the abdominal symptoms of irritable bowel syndrome.[11-13]

Gallstones

A formula containing menthol and related terpenes (menthone, pinene, borneol, cineole, and camphene) helps dissolve gallstones, as shown in several studies.[6-10] This nonsurgical approach to gallstone removal offers an effective alternative to surgery and has been shown to be safe even when consumed for prolonged periods of time (up to 4 years). Terpenes, like menthol, help dissolve gallstones by reducing bile cholesterol levels while increasing bile acid and lecithin levels in the gallbladder. As menthol is the major component of this formula, peppermint oil, especially if enteric-coated, may offer similar benefits.

The common cold

Menthol and peppermint oil are often employed in the treatment of the common cold, as components of topical nasal decongestants, cough and throat lozenges, ointments, salves, and inhalants. Whether the use of these products is of benefit has not been proven in clinical studies. However, their popularity appears to be based on their ability to ease breathing during the common cold. The best method of use for menthol or peppermint oil may be by applying commercial preparations on the upper chest during periods of rest, so that the vapors can be inhaled continuously.

Peppermint tea may also be of benefit during the common cold. Peppermint, as well as other members of the mint family, has demonstrated significant antiviral activity as well as a mild diaphoretic effect.[14] The most active antiviral components, the polyphenols, are concentrated in the tea.[2] Peppermint oil inhibits the growth of Newcastle disease virus, herpes simplex virus, and vaccina virus.

External analgesic

Menthol and related substances can be used as counterirritants in the treatment of arthritis, fibromyositis, tendinitis, and other inflammatory conditions involving the musculoskeletal system.

Dosage

Peppermint is most widely used as a tea (infusion), on its own or in combination with other herbs. The infusion is usually prepared with 1 to 2 teaspoons of the dried leaves per 8 ounces of water.

The dosage of peppermint oil administered in an enteric-coated capsule for the treatment of irritable bowel syndrome is 1–2 capsules (0.2 milliliter per capsule) three times daily between meals. This dosage is also appropriate in the treatment of gallstones.

Menthol as an external analgesic should be applied as a cream or ointment (containing 1.26–16 percent menthol) to the affected area no more than three or four times daily.

Toxicity

Peppermint herb is generally regarded as safe when used as a tea; however, hypersensitivity reactions have been reported. Adverse reactions to enteric-coated peppermint oil capsules are rare, but can include hypersensitivity reactions (skin rash), heartburn, bradycardia, and muscle tremor.

When applied topically, peppermint oil or menthol can induce contact dermatitis and hypersensitivity reactions. The likelihood of developing such a reaction increases when heating pads are used in conjunction with topically applied preparations containing menthol.[15]

The LD_{50} (50 percent lethal dose) of menthol in rats is 3,280 milligrams per kilogram. The fatal oral dose in humans is 1 gram per kilogram. Repeated high dose feeding of rats for 28 days with peppermint oil produced signs of dose-related brain lesions, but the dosage (40 milligrams per kilogram) far exceeds that used in humans.[1,16,17]

References

1. Briggs C: Peppermint: Medicinal herb and flavoring agent. *Can Pharm J* **129**, 89–92, 1993.
2. Duband F, *et al.*: The aromatic and polyphenolic composition of peppermint (*Mentha piperita*) tea. *Ann Pharm Franc* **50**, 146–155, 1992.
3. Giachetti D, Taddei E, and Taddei I: Pharmacological activity of essential oils on Oddi's sphincter. *Planta Medica* **54**, 389–392, 1988.
4. Hills JM and Aaronson PI: The mechanism of action of peppermint oil in gastrointestinal smooth muscle. *Gastroenterology* **101**, 55–65, 1991.
5. Hawthorne M, *et al.*: The actions of peppermint oil and menthol on calcium channel dependent processes in intestinal, neuronal, and cardiac preparations. *J Aliment Pharmacol Therap* **2**, 101–108, 1988.
6. Hordinsky BZ: Terpenes in the treatment of gallstones. *Minnesota Med* **54**, 649–651, 1971.
7. Bell GD and Doran J: Gallstone dissolution in man using an essential oil preparation. *Br Med J* **278**, 24, 1979.
8. Doran J, Keighley RB, and Bell GD: Rowachol—a possible treatment for cholesterol gallstones. *Gut* **20**, 312–317, 1979.
9. Ellis WR and Bell GD: Treatment of biliary duct stones with a terpene preparation. *Br Med J* **282**, 611, 1981.
10. Somerville KW, *et al.*: Stones in the common bile duct: Experience with medical dissolution therapy. *Postgrad Med J* **61**, 313–316, 1985.
11. Somerville K, Richmond C, and Bell G: Delayed release peppermint oil capsules (Colpermin) for the spastic colon syndrome: A pharmacokinetic study. *Br J Clin Pharmacol* **18**, 638–640, 1984.
12. Rees W, Evans B, and Rhodes J: Treating irritable bowel syndrome with peppermint oil. *Br Med J* **ii**, 835–836, 1979.
13. Lech U, *et al.*: Treatment of irritable bowel syndrome with peppermint oil. A double-blind study with a placebo. *Ugeskr Laeger* **150**, 2388–2389, 1988.
14. Kerrman EC and Kucera L: Antiviral substances in plants of the mint family (III). Peppermint (*Mentha piperita*) and other mint plants. *Proc Soc Exp Biol Med* **124**, 874–875, 1967.
15. Heng MC: Local necrosis and interstitial nephritis due to topical methyl salicylate and menthol. *Cutis* **39**, 442–444, 1987.
16. Olsen P and Thorup I: Neurotoxicity in rats dosed with peppermint oil and pulegone. *Arch toxicol* **7**(Suppl.), 408–409, 1984.
17. Thorup I, *et al.*: Short-term toxicity study in rats dosed with peppermint oil. *Toxicol Lett* **19**, 211–215, 1983.

29
Pygeum

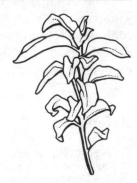

Key uses of *Pygeum*:

- Benign prostatic hyperplasia
- Prostatitis
- Male infertility
- Impotence

General description

Pygeum africanum, an evergreen tree native to Africa, can grow to a height of 120–150 feet. It has pendulous branches with thick, oblong-shaped, leather-like, mat-colored leaves and creamy white flowers. The fruit (drupe) resembles a cherry when ripe. The dark-brown to gray bark of the trunk is the part used for medicinal purposes.

Chemical composition

The major active components of the bark are fat-soluble compounds such as pentacyclic triterpenes, sterolic triterpenes, fatty acids, and esters of ferulic acid (Figure 29.1). The pentacyclic triterpenic components include ursolic acid (Figure 29.2), oleanolic acid, crataegolic acid, and their derivatives. The sterolic fraction is composed mainly of beta-sitosterol and beta-sitosterone (Figure 29.3). The fatty acids are twelve to twenty-four carbons in length (C_{12} to C_{24} and the important ferulic acid esters are those bound to *n*-tetracosanol and *n*-docosanol.[1–4]

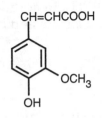

Figure 29.1 Ferulic acid

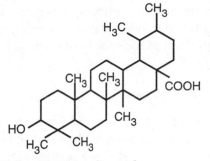

Figure 29.2 Ursolic acid

History and folk use

The powdered bark of *Pygeum africanum* is used by the natives of tropical Africa as a treatment for urinary disorders. It is often given with palm oil or milk.

Pharmacology

Pharmacological screening of various extracts prepared with solvents of differing degrees of polarity indicates that the highest activity is found in lipophilic extracts. This finding is interesting in light of pygeum's historical administration in oil-based media (palm oil or milk). Virtually all of the pharmacological research has featured a pygeum extract standardized to contain 14 percent triterpenes including beta-sitosterol and 0.5 percent *n*-docosanol. This extract has been extensively studied in both experimental animal studies and clinical trials with humans.

The primary target organ for pygeum's effects in males is the prostate. The three major active components of pygeum appear to exert different, yet

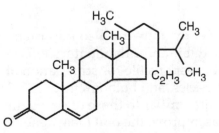

Figure 29.3 Beta-sitosterone

complementary, effects in benign prostatic hyperplasia (BPH). In addition, pygeum has been shown to enhance the secretions of the prostate and bulbourethral glands, both in terms of quantity and quality.

Ferulic acid esters

The esters of ferulic acid act primarily on the endocrine system. Studies in animals have shown that n-docosanol reduces levels of leutinizing hormone and testosterone while raising adrenal secretion of both adrenal androgens and corticosteroids.[5,6] n-Docosanol also significantly reduces serum prolactin levels. This reduction in prolactin is quite significant, as prolactin increases the uptake of testosterone and increases the synthesis of dihydrotestosterone within the prostate. The accumulation of testosterone within the prostate and its subsequent conversion to the more potent dihydrotestosterone is thought to be the major contributing factor to the hyperplasia of the prostatic cells observed in BPH.[7] Although traces of n-docosanol are present in pygeum, the esterification with ferulic acid results in greater bioavailability and activity.[2,4,8]

Fat-soluble components in pygeum exert a systemic cholesterol-lowering action and reduce the intraprostatic cholesterol content.[8] Breakdown products of cholesterol accumulate in prostate tissue affected with either BPH or cancer.[7] These metabolites of cholesterol initiate degeneration of prostatic cells, which can promote prostatic enlargement. Drugs that lower cholesterol levels exert a favorable influence on BPH, preventing the accumulation of cholesterol in the prostatic cells and limiting subsequent formation of damaging cholesterol metabolites. The lowering of intraprostatic cholesterol content is an important aspect of the pharmacology of pygeum.

The sterolic fraction is also endowed with competitive action against testosterone accumulation within the prostate. In addition, the sterols of pygeum have also been shown to reduce inflammation by preventing the intraprostatic formation of inflammatory prostaglandins.[8,9]

Other components

Other components of pygeum are also important. For example, the pentacyclic triterpenes exhibit antiinflammatory effects within the prostatic epithelium and may be responsible for stimulation of the secretory cells of the prostate, seminal vesicles, and bulbourethral glands.[8–10] And finally, the fatty acids components are similar to those of saw palmetto and may exert similar effects as well as improve the oral bioavailability of other components of the lipophilic extract.

Clinical applications

The pharmacological actions of the standardized pygeum extract support its use in prostate disorders, BPH in particular. Adding further support are the results from numerous clinical trials including more than 600 patients (Table 29.1).[11-34] Consistently, these studies demonstrate that pygeum effectively reduces the symptoms and clinical signs of BPH, especially in early cases.

Table 29.1 Results of the most significant open and double-blind studies of the last 20 years on outpatients treated with *Pygeum africanum* for 1 to 3 months[a]

				Percentage of patients showing reduction in:				
Ref.	Dosage (mg/day)	Days	No. of patients	Dysuria	Nocturia	Frequency	Res. Urine	Pros. Vol.
Open trials								
11	100	30	25	80	80	80	80	NC
12	100	30	25	72	NC	72	NC	NC
13	100	45	27	60	NC	71	NC	NC
14	75	60	20	64	NC	64	NC	NC
15	75	90	52	69	NC	NC	NC	NC
16	75	50	33	60	57	57	NC	—
17	50	30	55	85	85	85	NC	20
18	100	50	25	72	72	72	NC	25
19	100	60	19	90	85	70	20	NC
20	100	90	23	72	72	72	72	NC
21	75	90	35	94	94	94	94	—
22	100	75	30	—	—	—		
Double-blind trials								
23	100	60	60	77	70	57	23	—
24	75	60	50	88	88	88	88	88
25	100	60	77	85	NC	NC	NC	NC
26	100	60	30	—	—	48	—	—
27	150	45	47	—	70	—	76	NC
28	150	90	20	80	80	80	NC	NC
29	100	45	120	—	78	45	65	NC
30	100	45	104	89	89	89	NC	NC
31	200	60	39	75	75	75	NC	NC
32	200	60	20	—	—	—	—	—
34	200	60	40	70	70	70	70	70

[a]—, not measured; NC, no change

However, it must be pointed out that improvement is largely symptomatic, as the reduction in size of the prostate or the residual urine content of the bladder is modest. The results of the clinical trials on pygeum are given below, followed by a discussion of some of the most important aspects of these studies.

Benign prostatic hyperplasia

One of the major findings in evaluating the effectiveness of pygeum in BPH has been the high level of response to placebo. This is well demonstrated in one of the larger double-blind studies.[29] Similar to the results in other double-blind studies, pygeum extract was shown to be statistically superior to a placebo in reducing the major symptoms of BPH (nocturnal frequency, difficulty in starting micturition, and incomplete emptying of the bladder). However, there was a high percentage of response to the placebo (Table 29.2). It seems that simply taking a capsule provides relief to many sufferers.

Another study[28] highlights the importance of double-blind studies that feature objective and subjective findings. In the study, both patients and physicians rated the placebo and pygeum extract to be effective in improving subjective symptoms of daytime frequency, nighttime frequency, weak stream, after dribbling, hesitation, and interruption of flow. However, objective variables such as analysis of urine flow, frequency, and ultrasound measurements clearly demonstrated the superiority of pygeum over placebo.

One of the shortcomings of some of the clinical research on pygeum is the lack of objective measures such as urine flow rate (in milliliters per second), residual urine content, and prostate size. Studies that have used objective measurements show some good results.[34] For example, in one open trial, thirty patients with BPH given 100 milligrams of the pygeum extract per day for 75 days demonstrated significant improvements in objective parameters: maximum flow rate increased from 5.43 to 8.20 milliliters per second and the residual urine volume dropped from 76 to 33 milliliters.[22]

Table 29.2 Patients responding to placebo and pygeum

Symptom	Placebo group	Pygeum group
Nocturia	26/52 = 50%	44/56 = 78%
Daytime frequency	16/50 = 33%	27/54 = 50%
Incomplete voiding	14/40 = 35%	21/32 = 66%
Dribbling	15/34 = 44%	13/33 = 39%
Urine flow rate	11/43 = 26%	21/38 = 55%

Pygeum versus saw palmetto

The standardized fat-soluble extract of saw palmetto berries is another popular herbal treatment for BPH (see Chapter 34—Saw Palmetto). In a double-blind study comparing pygeum extract with an extract of saw palmetto, the saw palmetto extract produced a greater reduction of symptoms and was better tolerated.[35] In addition, the improvement in objective parameters, especially urine flow rate and residual urine content, is better in the clinical studies with saw palmetto. However, there may be circumstances in which pygeum is more effective than saw palmetto. For example, saw palmetto does not produce the same effects as pygeum on prostate secretion. Although the two extracts have somewhat overlapping mechanisms of actions, they can be used in combination.

Male infertility and impotence

Pygeum may improve fertility in cases in which diminished prostatic secretion plays a significant role. Pygeum has been shown to increase prostatic secretions and improve the composition of the seminal fluid.[36–38] Specifically, pygeum administration to men with decreased prostatic secretion has led to increased levels of total seminal fluid plus increases in alkaline phosphatase and protein. Pygeum appears to be most effective in cases in which the level of alkaline phosphatase activity is reduced (i.e., less than 400 international units [IU] per cubic centimeter) and there is no evidence of inflammation or infection (i.e., absence of white blood cells or IgA). The lack of IgA in the semen is a good predictor of clinical success. In one study, the patients with no IgA in the semen demonstrated an alkaline phosphatase increase from 265 to 485 IU per cubic centimeter.[36] In contrast, those subjects with IgA showed only a modest increase from 213 to 281 IU per cubic centimeter.

Among patients with BPH or prostatitis, pygeum extract can improve the capacity to achieve an erection, as determined by nocturnal penile tumescence in a double-blind clinical trial.[39] BPH and prostatitis are often associated with erectile dysfunction and other sexual disturbances. By improving the underlying condition, pygeum can presumably improve sexual function.

Dosage

The dosage of a lipophilic extract of *Pygeum africanum* standardized to contain 14 percent triterpenes including beta-sitosterol and 0.5 percent *n*-docosanol is 100 to 200 milligrams per day in divided doses. The crude herb is not used.

Toxicity

Acute and chronic toxicity tests in the rat and mouse have shown that the standardized extract of *Pygeum africanum* bark is nontoxic. Increasing the dosage from 1 to 6 grams per kilogram in the mouse and from 1 to 8 grams per kilogram in the rat caused no deaths within 48 hours. In chronic toxicity studies, dosing the animals with 60 to 600 milligrams per kilogram for 11 months did not produce any negative effects.

In human clinical trials, pygeum extract also demonstrated no significant toxicity. The most common side effect is gastrointestinal irritation resulting in symptoms ranging from nausea to severe stomach pains; however, the presence of these side effects rarely results in discontinuation of therapy.

References

1. Longo R and Tira S: Steroidal and other components of *Pygeum africanum* bark. *Il Farmaco* **38**, 288–292, 1982.
2. Martinelli EM, Seraglia R, and Pifferi G: Characterization of *Pygeum africanum* bark extracts by HRGC with computer assistance. *HRC & CC* **9**, 106–110, 1986.
3. Pierini N: Identification and determination of *n*-docosanol in *Pygeum africanum* bark extract and in medicinal specialties containing them. *Boll Chim Farm* **121**, 27–34, 1982.
4. Uberti E: HPLC analysis of *n*-docosyl ferulate in *Pygeum africanum* extracts and pharmaceutical formulations. *Fitotherapia* **41**, 342–347, 1990.
5. Muntzing J, *et al.*: Direct and indirect effects of docosanol, the active principle in Tadenan, on the rat prostate. *Invest Urol* **17**, 176–180, 1979.
6. Thieblot L: Preventive and curative action of *Pygeum africanum* extracts on experimental prostatic adenoma in the rat. *Therapie* **26**, 575–580, 1975.
7. Hinman F: *Benign Prostatic Hyperplasia*. Springer-Verlag, New York, 1983.
8. Bombardelli E: Methods, composition and compounds for the treatment of prostatic adenoma. European Patent Appl 8330491.3, June 10, 1985.
9. Marcoli M: Anti-inflammatory and antiedemigenic activity of extract of *Pygeum africanum* in the rat. *New Trends Androl Sci* **1**, 89, 1985.
10. Latalski M: The ultrastructure of the epithelium of bulbourethral glands after administration of *Pygeum africanum* extract. *Folia Morphol* **1**, 193–201, 1979.
11. Guillemin P: Clinical trials of V1326, or Tadenan, in prostatic adenoma. *Med Pract* **386**, 75–76, 1970.
12. Lange J and Muret P: Clinical trial of V1326 in prostatic disease. *Medicine* **11**, 2807–2811, 1970.
13. Wemeau L, Delmay J, and Blankaert J: Tadenan in prostatic adenoma. *Vie Medicale* January, 585–588, 1970.
14. Viollet G: Clinical experimentation of a new drug from prostatic adenoma. *Vie Medicale* June, 3457–3458, 1970.
15. Lhez A and Leguevague G: Clinical trials of a new lipid-sterolic complex of vegetal origin in the treatment of prostatic adenoma. *Vie Medicale* December, 5399–5404, 1970.
16. Thomas JP and Rouffilange F: The action of Tadenan in prostatic adenoma. *Rev Int Serv* **43**, 43–45, 1970.
17. Huet JA: Prostatic disease in old age. *Med Intern* **5**, 405–408, 1970.
18. Rometti A: Medical treatment of prostatic adenoma. *La Provence Medicale* **38**, 49–51, 1970.

19. Gallizia F and Gallizia G: Medical treatment of benign prostatic hypertrophy with a new phytothera-peutic principle. *Recent Med* **9**, 461–468, 1972.
20. Durval A: The use of a new drug in the treatment of prostatic disorders. *Minerva Urol* **22**, 106–111, 1970.
21. Pansadoro V and Benincasa A: Prostatic hypertrophy: Results obtained with *Pygeum africanum* extract. *Minerva Med* **11**, 119–144, 1972.
22. Zurita IE, Pecorini M, and Cuzzoni G: Treatment of prostatic hypertrophy with *Pygeum africanum* extract. *Rev Bras Med* **41**, 364–366, 1984.
23. Maver A: Medical therapy of the fibrous-adematose hypertrophy of the prostate with a new vegetal substance. *Minerva Med* **63**, 2126–2136, 1972.
24. Bongi G: Tadenan in the treatment of prostatic adenoma. *Minerva Urol* **24**, 129–139, 1972.
25. Doremieux J, Masson JC, and Bollack C: Prostatic hypertrophy, clinical effects and histological changes produced by a lipid complex extracted from *Pygeum africanum*. *J Med Strasbourg* **4**, 253–257, 1973.
26. Del Valio B: The use of a new drug in the treatment of chronic prostatitis. *Minerva Urol* **26**, 81–94, 1974.
27. Colpi G and Farina U: Study of the activity of chloroformic extract of *Pygeum africanum* bark in the treatment of urethral obstructive syndrome caused by non-cancerous prostapathy. *Urologia* **43**, 441–448, 1976.
28. Donkervoort T, *et al.*: A clinical and urodynamic study of Tadenan in the treatment of benign prosta-tic hypertrophy. *Urology* **8**, 218–225, 1977.
29. Dufour B and Choquenet C: Trial controlling the effects of *Pygeum africanum* extract on the functional symptoms of prostatic adenoma. *Ann Urol* **18**, 193–195, 1984.
30. Legramandi C, Ricci-Barbini V, and Fonte A: The importance of *Pygeum africanum* in the treatment of chronic prostatitis void of bacteria. *Gaz Medica Ital* **143**, 73–76, 1984.
31. Ranno S, *et al.*: Efficacy and tolerability in the treatment of prostatic adenoma with Tadenan 50. *Progresso Medico* **42**, 165–169, 1986.
32. Frasseto G, *et al.*: Study of the efficacy and tolerability of Tadenan 50 in patients with prostatic hyper-trophy. *Progresso Medico* **42**, 49–52, 1986.
33. Bassi P, *et al.*: Standardized extract of *Pygeum africanum* in the treatment of benign prostatic hypertro-phy. *Minerva Urol* **39**, 45–50, 1987.
34. Barlet A, *et al.*: Efficacy of *Pygeum africanum* extract in the medical therapy of urination disorders due to benign prostatic hyperplasia: Evaluation of objective and subjective parameters. A placebo-controlled double-blind multicenter study. *Wien Klin Wochenschr* **102**, 667–673, 1990.
35. Duvia R, Radice GP, and Galdini R: Advances in the phytotherapy of prostatic hypertrophy. *Med Praxis* **4**, 143–148, 1983.
36. Lucchetta G, *et al.*: Reactivation from the prostatic gland in cases of reduced fertility. *Urol Int* **39**, 222–224, 1984.
37. Menchini-Fabris GF, *et al.*: New perspectives of treatment of prostato-vesicular pathologies with *Pygeum africanum*. *Arch Int Urol* **60**, 313–322, 1988.
38. Clavert A, *et al.*: Effects of an extract of the bark of *Pygeum africanum* on prostatic secretions in the rat and man. *Ann Urol* **20**, 341–343, 1986.
39. Carani C, *et al.*: Urological and sexual evaluation of treatment of benign prostatic disease using *Pygeum africanum* at high dose. *Arch Ital Urol Nefrol Androl* **63**, 341–345, 1991.

30
St. John's wort

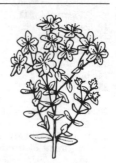

Key uses of St. John's wort:

* Depression
* Sleep disorders
* Viral infections

General description

St. John's wort (*Hypericum perforatum*) is a shrubby perennial plant with numerous bright yellow flowers. It is commonly found in dry, gravelly soils, fields, and sunny places. St. John's wort is native to many parts of the world, including Europe and the United States. It grows especially well in northern California and southern Oregon.

Chemical composition

The major compounds of interest in St. John's wort leaves and flowers are hypericin (Figure 30.1) and pseudohypericin. These compounds are typically found in very low concentrations ranging form 0.0095 to 0.466 percent in the leaves and as much as 0.24 percent in the flowers.[1]

Other active components include flavonoids (flowers, 16 percent, leaves, 12 percent; and whole herb, 9 percent), xanthones, phenolic carboxylic acids (caffeic, chlorogenic, ferulic, and gentisic acids), essential oils (whole herb content, 0.13 percent), carotenoids, alkanes, phloroglucinol derivatives, phytosterols, and medium-chain fatty acid alcohols.[1,2]

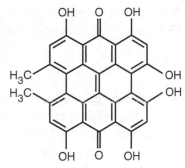

Figure 30.1 Hypericin

History and folk use

St. John's wort has a long history of folk use. Dioscorides, the foremost physician of ancient Greece, as well as Pliny and Hippocrates, administered St. John's wort in the treatment of many illnesses. Its Latin name, *Hypericum perforatum*, is derived from Greek and means "over an apparition," a reference to the belief that the herb was so obnoxious to evil spirits that a whiff of it would cause them to depart.

The naming of St. John's wort has its origins in folk traditions. One claims that red spots, symbolic of the blood of St. John, appeared on the leaves of the plant on the anniversary of the saint's beheading. Another comes from a common medieval belief that if one slept with a piece of the plant under his pillow on St. John's Eve, "the Saint would appear in a dream, give his blessing, and prevent one from dying during the following year."

Many people from the time of the ancient Greeks through the Middle Ages believed St. John's wort to have magical powers. Recent research using several components of St. John's wort is discovering the reasons behind some of the effects of the herb. From this research it appears that St. John's wort will continue to be a highly respected herb for many more years to come.

In Europe, St. John's wort has a long history of use, particularly as a folk remedy in the treatment of wounds, kidney and lung ailments, and depression.[?]

Pharmacology

St. John's wort extracts (primarily of the flowering tops) have shown a wide variety of effects in experimental and clinical studies. Some of the activities demonstrated include psychotropic, antidepressant, antiviral, and antibiotic effects as well as increased healing of wounds and burns.[1,2]

Antidepressant activity

Historically used as a nerve tonic, St. John's wort is now used widely as a mild to moderate antidepressant. This action appears to be based on the ability of hypericin and other components of St. John's wort to inhibit mono-amine oxidase (MAO) types A and B.[3,4] As a result of this inhibition the level within the brain increases of certain nerve impulse transmitters—those that maintain normal mood and emotional stability.

Extracts of St. John's wort have been tested in various animal models designed to study its antidepressant effects. In these studies, St. John's wort extract was found to enhance the exploratory activity of mice in a foreign environment, extend the narcotic sleeping time in a dose-dependent fashion, antagonize the effects of reserpine, and decrease aggressive behavior in socially isolated male mice.[5] These activities are consistent with the expected effects of antidepressant compounds.

Antiviral activity

In vitro studies have shown that hypericin and pseudohypericin exhibit strong antiviral activity against herpes simplex virus types 1 and 2 as well as influenza types A and B and vesicular stomatitis virus.[6] These compounds have also demonstrated remarkable antiviral activity against Epstein–Barr virus.[7]

A tremendous amount of excitement was generated when researchers from New York University Medical Center and the Weizmann Institute of Science in Israel demonstrated the antiretroviral activity of hypericin and pseudohypericin.[9] This preliminary study examined the effect of these compounds on two animal retroviruses, Friend leukemia virus and radiation leukemia virus, both in vitro and in vivo (in mice). The researchers found the effective dose of hypericin in mice to be 1.5 to 2.0 micrograms per milliliter. The researchers concluded:

> Hypericin and pseudohypericin display an extremely effective antiviral activity when administered to mice after retroviral infection. . . . The antiviral activity is remarkable both in its mechanism of action . . . and in the potency of one administration of a relatively small dose of the compounds. Availability . . . and the relatively convenient and inexpensive procedure for the extraction and purification of hypericin and pseudohypericin further enhance the potential of these compounds.

Later, two possible mechanisms were described to explain the antiviral activity of both hypericin and pseudohypericin.[10] The first concerned inhibition of assembly or processing of intact virions from infected cells—the virions released contained no detectable reverse transcriptase activity. Second, these compounds also directly inactivated mature and properly assembled retroviruses.

The antiviral activity of hypericin against human immunodeficiency virus (HIV) appears to require light to activate the hypericin.[10,11] A sufficient concentration of hypericin is required as well, as entry of hypericin into infected cells depends on its concentration in the blood. At sufficient concentrations, hypericin incubated with HIV-infected whole blood decreases culturable HIV, indicating significant antiviral activity.[12]

Antibacterial activity

St. John's wort extracts have broad-spectrum antimicrobial activity against both gram-negative and gram-positive bacteria.[13] The organisms studied included *Staphylococcus aureus*, *Streptococcus mutans*, *Proteus vulgaris*, *Escherichia coli*, and *Pseudomonas aeruginosa*.

Clinical applications

The primary use of St. John's wort is in the treatment of depression. It may also be of benefit in the treatment of chronic viral infections and, topically, in various skin products.

Depression

The standardized extract of St. John's wort (containing 0.14 percent hypericin) has significant support in the treatment of mild to moderate depression. The official German Commission E monograph for St. John's wort lists psychovegetative disturbances, depressive states, fear, and nervous disturbances as clinical indications for the extract.

The clinical evelution of St. John's wort extract began with an initial clinical study of six depressed women, aged 55 to 65 years. The study measured the change in urinary metabolites of noradrenaline and dopamine following administration of a standardized extract of St. John's wort (0.14 percent hypericin content).[14] Researchers found a significant increase in the metabolite 3-methoxy-4-hydroxyphenylglycol, a marker commonly used to evaluate the efficacy of antidepressant therapy. A follow-up study by the same researchers involved fifteen women with depression taking the same standardized extract. The results demonstrated a significant improvement in symptoms of anxiety, apathy, hypersomnia and insomnia, anorexia, psychomotor retardation, depression, and feelings of worthlessness. No side effects were observed.

Since this initial study, there have been more than twenty-six double-blind controlled studies with the standardized St. John's wort extract (0.3% hypericin).[1,15-18] The results from these studies indicate that this St. John's wort extract at a dosage of 300 milligrams three times daily is as effective in relieving symptoms of depression as standard antidepressants but is much better tolerated with fewer side effects.

AIDS and other viral infections

Research suggests that St. John's wort may be a useful adjunctive treatment for herpes simplex, mononucleosis, and influenza, although further human studies are needed to establish the optimal dosage of the standardized extract. Combined with its antidepressant activity, St. John's wort also appears to be a promising treatment for chronic fatigue syndrome.

The greatest promise of St. John's wort, however, may be in the treatment of acquired immunodeficiency syndrome (AIDS). In response to the results of *in vitro* and animal studies, many AIDS patients began self-administering St. John's wort. Although most patients reported feeling better with a more positive outlook, more energy, and less fatigue, it was not known to what degree this was due to a placebo effect.[19,20] To better determine the benefits, a number of trials evaluated the efficacy of standardized extracts of St. John's wort in the treatment of HIV-infected individuals.

In one study, St. John's wort extracts providing approximately 1 milligram of hypericin per day were studied in thirty-one patients.[21] Baseline and four monthly measurements, including physical examination, T cell subsets, and other laboratory parameters, were performed. Concomitant use of azidothymidine (AZT) and other treatments was permitted. The results of the study were encouraging. In the subgroup of ten patients who took no AZT either before or during the study ("AZT virgins"; none had AIDS), the mean helper T cell count increased 13 percent from baseline after 1 month on St. John's wort and maintained this increase for 4 months. These increases were not statistically significant; in contrast, helper T cell counts of the ten patients using AZT throughout the study fell significantly after an initial mild rise. Toxicities were limited to reversible liver enzyme elevations in five patients, with all levels returned to baseline after 1 month without St. John's wort extract.

In another open pilot study, eighteen HIV patients (three classified as CDC [Centers for Disease Control, Atlanta, GA] II, eight as CDC III, four as CDC IV B, and three as CDC IV C1) were treated solely with standardized St. John's wort extract (weekly intravenous injection and daily oral intake) providing a daily intake of 2 milligrams of hypericin.[22] The sixteen patients with good compliance showed stable or even increasing absolute helper T cell counts over the 40 months of observation. Also, the helper-to-suppressor T cell ratio showed an improvement in the majority of these patients. Clinically, it was noteworthy that only two of these sixteen patients encountered an opportunistic infection during the 40 months of observation. The remaining fourteen patients remained clinically stable and are active in work and life. This steady state situation also correlated with stable values for hemoglobin, leukocytes, and platelets. Furthermore, none of the usual viral complications due to cytomegalovirus (CMV), herpes virus, or Epstein–Barr (EBV) were encountered in these sixteen patients.

Despite these good preliminary results the trials proved disappointing, as significant blood levels of hypericin could not be achieved using the extract either orally or intravenously. The standardized extract for the treatment of HIV infection has since been replaced by an intravenously administered synthetic hypericin. Preliminary studies are again producing encouraging results with good safety, although photosensitivity may occur (see Toxicity).[23,24]

Topical applications

St. John's wort has long been used as a wound healing substance. Scientific studies have demonstrated antibacterial and wound healing activity.[2] St. John's wort preparations have also been used in burns, as a sunscreen, and in the treatment of muscular pain.[2] Oily preparations are preferred for topical applications.

Dosage

The best preparation to use appears to be the St. John's wort extract standardized to contain 0.3% hypericin. The recommended dosage of this extract as an antidepressant is 300 milligrams three times daily. Each dose should be taken with meals.

Toxicity

St. John's wort can cause severe photosensitivity in animals grazing extensively on the plant. The term *hypericism* describes a skin disease found in animals who graze on large quantities of St. John's wort. However, reports of photosensitivity in humans are rare and have been limited to those taking excessive quantities for HIV infection. St. John's wort is unlikely to be toxic to humans when used at recommended medicinal doses. However, those individuals with AIDS who take larger amounts of St. John's wort extracts (or hypericin) have developed photosensitivity.[24]

Because of the possibility of photosensitivity, some herbalists recommend that individuals, especially those with fair skin, avoid exposure to strong sunlight and other sources of ultraviolet light when using St. John's wort.[2]

Those taking St. John's wort should also avoid foods and medications that are known to interact negatively with MAO-inhibiting drugs. Tyramine-containing foods (cheeses, beer, wine, pickled herring, yeast, etc.) and drugs such as L-dopa and 5-hydroxytryptophan should be avoided. St. John's wort should also be taken with food, as it may cause mild gastric upset in sensitive individuals.

References

1. Morazzoni P and Bombardellie E: *Hypericum perforatum*. Indena, Milan, Italy, 1994.
2. Hobbs C: St. John's wort, *Hypericum perforatum* L. HerbalGram **18/19**, 24–33, 1989.
3. Suzuki O, *et al.*:Inhibition of monoamine oxidase by hypericin. *Planta Medica* **50**, 272–274, 1984.
4. Holzl J, Demisch L, and Gollnik B: Investigations about antidepressive and mood changing effects of *Hypericum perforatum*. *Planta Medica* **55**, 643, 1989.
5. Okpanyi VSN and Weischer ML: Tierexperimentelle Untersuchungen zur psychotropen Wirksamkeit eines Hypericum-extraktes. *Arzneimittel-Forsch* **37**, 10–13, 1987.
6. Muldner VH and Zoller M: Antidepressive wirkung eines auf den wirkstoffkomplex hypericin standardisierten hypericum-extrakes. *Arzneimittel-Forsch* **34**, 918, 1984.
7. Lavie D: Antiviral pharmaceutical compositions containing hypericin or pseudohypericin. European Patent Application No. 87111467.4, filed 8/8/87, European Patent Office. Publ No: 0 256 A2. 175–177, 1987.
8. Someya H: Effect of a constituent of *Hypericum erectum* on infection and multiplication of Epstein-Barr virus. *J Tokyo Med Coll* **43**, 815–826, 1985.
9. Meruelo D, Lavie G, and Lavie D: Therapeutic agents with dramatic antiretroviral activity and little toxicity at effective doses: Aromatic polycyclic diones hypericin and pseudohypericin. *Proc Natl Acad Sci USA* **85**, 5230–5234, 1988.
10. Lavie G, *et al.*: Studies of the mechanism of action of the antiretroviral agents hypericin and pseudohypericin. *Proc Natl Acad Sci USA* **86**, 5963–5967, 1989.
11. Degar S, *et al.*: Inactivation of the human immunodeficiency virus by hypericin: Evidence for photochemical alterations of p24 and a block in uncoating. *AIDS Res Hum Retroviruses* **8**, 1929–1936, 1992.
12. Valentine FT, *et al.*: Synthetic hypericin enters blood lymphocytes and monocytes in vitro and decreases culturable HIV in blood obtained from infected individuals. *Int Conf AIDS* **7**, 97, 1991 [Abstract No. W.A.1022]
13. Barbagallo C and Chisari G: Antimicrobial activity of three *Hypericum* species. *Filoterapia* **58**, 175–177, 1987.

14. Muldner VH and Zoller M: Antidepressive effect of a hypericum extract standardized to the active hypericine complex. *Arzneimittel-Forsch* **34**, 918–920, 1984.
15. Schmidt U and Sommer H: St. John's wort extract in the ambulatory therapy of depression. Attention and reaction ability are preserved. *Forschr Med* **111**, 339–342, 1993.
16. Johnson D: Effects of St. John's wort extract Jarsin. Paper presented at the 4th International Congress on Phytotherapy. Munich, Germany. September 10–13, 1992. [Abstract SL53]; Woelk H: Multicentric practice-study analyzing the functional capacity in depressive patients. Paper presented at the 4th International Congress on Phytotherapy. Munich, Germany. September 10–13, 1992. [Abstract SL54]; Sommer H. Improvement of psychovegetative complaints by hypericum. Paper presented at the 4th International Congress on Phytotherapy. Munich, Germany. September 10–13, 1992. [Abstract SL55]
17. Schlich D, Brauckmann F, and Schenk N: Treatment of depressive conditions with hypericum. *Psychol* **13**, 440–444, 1987.
18. Harrer G and Sommer H: Treatment of mild/moderate depressions with Hypericum. *Phytomed* **1**, 3–8, 1994.
19. James JS: *AIDS Treatment News.* Issue 74, February 24, 1989.
20. James JS: *AIDS Treatment News.* Issue 91, November 17, 1989.
21. Cooper WC and James J: An observational study of the safety and efficacy of hypericin in HIV+ subjects. *Int Conf AIDS* **6**, 369, 1990. [Abstract 2063]
22. Steinbeck-Klose A and Wernet P: Successful long term treatment over 40 months of HIV-patients with intravenous Hypericin. *Int Conf AIDS* **9**(1), 470, 1993. Abstract PO-B26-2012]
23. Furner V, Bek M, and Gold J: A phase I/II unblinded dose ranging study of hypericin in HIV-positive subjects. *Int Conf AIDS* **7**, 199, 1991. [Abstract W.B.2071]
24. Gulick R, *et al.*: Human hypericism: A photosensitivity reaction to hypericin (St. John's wort). *Int Conf AIDS* **8**, B90, 1992. [Abstract PoB 3018]

31
Sarsaparilla

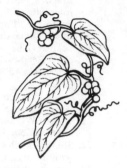

Key uses of sarsaparilla:

- Psoriasis
- Eczema
- General tonic

General description

Sarsaparilla (*Smilax sarsaparilla*) is a tropical American perennial plant. Its long slender root and short, thick rhizomes produce a vine that trails on the ground and climbs by means of tendrils growing in pairs from the petioles of the alternate, obicular to ovate, evergreen leaves. The root is the part of the plant utilized for medicinal purposes.

Chemical composition

Sarsaparilla contains 1.8–2.4 percent steroid saponins, including sarsaponin; smilasaponin; and sarsaparilloside and its aglycones sarsasapogenin, smilagenin, and pollinastanol. Other constituents include starch, resins, and a trace of volatile oil.[1]

History and folk use

Sarsaparilla's medicinal use has been as a tonic and blood purifier. Tonics are defined as agents[2] ". . . which permanently exalt the energies of the body at large, without vitally affecting any one organ in particular. . . ." In short, tonics tone the whole system.

A blood purifier or depurative refers to an agent that cleanses and purifies the system.[2] Sarsaparilla's reputation in this regard probably stems from its importation from the Caribbean and South America to Europe in the sixteenth century for the treatment of syphilis.[3]

As discussed in Chapter 1, a French physician, Nicholas Monardes, published a comprehensive account of sarsaparilla and several other "new" drugs in the treatment of syphilis in 1574. Many Europeans at the time believed that syphilis had come to Europe from the West Indies with Columbus's sailors, and because there was a general belief that whatever disease was native to a country might be cured by the medicinal herbs growing in that region, it was only natural for sarsaparilla to become a popular remedy. Furthermore, the standard treatment for syphilis, mercury, often resulted in greater morbidity and mortality than the disease itself.

Sarsaparilla was a welcome alternative, but despite initial excitement, Monardes's sarsaparilla cure sank in favor. This was probably due to other aspects of the cure, which included confinement to a warm room for 30 days, followed by forty days of abstinence from both wine and sexual intercourse.[3]

However, sarsaparilla continued to be used in the treatment of syphilis. During military operations in Portugal in 1812, a British Inspector General of Hospitals noted that the Portuguese soldiers suffering from syphilis who used sarsaparilla recovered much faster and more completely than their British counterparts, who were treated with mercury.[3]

Sarsaparilla was also used by the Chinese in the treatment of syphilis. Clinical observations in China demonstrated that sarsaparilla is effective, according to blood tests, in about 90 percent of acute cases and 50 percent of chronic cases.[1,4]

Although sarsaparilla was clearly more beneficial in the treatment of syphilis, it was mercury that established itself as the standard treatment for over four and a half centuries. It has been stated that "the use of mercury in the treatment of syphilis may have been the most colossal hoax ever perpetrated" in the history of medicine. Mercury represented a new kind of medicine, one formulated and prepared in a laboratory using the new techniques of chemistry. It helped prepare the way for future use of drugs rather than herbal medicines.[3]

An interesting note is that sarsaparilla species have been used all over the world in many different cultures for the same conditions, namely gout, arthritis, fevers, digestive disorders, skin disease, and cancer.[1]

Pharmacology

The mechanism of action of sarsaparilla is largely unknown, although the plant does contain several saponins and has been shown to be clinically effective in the treatment of psoriasis.[1,5,6] This evidence points to a possible effect on binding of cholesterol and bacterial toxins in the intestines.

Endotoxin binding

Evidence seems to support sarsaparilla as an endotoxin binder. Endotoxins are cell wall constituents of bacteria that are absorbed from the gut. Normally, the liver filters out these and other gut-derived compounds before they reach the general circulation. If the amount of endotoxin absorbed is excessive or if the liver is not functioning adequately, the liver can become overwhelmed, and endotoxins will spill into the blood.[7]

If endotoxins are allowed to circulate, activation of the alternate complement system occurs. This system plays a critical role in aggravating inflammatory processes, and activation of complement is responsible for much of the inflammation and cell damage that occurs in many diseases, including gout, arthritis, and psoriasis,

For example, individuals with psoriasis have been shown to have high levels of circulating endotoxins. Binding of endotoxin in the gut is associated with clinical improvement in these individuals. In a controlled study of ninety-two patients, an endotoxin-binding saponin (sarsaponin) from sarsaparilla greatly improved the psoriasis in 62 percent of the patients and resulted in complete clearance in 18 percent.[6]

In further support of sarsaparilla's effect as a binder of endotoxin is its historical use in the treatment of fever, as absorbed endotoxins produce fever.[7] Sarsaparilla also exhibits some antibiotic activity, but this is probably secondary to its endotoxin-binding action.[1]

Clinical applications

Despite sarsaparilla's long historical use, there is little scientific information about the plant. From the limited information available it appears that sarsaparilla's medicinal effects occur as it binds bacterial endotoxins in the gut, rendering them unabsorbable. This greatly reduces stress on the liver and other organs and is probably responsible for sarsaparilla's historical use as a tonic and blood purifier. This ability to bind endotoxins is also the probable reason why sarsaparilla is reported to be effective in many cases of psoriasis, gout, and arthritis.

The "testosterone controversy"

Sarsparilla has been widely touted as a "sexual rejuvenator," with some commercial suppliers even claiming that it is a rich source of human testosterone. The fact is, although sarsaparilla may have good tonic effects there is no actual testosterone in the plant. It is unlikely that the steroid-like substances in sarsaparilla are absorbed to any great degree. It is also unlikely that sarsaparilla has any significant "anabolic" effects, as no published evidence supports the contention that it increases muscle mass.

The confusion arises because the sarsaparilla saponin, sarsasapogenin, can be synthetically transformed in the laboratory to testosterone. However, it is extremely unlikely that this reaction could take place in the human body.

Dosage

Sarsaparilla can be used at the following dosages as a "blood purifier" and tonic as well as for conditions associated with high endotoxin levels, most notably psoriasis, eczema, arthritis, and ulcerative colitis. Doses should be taken three times daily:

- Dried root: 1–4 grams or by decoction
- Liquid extract (1:1): 8–12 milliliters (2 to 3 teaspoons)
- Solid extract (4:1): 250 milligrams

Toxicity

No adverse effects have been reported; however, problems could arise if large doses are used for a long period of time.

References

1. Leung AY: *Encyclopedia of Common Natural Ingredients Used in Food, Drugs and Cosmetics.* John Wiley & Sons, New York, 1980.
2. Felter HW: *The Eclectic Materia Medica, Pharmacology and Therapeutics.* Eclectic Medical Publications, Portland, OR, 1983.
3. Griggs B: *Green Pharmacy: A History of Herbal Medicine.* Jill Norman & Hobhouse, London, 1981.
4. Bensky D and Gamble A: *Chinese Herbal Medicine Materia Medica.* Eastland Press, Seattle, WA, 1986.
5. Duke JA: *Handbook of Medicinal Herbs.* CRC Press, Boca Raton, FL, 1985.
6. Thurman FM: The treatment of psoriasis with sarsaparilla compound. *New Engl J Med* **227**, 128–133, 1942.
7. Pizzorno JE and Murray MT: *A Textbook of Natural Medicine.* JBC Publications, Seattle, WA, 1987, Chapter IV (Alternate Complement Pathway) and Chapter IV (Bowel Toxemia).

32
Saw palmetto

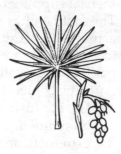

Key use of saw palmetto:

• Benign prostatic hyperplasia

General description

Saw palmetto (*Serenoa repens*) is a small palm tree native to the West Indies and the Atlantic coast of North America from South Carolina to Florida. The plant grows from 6 to 10 feet high with a crown of large, 2- to 4-foot high, spiny-toothed leaves that form a circular, fan-shaped outline. The berries are used for medicinal purposes. The deep red-brown to black berries are wrinkled, oblong, and 0.5 to 1 inch long with a diameter of 0.5 inch.[1]

Chemical composition

The saw palmetto berries contain about 1.5 percent of a fruity-smelling oil containing saturated and unsaturated fatty acids and sterols.[1] About 63 percent of this oil is composed of free fatty acids including capric, caprylic, caproic, lauric, palmitic, and oleic acids. The remaining portion is composed of ethyl esters of these fatty acids and sterols, including beta-sitosterol and its glucoside. The lipid-soluble compounds are thought to be the major pharmacological components. Other components of the berries include carotenes, lipase, tannins, and sugars.

The purified fat-soluble extract is used medicinally and contains between 85 and 95 percent fatty acids and sterols. It is made up predominantly of a complex mixture of saturated and unsaturated free fatty acids, their methyl and ethyl esters (approximately 7 percent), long-chain alcohols in free and esterified form, and various free and esterified sterol derivatives.

The free fatty acids in this extract are identified by gas chromatography and mass spectrometry as caproic acid (six-carbon chain, C_6), capric acid (C_8), caprylic acid (C_{10}), lauric acid (C_{12}), myristic acid (C_{14}), isomyristic acid (C_{14}), palmitic acid (C_{16}), oleic acid ($C_{18:1}$), and stearic acid (C_{18}). Lauric and myristic acid are the major fatty acids, accounting for approximately 30 percent of the fatty acid content.

The identified alcohols include those with n-C_{22}, n-C_{23}, n-C_{24}, n-C_{26}, n-C_{28}, and n-C_{30} chains, phytol, farnesol, and geranylgeraniol, in addition to high molecular weight unsaturated polyphenols.

The sterolic fraction is composed of beta-sitosterol, stigmasterol, cycloartenol, lupeol, lupenone, and 24-methylcycloartenol. Many of these sterols are esterified with the fatty acids of the extract.

History and folk use

The American Indians used saw palmetto berries in the treatment of genitourinary tract disturbances and as a tonic to support the body nutritionally. It was administered to men to increase the function of the testicles and relieve irritation in mucous membranes, particularly those of the genitourinary tract and prostate. It has been given to women with disorders of the mammary glands: long-term use was reputed to slowly cause the mammae to enlarge. Many herbalists consider it to be an aphrodisiac.[1]

Pharmacology

A standardized liposterolic (fat-soluble) saw palmetto berry extract demonstrates numerous pharmacological effects relating to its primary clinical application in the treatment of the common disorder of the prostate gland—benign prostatic hyperplasia (BPH). Benign prostatic hyperplasia is thought to be caused by an accumulation of testosterone in the prostate. Once within the prostate, testosterone is converted to the more potent hormone dihydrotestosterone (DHT). This compound stimulates the cells to multiply excessively, eventually causing the prostate to enlarge.

The primary therapeutic action of saw palmetto extract in the treatment of BPH is to inhibit the intraprostatic conversion of testosterone to DHT, and to inhibit DHT's intracellular binding and transport.[2,3] However, a more recent clinical study has shed light on another mechanism of action—an antiestrogenic effect. Estrogen contributes to BPH because it inhibits the hydroxylation and subsequent elimination of DHT.

A double-blind, placebo-controlled study was performed on thirty-five men with BPH; eighteen were given the saw palmetto extract at 160 milligrams twice daily and seventeen were given a placebo.[4] At the end of the 90-day study, androgen, estrogen, and progesterone receptors from prostate tissue samples were evaulated by two different techniques. The results of the steroid evaluation indicated that the men receiving the saw palmetto extract had significantly lower cytosol (cellular) and nuclear (control center for the cell) receptor values for estrogen and progesterone compared to the placebo group. Since the progesterone receptor content is linked to estrogenic activity, the results of the evaluation imply that the saw palmetto extract exerts significant antiestrogenic effect.

The results from the androgen receptor analysis were quite interesting: there was no change in the number of cytosol androgen receptors, but the number of nuclear androgen receptors was significantly lower in the saw palmetto group (60 percent of the placebo group were positive for the nuclear receptor compared to 10 percent in the saw palmetto group). These results indicate that the saw palmetto extract probably competively blocks the translocation of the cytosol androgen receptor to the nucleus. In other words, it blocks the transport of the cytosol receptor to the nucleus.

The overall results of the study indicate that the standardized extract of saw palmetto exerts both antiandrogenic and antiestrogenic activities. Preliminary analysis of the extract indicates that separate fractions are responsible for these effects. Researchers in this study[4] concluded: "it cannot be excluded, however, that the primary effect is antiestrogenic and that the inactivation of androgen receptors and progesterone receptors and of the 5-alpha-reductase activity is secondary to the estrogen receptor blockade."

Clinical applications

Currently, the primary clinical application of saw palmetto berries (specifically the fat-soluble extract) is in the treatment of BPH. On the basis of its pharmacology, this extract may also be of benefit in conditions of androgen excess in women, such as hirsutism and polycystic ovarian disease.

Benign prostatic hyperplasia

Approximately 50 to 60 percent of men between 40 and 59 years of age have BPH. This disorder is characterized by increased urinary frequency, nighttime awakening to empty the bladder, and reduced force and caliber of urination.

Finasteride (Proscar) is currently the only approved drug in the treatment of BPH. It works by inhibiting the activity of an enzyme, 5-alpha-reductase, involved in testosterone metabolism. Finasteride blocks the transformation of testosterone to dihydrotestosterone, a very potent hormone derived from testosterone. Dihydrotestosterone is responsible for the overproduction of prostate cells, which ultimately results in prostatic enlargement.

Although Proscar has received much attention, it is much less effective (on the basis of results of the clinical trials) than the extract of saw palmetto. Fewer than 50 percent of patients on Proscar will experience clinical improvement after taking the drug for 1 year and it must be taken for at least 6 months before any improvement can be expected. Proscar costs about $75 dollars a month. Merck, the manufacturer of Proscar, has predicted sales will soon reach $1 billion dollars annually. However, men with prostate enlargement would receive far better results from saw palmetto.

Numerous studies on the saw palmetto extract have shown it to be effective in nearly 90 percent of patients (Table 32.1), usually in a period of 4 to 6 weeks.[5-16] In contrast, Proscar is effective in reducing the symptoms in less than 50 percent after taking the drug for 1 year. To illustrate saw palmetto extract's superiority over Proscar, let's look at the effect of both on the maximum urine flow rate, a good indicator of bladder neck obstruction due to an enlarged prostate. The data in Table 32.1 are based on pooled data from clinical studies.

In one of the larger double-blind studies involving 110 outpatients suffering from BPH, impressive clinical results were obtained.[14] Nocturia

Table 32.1 Effect of saw palmetto versus Proscar on urine flow rate

| | Urine flow rate (ml/sec) when using | |
Time of measurement	Saw palmetto extract	Proscar
Initial	9.53	9.6
3 months	13.15[a]	10.4
12 months	[b]	11.2
Percent increase	38% in 3 months	16% in 12 months

[a]Many studies on the saw palmetto extract were less than 90 days in duration; final measurements were calculated as 90-day measurements.
[b]There are no long-term studies on saw palmetto extract, yet the effects at 3 months (or less) are obviously superior to those of Proscar.

decreased by over 45 percent, flow rate (in milliliters per second) increased by over 50 percent, and postmicturition residue (in milliliters) decreased by 42 percent in the group receiving the *Serenoa repens* extract. In contrast, those on placebo showed no significant improvement in nocturia or flow rate, and postmicturition residue actually worsened.

Significant improvements were also noted in self-rating by the patients and global rating by the physicians. Of the fifty treated subjects completing the 30-day study, physicians rated fourteen as greatly improved, thirty-one as improved, and only five as unchanged or worsened. In contrast, no subjects in the placebo group had greatly improved, sixteen showed some improvement, and twenty-eight remained unchanged or worsened.

From Table 32.2, it is apparent that the liposterolic extract of saw palmetto berries is quite effective in the treatment of BPH.

Although the saw palmetto extract has shown excellent results in numerous double-blind, placebo-controlled clinical trials (Table 32.2), results from a recent open multicenter study are perhaps the most interesting.[16] The results corroborate those from numerous double-blind, controlled studies showing that the liposterolic extract of saw palmetto (*Serenoa repens*) standardized to contain 85 to 95 percent fatty acids and sterols is an effective treatment for BPH. In fact, the results produced in the trial once again demonstrated the superiority of saw palmetto extract over finasteride (Proscar). While Proscar typically takes up to a year to produce any significant benefit, the saw palmetto extract produces better results in a much shorter period of time. Most patients achieve some relief of symptoms within the first 30 days of treatment with the saw palmetto extract.

A total of 305 patients fulfilled inclusion criteria.[16] Each patient was given a dosage of 160 milligrams twice daily. The subjective evaluations of treatment made by patients after 45 and 90 days of treatment were quite favorable. After 45 days, 83 percent of patients estimated the drug was effective. After 90 days, the percentage increased to 88 percent. Similarly, global evaluations made by physicians after 45 and 90 days demonstrated 81 and 88 percent effectiveness, respectively. There were no serious adverse reactions reported.

The objective evaluations demonstrated remarkable improvements in all measurements. Maximum urinary flow (in milliliters per second) increased from 9.78 to 12.19; mean urinary flow rate (in milliliters per second) increased from 5.83 to 7.41; prostatic volume (in cubic millimeters) decreased from 40,348 to 36,246; and the international prostate symptom score decreased from 19 to 12.4.

While these improvements are impressive, perhaps the most impressive changes occurred in the Quality of Life scores.

Table 32.2 Clinical studies demonstrating the efficiency of *Serenoa repens*[a] in benign prostatic hyperplasia

Ref.	Type of study	No. of patients	Length of study	Results
5	Double blind	22	60 days	Significant difference for: volume voided, maximum flow, mean flow, dysuria, nocturia
6	Open	47	4 months	Significant difference for: dysuria, nocturia, urine flow
7	Open	40	30–90 days	Significant difference for: dysuria, nocturia, volume of prostate, voiding rate, residual urine
8	Double blind	30	30 days	Significant difference for: number of voidings, strangury, maximum and mean urine flow, residual urine
9	Open	14	1–2 months	Significant difference for: dysuria, perineal heaviness, nocturia, volume of urine per voiding, interval between two diurnal voidings, sensation of incomplete voiding
10	Controlled trial vs. *Pygeum africanum*	30	30 days	Significant difference for: voiding rate
11	Double blind	30	31–90 days	Significant difference for: frequency, urine flow measurement
12	Double blind	168	60–90 days	Significant difference for: dysuria, frequency, residual urine
13	Open	32	4 weeks	Significant difference for: dysuria, nocturia, volume of prostate, voiding rate
14	Double blind	110	28 days	Significant difference for: dysuria, nocturia, flow measurement, residual urine
15	Double blind	40	3 months	Significant difference for: dysuria, nocturia, residual urine
16	Open	305	3 months	Significant difference for: maximum urine flow, prostate volume, and international prostate score

*Dose, 320 mg/day.

Quality of Life scores—day 0 of study

Unsatisfied	43.8%
Mitigated	22.7%
Unhappy	18.5%
Satisfied	9.7%
Happy	2.3%
Hopeless	2.3%
Delighted	0.6%

Quality of Life scores—day 90 of study

Satisfied	36.8%
Happy	24%
Mitigated	20.9%
Unsatisfied	9.5%
Delighted	5.4%
Unhappy	2.4%
Hopeless	1.0%

These improvements in Quality of Life scores demonstrate just how powerful an effect bothersome symptoms such as nocturia can have on an individual's mental outlook.

Another important finding was that the saw palmetto extract had no demonstratable effect on serum prostatic specific antigen levels.

Dosage

To achieve the benefit with saw palmetto, it is essential that fat-soluble saw palmetto extracts standardized to contain 85–95 percent fatty acids and sterols be used at the recommended dosage of 160 milligrams twice daily. A similar dose of active compounds using crude berries, fluid extracts, and tinctures cannot be achieved.

Toxicity

Saw palmetto extract is completely safe, as no significant side effects have ever been reported in the clinical trials of the extract or with saw palmetto berry ingestion. Detailed toxicology studies on the extract have been carried out on mice, rats, and dogs and indicate that the extract has no toxic effects.

References

1. Duke JA: *Handbook of Medicinal Herbs*. CRC Press, Boca Raton, FL, 1985, p. 118.
2. Carilla E, *et al.*: Binding of Permixon, a new treatment for prostatic benign hyperplasia, to the cytosolic androgen receptor in the rat prostate. *J Steroid Biochem* **20**, 521–523, 1984.
3. Sultan C, *et al.*: Inhibition of androgen metabolism and binding by a liposterolic extract of *Serenoa repens* B in human foreskin fibroblasts. *J Steroid Biochem* **20**, 515–519, 1984.
4. Di Silverio F, *et al.*: Evidence that *Serenoa repens* extract displays antiestrogenic activity in prostatic tissue of benign prostatic hypertrophy. *Eur Urol* **21**, 309–314, 1992.
5. Boccafoschi and Annoscia S: Comparison of *Serenoa repens* extract with placebo by controlled clinical trial in patients with prostatic adenomatosis. *Urologia* **50**, 1257–1268, 1983.
6. Cirillo-Marucco E, *et al.*: Extract of *Serenoa repens* (Permixon®) in the early treatment of prostatic hypertrophy. *Urologia* **5**, 1269–1277, 1983.
7. Tripodi V, *et al.*: Treatment of prostatic hypertrophy with *Serenoa repens* extract. *Med Praxis* **4**, 41–46, 1983.
8. Emili E, Lo Cigno M, and Petrone U: Clinical trial of a new drug for treating hypertrophy of the prostate (Permixon). *Urologia* **50**, 1042–1048, 1983.
9. Greca P and Volpi R: Experience with a new drug in the medical treatment of prostatic adenoma. *Urologia* **52**, 532–535, 1985.
10. Duvia R, Radice GP, and Galdini R: Advances in the phytotherapy of prostatic hypertrophy. *Med Praxis* **4**, 143–148, 1983.
11. Tasca A, *et al.*: Treatment of obstructive symptomatology caused by prostatic adenoma with an extract of *Serenoa repens*. Double-blind clinical study vs. placebo. *Minerva Urol Nefrol* **37**, 87–91, 1985.
12. Cukier, *et al.*: Permixon versus placebo. *C R Ther Pharmacol Clin* **4**(25), 15–21, 1985.
13. Crimi A and Russo A: Extract of *Serenoa repens* for the treatment of the functional disturbances of prostate hypertrophy. *Med Praxis* **4**, 47–51, 1983.
14. Champlault G, Patel JC, and Bonnard AM: A double-blind trial of an extract of the plant *Serenoa repens* in benign prostatic hyperplasia. *Br J Clin Pharmacol* **18**, 461–462, 1984; Champault G, *et al.*: Medical treatment of prostatic adenoma. Controlled trial: PA 109 vs placebo in 110 patients. *Ann Urol* **18**, 407–410, 1984.
15. Mattei FM, Capone M, and Acconcia A: *Serenoa repens* extract in the medical treatment of benign prostatic hypertrophy. *Urologia* **55**, 547–552, 1988.
16. Braeckman J: The extract of *Serenoa repens* in the treatment of benign prostatic hyperplasia: A multicenter open study. *Curr Ther Res* **55**, 776–785, 1994.

33

Siberian ginseng

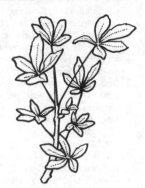

Key uses of Siberian ginseng:

- Stress and fatigue
- Atherosclerosis
- Impaired kidney function

General description

Siberian ginseng (*Eleutherococcus senticosus*) is a shrub, usually 1.5–2.6 meters in height, with erect, spiny shoots (4–6 centimeters in diameter) covered with light gray or brownish bark. The leaves are long-petioled in a compound palmate configuration. The leaflets (five) are elliptic and finely serrated at the margins on both sides with scattered, minute spinules along the veins.[1,2]

Siberian ginseng grows abundantly in parts of the Soviet Far East, Korea, China, and Japan, north of latitude 38. Its distribution is actually much greater than that of *Panax ginseng*.[1]

The root is the most widely used medicinal part, with the highest concentration of biologically active substances occurring in the fall, just before defoliation. The leaves are also used medicinally. The highest concentration of biologically active substances occurs in July, just before flowering.

Chemical composition

The initial chemical report on Siberian ginseng was published in 1965 by members of the Institute of Biologically Active Substances (Vladivostok,

Russia.[1] Seven compounds, termed eleutherosides A–G, were isolated from a physiologically active fraction of the methanol extract of Siberian ginseng. The total eleutheroside content of the root is in the range of 0.6–0.9 percent; in the stems the range is 0.6–1.5 percent. *Note*: Thin-layer chromatographic analysis has shown that the ginsenosides characteristic of *Panax* species (American, Chinese, Korean, and Japanese ginsengs) are not present in the roots of *Eleutherococcus senticosus*.

History and folk use

The ginseng plants, that is, members of the family Araliaceae, including *Eleutherococcus senticosus*, are among the most honored and ancient of all medicinal herbs. Their use in Chinese herbal medicine dates back more than 4,000 years.[1-3] Confusion has arisen at times over the lack of specificity in ancient documents with regard to exactly what member of the ginseng family was being prescribed. However, the value of Siberian ginseng as a medicinal agent was certainly known to the Chinese, as is evident by the following Chinese ode to Wujia (*Eleutherococcus senticosus*):[3]

Ode to Wujia

From earth and heavens the quintessence originates,
Five folioles clustering your leaves,
And pretty little thorns wrapped whole your shoots;
Oh what a jackal's gaunt leg looks much alike.
How wonderful is Winzhang-grass, the Eleuthero-ginseng
Dispensing in liquor for drinking,
And decocting with burnet for daily using, It will keep your virgin face
   younger
And prolong your life for ever and ever;
Even if a cartload of gold and jewels,
That can not estimate your price of nature

Ye Zhishen (Qing Dynasty)

In summary, the Chinese believe that regular use of Siberian ginseng will increase longevity, improve general health, improve the appetite, and restore memory.

Despite a long history of use by the Chinese herbalists (references date back to 2000 B.C.), the Russians have their own history of Siberian ginseng and even go so far as to say, "*Eleutherococcus* was not known in Oriental folk medicine."[1] The Russian history of Siberian ginseng begins in 1855 when a pair of Russian scientists, C. I. Maximovich and L. Shrenk, traveled from St. Petersburg (now Leningrad) to the Ussuri region of Russia on the Amur river. It was in this area that Maximovich observed a vast thicket of unusual plants with leaves resembling horse chestnut and young shoots resembling ginseng. Unable to identify the plant, the two scientists brought it back to St. Petersburg for classification. The plant was given the genus name of *Eleuthero* or "free-berried shrub" and the species name of *senticosus*, which means "thorny" in Latin.

Siberian ginseng remained largely unknown to Russians for roughly 100 years after Maximovich's discovery. It wasn't until the middle of the twentieth century that Siberian ginseng was "discovered," when Russian scientists began investigating substances that produce a "state of nonspecific resistance" on the body. Substances with this effect were termed *adaptogens*. As defined by Brekhman in 1958, an adaptogen is a substance that (1) must be innocuous and cause minimal disorders in the physiological functions of an organism, (2) must have a nonspecific action (i.e., it should increase the resistance to adverse influences by a wide range of physical, chemical, and biochemical factors), and (3) usually has a normalizing action irrespective of the direction of the pathological state (alterative action).[1,4]

Brekhman's research with adaptogens began with *Panax ginseng*, since this was the best known natural adaptogen. After confirming the adaptogenic action of panax in human studies, Brekhman began searching for an alternative to this plant because of the difficulty in obtaining *Panax ginseng* and its expense. Initially, all six species of Araliaceae native to Russia were investigated, but Siberian ginseng appeared to be the most promising. Numerous studies have been done on Siberian ginseng since the late 1950s, with the overwhelming majority being done in the Soviet Union.[1-8]

Pharmacology

As mentioned above, a number of experimental and clinical studies have demonstrated that Siberian ginseng does possess adaptogenic properties; that is, the ability to increase nonspecific body resistance to stress, fatigue, and disease. Further experimental and clinical research supports additional therapeutic applications of *Eleutherococcus senticosus*.

Adaptogenic activity

An important characteristic of an adaptogen is its ability to "normalize" irrespective of the direction of pathology. *Eleutherococcus senticosus* has been shown in experimental models to do just this.[1-7] Similar results have been obtained with *Panax ginseng*.

Another important action of adaptogens is to inhibit the alarm phase (fight or flight response) of the stress reaction. The action of Siberian ginseng was similar to that of *Panax ginseng* in experiments designed to demonstrate an antialarm action. Specifically, Siberian ginseng increases the swimming time of rats, reduces activation of the adrenal cortex in response to stress (alarm phase reaction), and prevents stress-induced damage to the thymus gland and lymphatic system.[1-7]

In addition to its confirmed adaptogenic activity, Siberian ginseng also demonstrates a protective and medicinal action in animals exposed to both single and prolonged X-ray radiation. In one study, both *Eleutherococcus senticosus* and *Panax ginseng* doubled the life span of rats exposed to prolonged radiation (total doses of 1,620 to 7,000 rads). When Siberian ginseng was combined with antibiotics the life span of irradiated rats (60 days; total dose, 3,000 rads) increased threefold.[8]

These results suggest that Siberian ginseng may protect against harmful radiation and act as an aid in the radiation therapy of cancer patients. The latter suggestion is further supported by studies of Siberian ginseng that have demonstrated an inhibition of cancer.[1,4]

As evident from the discussion of Siberian ginseng's adaptogenic activities above, Siberian ginseng shares many common features with *Panax ginseng*. In addition to the adaptogenic activities discussed above, Siberian ginseng, like *Panax ginseng*, has been shown to increase resistance to infection in animals, reduce cholesterol biosynthesis in the liver; increase reproductive capacity and sperm counts in bulls, possess significant antioxidant activity, and stimulate protein synthesis and cellular repair enzymes.[1]

Clinical applications

Siberian ginseng possesses significant adaptogenic action. Currently, its use can be recommended as a general tonic. Because of its nonspecific mechanisms of action, Siberian ginseng has a broad range of clinical applications.

Siberian ginseng as an adaptogen in normal and stressed individuals

Farnsworth and colleagues[1] have reviewed data on an *Eleutherococcus senticosus* root extract (33 percent ethanol) that has been administered to more than 2,100 healthy human subjects in clinical trials for the purpose of evaluating the adaptogenic effects of Siberian ginseng. These studies indicated that Siberian ginseng (1) increased the ability of humans to withstand many adverse physical conditions (i.e., heat, noise, motion, work load increase, exercise, and decompression), (2) increased mental alertness and work output, and (3) improved the quality of work produced under stressful conditions and athletic performance.

The studies included both male and female subjects ranging in age from 19 to 72 years. Doses of the 33 percent ethanol (fluid) extract of *Eleutherococcus senticosus* roots ranged from 2.0 to 16.0 milliliters, one to three times a day, for periods up to 60 consecutive days. In multiple dosing regimens, there is usually a 2- to 3-week interval between courses.

Siberian ginseng as an adaptogen in disease processes

Farnsworth *et al.*[1] have also reviewed data on an *Eleutherococcus senticosus* root extract (33 percent ethanol) that has been administered to more than 2,200 human subjects in clinical trials for the purpose of evaluating the "adaptogenic" effects of Siberian ginseng in disease states. A variety of illnesses were included in these studies, including angina, hypertension, hypotension, acute pyelonephritis, various types of neuroses, acute craniocerebral trauma, rheumatic heart disease, chronic bronchitis, and cancer.

Siberian ginseng appears to be effective in atherosclerotic conditions as evidenced by its ability to lower elevated serum cholesterol, reduce blood pressure, and eliminate angina symptoms in human subjects. Its action on blood pressure is truly adaptogenic, as Siberian ginseng has also been shown to increase blood pressure in subjects with low blood pressure.[1]

Its effect in regulating blood pressure may be indicative of improved kidney function since it has been demonstrated that patients with acute kidney infection given Siberian ginseng extract demonstrate improved kidney function.[1]

Siberian ginseng appears to have some action on the brain as well, because it has consistently demonstrated an ability to increase the sense of well-being regardless of the psychological complaint (insomnia, hypochondriasis, various neuroses, etc.). A possible explanation of this effect is an improvement in balance between the various biogenic amines (serotonin, dopamine, norepinephrine, epinephrine, etc.), which act as transmitters in the nervous system, as Siberian ginseng extract administered to rats has been shown to increase biogenic amine content in the brain, adrenals, and urine.[1]

Siberian ginseng in chronic fatigue syndrome

One of the more popular uses of Siberian ginseng is in the treatment of "chronic fatigue syndrome" (CFS). Although a newly defined illness, CFS has been around a long time. Chronic fatigue syndrome can be a debilitating illness characterized by persistent fatigue along with other symptoms including low-grade fever, frequent sore throats, joint and muscle pain, and various neuro/psychological symptoms including depression.

Central to CFS is a disturbed immune system. While research has focused on trying to identify a specific infectious organism, CFS is more likely due to a general immune system failure.

Effective treatment of CFS must be comprehensive and address underlying factors that contribute to the weakened status of the immune system. However, Siberian ginseng appears to address the fatigue, decreased sense of well being, and impaired immune functions.

In regard to immune function, Siberian ginseng has been shown to exert a number of beneficial effects that may be useful in the treatment of chronic fatigue syndrome. In one double-blind study, thirty-six healthy subjects received either 10 milliliters of a Siberian ginseng fluid extract or placebo daily for 4 weeks.[9] The group receiving the Siberian ginseng demonstrated significant improvements in a variety of immune system parameters. Most notable were a significant increase in helper T cells and an increase in natural killer cell activity. Both of these effects could be put to good use in the treatment of chronic fatigue syndrome.

Dosage

The standard dosage of the 33 percent ethanol extract (fluid extract) of *Eleutherococcus senticosus* roots used in the majority of studies ranged from 2.0 to 4.0 milliliters (up to 16.0 milliliters), one to three times a day, for periods up to 60 consecutive days. In multiple dosing regimens, there is usually a 2- to 3-week interval between courses.[1,4] Doses to be administered three times a day are as follows:

- Dried root: 2–4 grams
- Tincture (1:5): 10–20 milliliters
- Fluid extract (1:1): 2.0–4.0 milliliters
- Solid (dry powdered) extract (20:1, containing more than 1 percent eleutheroside E: 100–200 milligrams

Toxicity

Toxicity studies in animals have demonstrated that Siberian ginseng extracts are virtually nontoxic. The LD_{50} (50 percent lethal dose) of the 33 percent ethanol extract of Siberian ginseng is 14.5 milliliters per kilogram in mice and greater than 20.0 milliliters per kilogram, and no long-term toxicity was observed in rats administered the 33 percent ethanol extract of Siberian ginseng at a daily dose of 5.0 milliliters per kilogram.[1]

In human studies it was demonstrated that Siberian ginseng extracts (33 percent ethanol) are extremely well tolerated and side effects are quite infrequent. However, side effects often reported at higher dosages (4.5–6.0 milliliters three times daily) include insomnia, irritability, melancholy, and anxiety. Individuals with rheumatic heart disease have reported pericardial pain, headaches, palpitations, and elevations in blood pressure following the administration of Siberian ginseng.[1]

References

1. Farnsworth NR, *et al.*: Siberian ginseng (*Eleutherococcus senticosus*): Current status as an adaptogen. *Econ Med Plant Res* **1**, 156–215, 1985.
2. Leung AY: *Encyclopedia of Common Natural Ingredients Used in Food, Drugs and Cosmetics.* John Wiley & Sons, New York, 1980, pp. 186–189.
3. Duke JA: *Handbook of Medicinal Herbs.* CRC Press, Boca Raton, FL, 1985, pp. 337–338.
4. Baranov AI: Medicinal uses of ginseng and related plants in the Soviet Union: Recent trends in the Soviet literature. *J Ethnopharmacol* **6**, 339–353, 1982.
5. Brekhman II and Dardymov IV: New substances of plant origin which increase nonspecific resistance. *Annu Rev Pharmacol* **9**, 419–430, 1969.
6. Brekhman II and Dardymov IV: Pharmacological investigation of glycosides from ginseng and *Eleutherococcus. Lloydia* **32**, 46–51, 1969.
7. Brekhman II and Kirillov OI: Effect of *Eleutherococcus* on alarm-phase of stress. *Annu Rev Pharmacol* **8**, 113–121, 1969.
8. Ben-Hur E and Fulder S: Effect of *P. ginseng* saponins and *Eleutherococcus* S. on survival of cultured mammalian cells after ionizing radiation. *Am J Chin Med* **9**, 48–56, 1981.
9. Bohn B, Nebe CT, and Birr C: Flow-cytometric studies with *Eleutherococcus senticosus* extract as an immunomodulatory agent. *Arzneimittel-Forsch* **37**, 1193–1196, 1987.

34
Tea tree oil

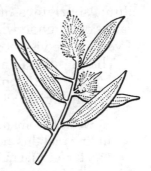

Key uses of tea tree oil:

- Topical antiseptic
- Fungal nail infections
- Acne
- Vaginal infections

General description

The tea tree (*Melaleuca alternifolia*) is a small tree native to only one area of the world: the northeast coastal region of New South Wales, Australia. The leaves (the portion of the plant that is used medicinally) are the source of a valuable therapeutic oil. Although there are more than fifty members of the *Melaleuca* genus, the oil from the leaf of *Melaleuca alternifolia* has received the most research attention.

Chemical composition

Tea tree leaves contain an oil (about 1.8 percent) obtained via steam distillation.[1] This oil contains more than forty-eight compounds, but is chiefly composed of 1-terpinen-4-ol, 1,8-cineol, gamma-terpinene, *p*-cymene, and and other terpenes.[2] The Australian Standard (AS 2782-1985) for "Oil of Melaleuca (Terpinen-4-ol type)" sets a minimum content of terpinen-4-ol at 30 percent and a maximum 1,8-cineol content of 15 percent.[1]

History and folk use

The medicinal properties of crushed tea tree leaves were known to the Bund-jalung aborigines of northern New South Wales, Australia. In fact, the waters of a lagoon where tea tree leaves had fallen and decayed for hundreds of years were viewed as having tremendous healing properties.[1]

The popular name of "tea tree" was first reported in 1777 in Captain Cook's account of his second voyage entitled *A Voyage to the South Pole* (quoted in Altman):[1]

> . . . we at first made it [some beer] of a decoction of the spruce leaves; but finding that this alone made the beer too astringent, we afterwards mixed with it an equal quantity of the tea plant (a name it obtained in my former voyage from our using it as tea then, as we also did now), which partly destroyed the astringency of the other, and made the beer exceedingly palat-able, and esteemed by everyone on board.

The leaves of *Melaleuca alternifolia* were also used by the early settlers of Australia to make tea, hence the further use of the popular name of "tea tree."[1]

The first report of the tea tree's medicinal use appeared in the *Medical Journal of Australia* in 1930.[3] A surgeon in Sydney reported impressive results using a solution of tea tree oil to clean surgical wounds. According to the author:

> The results obtained in a variety of conditions when it [tea tree oil] was first tried were most encouraging, a striking feature being that it dissolved pus and left the surface of infected wounds clean so that its germicidal action became more effective without any apparent damage to the tissues. This was something new, as most efficient germicides destroy tissue as well as bacteria. . . .

During World War II, tea tree oil was issued to soldiers to use as a disin-fectant. The Australian Army went so far as to commandeer supplies of the oil and exempt leaf cutters from national service in order to maintain pro-duction. The production of tea tree oil during World War II was regarded as an "essential" industry.[1]

After World War II, the tea tree oil industry stagnated for more than 30 years. There were a number of reasons for this, including the general trend away from natural medicines toward synthetic medical drugs. However, during the late 1970s and early 1980s, the Australian tea tree oil industry was reborn as successful plantations growing *Melaleuca alternifolia* were established.[1]

Tea tree oil has been used to treat acne, aphthous stomatitis, tinea pedis (athlete's foot), boils, burns, carbuncles, corns, gingivitis, herpes, impetigo, infections of the nail bed, insect bites, lice, mouth ulcers, psoriasis, root canal treatment, ringworm, sinus infections, pharyngitis, skin and vaginal infections, thrush, and tonsillitis.[1]

A variety of tea tree oil-based cosmetic products exist in the market place including toothpastes, shampoos and conditioners, creams, hand and body lotions, soaps, gels, liniments, and nail polish removers.

Pharmacology

Tea tree oil possesses significant antiseptic properties and is regarded by many as the ideal skin disinfectant. This claim is supported by its efficacy against a wide range of organisms, and by its good penetration and lack of irritation to the skin.[1] The therapeutic uses of tea tree oil are based largely on its antiseptic and antifungal properties.

Organisms inhibited by tea tree oil[1,7,8]

- *Candida albicans*
- *Propionibacterium acnes*
- *Pseudomonas aeruginosa*
- *Staphylococcus aureus*
- *Streptococcus pyrogenes*
- *Trichomonas vaginalis*
- *Trichophyton mentagrophytes*

Clinical applications

The historical uses of tea tree oil demonstrate its wide range of applications as an antiseptic. Three of the more popular and documented uses are in the treatment of skin infections, vaginal infections, and common foot complaints. These clinical applications are discussed below.

Skin infections

Tea tree oil is useful in a broad range of dermal infections, not only because of its broad-spectrum antiseptic properties, but also because of its capacity to mix with sebaceous secretions and penetrate the epidermis.

A clinical trial in patients with furuncles demonstrated that tea tree oil encouraged more rapid healing without scarring, compared to matched controls.[5] Presumably the positive clinical effects were due to the oil's germicidal activity against *Staphylococcus aureus*. The method of application included cleaning the site, followed by painting the surface of the furuncle freely with tea tree oil two or three times a day.

For most skin infections, the most effective treatment appears to be direct application of full-strength, undiluted oil at the site of infection. If irritation occurs, diluted preparations may be tried.

Acne   A topical application of tea tree oil is a suitable alternative to benzoyl peroxide preparations. In one study, 124 patients with mild to moderate acne randomly received either a 5 percent gel of tea tree oil or a 5 percent benzoyl peroxide lotion to be applied topically daily. After 3 months, both treatments produced a significant improvement in mean number of both noninflamed and inflamed lesions—only with noninflamed lesions was benzoyl peroxide found to be more effective. Importantly, side effects (dryness, pruritis, stinging, burning, and skin redness) were reported less frequently with tea tree oil (44 percent versus 79 percent).[6]

Common foot problems

Tea tree oil, in emollient form (8 percent tea tree oil) or in solution (40 percent), can be massaged into the feet daily for the treatment of tinea pedis, foot irritation, and bromhidrosis (severely foul-smelling feet).

One author concluded after 6 years of using different concentrations and preparations that tea tree oil eradicates or improves the symptoms of tinea pedis when used daily by the patient at home.[7] He also reported that even undiluted forms had little effect on onychomycosis (i.e., fungal nail infection). Diluted tea tree oil in solution reduced foot irritation and promoted wound healing in cases of surgical incision of corns, calluses, bunion, and hammertoes, and was extremely effective in diminishing bromhidrosis.

Fungal nail infection   Fungal nail infections (onychomycosis) are the most frequent cause of nail disease, affecting approximately 2 to 13 percent of the population. Standard medical treatments include debridement, topical antifungals, and systemic antifungals. All current therapies have high recurrence rates. Oral therapy has the added disadvantages of high cost and potentially serious adverse effects. A recent study compared the efficacy and tolerability of a topical application of 1 percent clotrimazole solution to that of 100 percent tea tree oil for the treatment of toenail onychomycosis.[8]

The 117 patients received a twice-daily application of either 1 percent clotrimazole (CL) solution or 100 percent tea tree (TT) oil for 6 months. Debridement and clinical assessment were performed at 0, 1, 3, and 6 months. Cultures were obtained at 0 and 6 months. Each patient's subjective assessment was also obtained 3 months after the conclusion of therapy. After 6 months of therapy, the two treatment groups were comparable, based on culture cure (CL = 11 percent, TT = 18 percent) and clinical assessment documenting partial or full resolution (CL = 61 percent, TT = 60 percent). Three months later, about half of each group reported continued improvement or resolution (CL = 55 percent; TT = 56 percent). These results indicate that topical therapy with tea tree oil, in conjunction with debridement, provides excellent improvement in nail appearance and symptomatology.

Vaginal infections

Tea tree oil demonstrates germicidal activity against a number of common vaginal pathogens and opportunistic organisms including *Trichomonas vaginalis* and *Candida albicans*.[9,10]

A 40 percent solution of tea tree oil emulsified with isopropyl alcohol and water was found in a clinical study to be highly effective for the treatment of cervicitis, chronic endocervicitis, trichomonal vaginitis, and vaginal candidiasis.[8] Weekly in-office treatment (usually four to six were necessary) involved thorough washing of the perineum, labia, and vagina with a suitable scrub (the commercial product phisohex was used in the study). After drying, the affected areas were washed with a 1 percent tea tree oil solution. This was followed by insertion of a tampon (three 4×4 inch sponges) saturated with the 40 percent tea tree oil solution. Patients were instructed to remove the tampon in 24 hours.

For infectious processes, that is, trichomonas and candidiasis, daily vaginal douches containing 1 quart of water with a 0.4 percent concentration of the oil were prescribed. No irritation, burning or other side effects were reported or observed with either the office applications or the douches.

Dosage

A number of commercial products contain tea tree oil. Tea tree oil can be used as a topical antiseptic for reducing microbial counts in wounds, surgical incisions, and skin and vaginal infections. In addition, tea tree leaves can be used to make a tea that may be of benefit in cases of sore throat, tonsillitis, sinus infections, and colitis.

Toxicity

Tea tree oil is extremely safe for use as a topical antiseptic. However, the oral ingestion of tea tree oil cannot be recommended, as this could lead to a toxic reaction. However, folk use suggests that oral ingestion of tea from the leaves is safe.

References

1. Altman PM: Australian tea tree oil. *Aust J Pharm* **69**, 276–278, 1988.
2. Swords G and Hunter GLK: Composition of Australian tea tree oil (*Melaleuca alternifolia*). *J Agric Food Chem* **26**, 734–737, 1978.
3. Humphery EM: A new Australian germicide. *Med J Aust* **1**, 417–418, 1930.
4. Leung AY: *Encyclopedia of Common Natural Ingredients Used in Food.* John Wiley & Sons, New York, 1980.
5. Feinblatt HM: Cajeput-type oil for the treatment of furunculosis. *J Natl Med Assoc* **52**, 32–34, 1960.
6. Bassett IB, *et al.*: A comparative study of tea-tree oil versus benzoyl peroxide in the treatment of acne. *Med J Aust* **153**, 455–458, 1990.
7. Walker M: Clinical investigation of Australian *Melaleuca alternifolia* oil for a variety of common foot problems. *Curr Podiatry* **18**, 30–35, 1972.
8. Buck DS, Nidorf DM, and Addino JG: Comparison of two topical preparations for the treatment of onychomycosis: *Melaleuca alternifolia* (tea tree) oil and clotrimazole. *J Fam Pract* **38**, 601–605, 1994.
9. *Melaleuca alternifolia* Essential Oils Data Search, Vancouver, WA, 1985.
10. Pena EF: *Melaleuca alternifolia* oil. *Obstet Gynecol* **19**, 793–795, 1962.

35
Turmeric

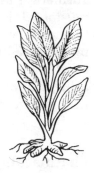

Key uses of turmeric and curcumin:

- Antioxidant
- Cancer prevention and treatment adjunct
- Gallstones
- Inflammatory conditions
- Irritable bowel syndrome
- Liver disorders

General description

Turmeric (*Curcuma longa*) is a perennial herb of the ginger family that is extensively cultivated in India, China, Indonesia, and other tropical countries. It has a thick rhizome from which arise large, oblong, long-petioled leaves. The rhizome is the part used; it is usually cured (boiled, cleaned, and sun-dried) and polished.[1]

Chemical composition

Turmeric contains 0.3–5.4 percent curcumin; an orange-yellow volatile oil (4–14 percent) composed mainly of turmerone, atlantone, and zingiberone; sugars (28 percent glucose, 12 percent fructose, and 1 percent arabinose); resins; protein; vitamins; and minerals.[1,2]

History and folk use

Turmeric is the major ingredient of curry powder and is also used in prepared mustard. It is extensively used in foods both for its color and flavor. In addition, turmeric is used in both the Chinese and Indian (Ayurvedic) systems of medicine as an antiinflammatory agent and in the treatment of numerous conditions, including flatulence, jaundice, menstrual difficulties, bloody urine, hemorrhage, toothache, bruises, chest pain, and colic.[1] Turmeric poultices are often applied locally to relieve inflammation and pain.

Pharmacology

Turmeric and its derivatives exert a great deal of pharmacological activity.[2] Although a number of components have demonstrated activity, the volatile oil components and curcumin are believed to be the most active components. Turmeric is an effective antioxidant, anticarcinogenic, antiinflammatory, cardiovascular, hepatic, gastrointestinal, and antimicrobial agent.

Antioxidant effects

Turmeric extracts exert significant antioxidant activity. Although both water and fat-soluble extracts are effective antioxidants in various *in vitro* and *in vivo* models, curcumin is the most potent component.[3-7] The antioxidant activity of curcumin is comparable to standard antioxidants such as vitamins C and E, butylated hydroxyanisole (BHA), and butylated hydroxytoluene (BHT).[3,4] Because of its bright yellow color and antioxidant properties against lipid peroxidation, curcumin is used in butter, margarine, cheese, and other food products.

Curcumin combats active oxygen species slightly less well than vitamin C, but better than vitamin E and superoxide dismutase. Against hydroxyl radicals, curcumin offers greater effectiveness than these vitamins.[3-5] The antioxidant properties of turmeric are not due to curcumin alone, as the aqueous extract of turmeric is more effective against superoxide than is curcumin, and is much stronger in inhibiting oxidative damage to DNA.[6,7]

Anticancer effects

The anticancer effects of turmeric and curcumin have been demonstrated at all steps of cancer formation: initiation, promotion, and progression. In addition to inhibiting the development of cancer, data obtained from several studies suggest that curcumin can also promote cancer regression.

Turmeric and curcumin are nonmutagenic[8] and suppress the mutagenicity of several common mutagens[9] (cigarette smoke condensates, benzopyrene, DMBA, etc.), as do chili and capsaicin.[10] Turmeric and curcumin also exert impressive anticancer effects against a number of chemical carcinogens in a wide range of cell types in both *in vitro* and *in vivo* studies.[11-18] Curcumin has demonstrated an impressive ability to reduce the levels of urinary mutagens.[19,20]

The protective effects of turmeric and its derivatives are only partially explained by its direct antioxidant and free radical-scavenging effects. It also inhibits nitrosamine formation, enhances the body's natural antioxidant system, increases the levels of glutathione and other nonprotein sulfhydryls, and acts directly on several enzymes and genetic material.

Antiinflammatory effects

The volatile oil fraction of *Curcuma longa* possesses antiinflammatory activity in a variety of experimental models (e.g., Freund's adjuvant-induced arthritis, formaldehyde- and carrageenan-induced paw edema, and cotton pellet and granuloma pouch tests).[21,22] Its effects in these studies were comparable to those of cortisone and phenylbutazone.

Even more potent in acute inflammation is curcumin.[23-25] Curcumin is as effective as cortisone or phenylbutazone in models of acute inflammation, but only half as effective in chronic models. However, while phenylbutazone and cortisone are associated with significant toxicity, curcumin displays virtually no toxicity (see Toxicity, below).

The ranking, in order of potency, of curcumin analogs, cortisone, and phenylbutazone in carrageenan-induced paw edema is as follows:[24,25]

Sodium curcuminate > tetrahydrocurcumin > curcumin >
cortisone > phenylbutazone > triethylcurcumin

Sodium curcuminate can be produced by mixing turmeric with slaked lime. This mixture, applied as a poultice, is an ancient household remedy for sprains, muscular pain, and inflamed joints.[25]

Curcumin's counterirritant effect may also be a major factor in its topical antiinflammatory action.[24] Capsaicin, a similar pungent principle from *Capsicum frutescens,* has been shown to be quite effective as a topical pain reliever in cases of postherpetic neuralgia and arthritis. Both capsaicin and curcumin deplete nerve endings of substance P, the neurotransmitter of pain receptors.[26]

Used orally, curcumin exhibits many direct antiinflammatory effects, including inhibition of leukotriene formation; inhibition of platelet aggregation; promotion of fibrinolysis; inhibition of neutrophil response to various stimuli involved in the inflammatory process; and stabilization of cell membranes, thereby preventing the release of inflammatory mediators.[2,23,24,27-29]

In addition to its direct antiinflammatory effects, curcumin also appears to exert some indirect effects. In models of chronic inflammation, curcumin is much less active in animals from which the adrenal glands have been removed. Possible mechanisms of action include (1) stimulation of the release of adrenal corticosteroids, (2) "sensitizing" or priming cortisol receptor sites, thereby potentiating cortisol action, and (3) increasing the half-life of endogenous cortisol through alteration of hepatic degradation.

Cardiovascular effects

The effects of turmeric and curcumin on the cardiovascular system include lowering of cholesterol levels[30,31] and inhibition of platelet aggregation.[32,33] This is of great significance in preventing atherosclerosis and its complications.

In rats fed a diet containing as little as 0.1 percent curcumin and cholesterol, cholesterol levels fell to one-half those in rats fed cholesterol and no curcumin.[30] This indicates that even at small doses, curcumin may be effective.

Curcumin's cholesterol-lowering actions include interfering with intestinal cholesterol uptake, increasing the conversion of cholesterol into bile acids, and increasing the excretion of bile acids via its choleretic effects.[30,31,34]

Turmeric and curcumin may inhibit platelet aggregation by inhibiting the formation of thromboxanes (a promoter of aggregation) while simultaneously increasing prostacyclin (an inhibitor of aggregation).[32,33]

Hepatic effects

Curcumin has exhibited hepatoprotection similar to that of glycyrrhizin and silymarin against carbon tetrachloride- and galactosamine-induced liver injury.[2,35] This protection is largely a result of its potent antioxidant activity.

The antioxidant and hepatoprotective effects alone would support turmeric's historical use in liver disorders; however, turmeric and curcumin also exert antiinflammatory and choleretic effects. The increases in liver enzymes, SGOT and SGPT, commonly seen in experimental models of inflammation have been prevented by curcumin.[23]

Curcumin is an active choleretic, increasing bile acid output by over 100 percent.[2] In addition to increasing biliary excretion of bile salts, cholesterol, and bilirubin, curcumin also increases the solubility of bile.[34] This suggests a benefit in the prevention and treatment of cholelithiasis.

Gastrointestinal effects

Turmeric and its components exert a number of beneficial effects on the gastrointestinal system. Turmeric's long use as a carminative has received significant research support.[2] Specifically, curcumin has been shown to inhibit gas formation by *Clostridium perfringens* in rats given diets rich in flatulence-producing foods. In addition, sodium curcuminate has been shown to inhibit intestinal spasm, and another compound from turmeric (*p*-tolymethylcarbinol) has been shown to increase the secretion of secretin, gastrin, bicarbonate, and pancreatic enzymes.[2]

As a component of curries and spicy foods, there is some concern that turmeric may be irritating to the stomach. However, several studies have shown turmeric to be beneficial to gastric integrity. Turmeric and curcumin increase the mucin content of the stomach and exert gastroprotective effects against ulcer formation induced by stress, alcohol, indomethacin, pyloric ligation, and reserpine.[2,36] However, at high doses curcumin or turmeric may be ulcerogenic (see Toxicity, below).

Antimicrobial effects

Alcohol extracts and the essential oil of *Curcuma longa* were shown in one study to inhibit the growth of most organisms occurring in cholecystitis, that is, *Sarcina*, *Gaffkya*, *Corynebacterium*, and *Clostridium*.[2] Other microorganisms that are inhibited include *Staphylococcus*, *Streptococcus*, *Bacillus*, *Entamoeba histolytica*, and several pathogenic fungi.[2,37] The concentrations used in these studies were relatively high: 0.5–5.0 milligrams per milliliter of the alcohol extract and essential oil, and 5–100 micrograms per milliliter of curcumin.

Clinical applications

Turmeric and curcumin are applied clinically as a cancer preventative and treatment adjunct, and in the treatment of inflammation, atherosclerosis, liver disorders, cholelithiasis, and irritable bowel syndrome.

Cancer prevention and treatment adjunct

As discussed above, turmeric and curcumin have demonstrated significant protective effects against cancer development in experimental studies in animals. There is also some human research showing similar results.

In one human study, sixteen chronic smokers were given 1.5 grams of turmeric daily while six nonsmokers served as a control group.[19] At the end of the 30-day trial, the smokers receiving the turmeric demonstrated significant reduction in the level of urinary-excreted mutagens. These results are quite significant, as the level of urinary mutagens is thought to correlate with the systemic load of carcinogens and the efficacy of detoxification mechanisms. Owing to widespread exposure to smoke, aromatic hydrocarbons, and other environmental carcinogens, the frequent use of turmeric as a spice appears warranted. In addition, there may be instances when supplementation with curcumin is also appropriate.

Turmeric extracts and curcumin have demonstrated direct antitumor results in a number of experimental models of skin and epithelial cancers.[15,38] This effect has also been substantiated in a human study.[39] Sixty-two patients with either ulcerating oral or cutaneous squamous cell carcinomas who had failed to respond to standard treatments such as surgery, radiation, and chemotherapy were given either an ethanol extract of turmeric (for oral cancer) or an ointment containing 0.5 percent curcumin in petroleum jelly. The ointment or extract was applied topically three times daily. At the end of the 18-month study, the treatment was found to have been effective in reducing the smell of the lesion (90 percent), itching and exudate (70 percent), pain (50 percent), and the size of the lesion (10 percent). Although not spectacular results, it must be pointed out that this patient population had failed to respond to standard medical treatment.

It appears that while more human studies are needed on the use of turmeric and curcumin in cancer, ample evidence supports their use in cancer prevention and as an adjunct in an overall cancer treatment plan.

Inflammation

Curcuma longa has been used in Ayurvedic medicine, both locally and internally, in the treatment of sprains and inflammation. This use seems to be substantiated not only by the experimental studies described above, but also by clinical investigations.[40,41]

In one double-blind cross-over clinical trial in patients with rheumatoid arthritis, curcumin (1,200 milligrams per day) was compared to phenylbutazone (300 milligrams per day). The improvements in the duration of morning stiffness, walking time, and joint swelling were comparable in both groups.[40] However, it must be pointed out that while phenylbutazone is associated with significant adverse effects, curcumin has not been shown to produce any side effects at the recommended dosage level.

In another study which used a new human model—the postoperative inflammation model—for evaluating nonsteroid antiinflammatory drugs

(NSAIDs), curcumin was again shown to exert an antiinflammatory action comparable to that of phenylbutazone.[41] While curcumin has an antiinflammatory effect similar to phenylbutazone and various NSAIDs, it does not possess direct pain-relieving action.

The results of these studies indicate that turmeric or curcumin may provide benefit in the treatment of inflammation. Furthermore, the safety and excellent tolerability of curcumin compared to standard drug treatment are major advantages.

Dosage

On the basis of the evidence presented above, turmeric should be consumed liberally in the diet. When specific medicinal effects are desired, higher doses of turmeric can be given or extracts of *Curcuma longa* or curcumin can be used.

The recommended dosage for curcumin as an antiinflammatory is 400 to 600 milligrams three times a day. To achieve a similar amount of curcumin in the form of turmeric would require a dosage of 8,000 to 60,000 milligrams three times a day.

Because the absorption of orally administered curcumin may be limited (pharmacokinetic studies in animals show that 40 to 85 percent of an oral dose of curcumin passes through the gastrointestinal tract unchanged),[42–44] curcumin is often formulated in conjunction with an equal amount of bromelain, which may possibly enhance absorption. In addition, bromelain also has significant antiinflammatory effects.

Curcumin–bromelain combinations are best taken on an empty stomach 20 minutes before meals or between meals.

Providing curcumin in a lipid base such as lecithin, fish oils, or essential fatty acids may also increase absorption. This combination is probably best absorbed when taken with meals.

Toxicity

Toxicity reactions have not been reported at standard dosage levels. The oral LD_{50} (50 percent lethal dose) for turmeric, its alcohol extracts, and curcumin has not been determined, because curcumin fed to mice, rats, guinea pigs, and monkeys at 2.5 grams per kilogram, and sodium curcuminate fed to rats at 3.0 grams per kilogram, resulted in neither mortality nor genetic damage.[2,42–44] At high doses curcumin or turmeric may damage the gastrointestinal system because curcumin, at doses of 100 milligrams per kilogram body weight, was ulcerogenic in rats.[2]

References

1. Leung A: *Encyclopedia of Common Natural Ingredients Used in Food, Drugs, and Cosmetics.* John Wiley & Sons, New York, 1980, pp. 313–314.
2. Ammon HPT and Wahl MA: Pharmacology of *Curcuma longa. Planta Medica* **57**, 1–7, 1991.
3. Sharma OP: Antioxidant properties of curcumin and related compounds. *Biochem Pharmacol* **25**, 1811–1825, 1976.
4. Toda S, *et al.*: Natural antioxidants: Antioxidative compounds isolated from rhizome of *Curcuma longa L. Chem Pharmacol Bull* **33**, 1725–1728, 1985.
5. Zhao B, *et al.*: Scavenging effect of extracts of green tea and natural antioxidants on active oxygen radicals. *Cell Biophys* **14**, 175–185, 1989.
6. Shalini VK and Srinivas L: Lipid peroxide induced DNA damage: Protection by turmeric (*Curcuma longa*). *Mol Cell Biochem* **77**, 3–10, 1987.
7. Srinivas L and Shalini VK: DNA damage by smoke: Protection by turmeric and other inhibitors of ROS. *Free Radical Biol Med* **11**, 277–283, 1991.
8. Jensen NJ: Lack of mutagenic effect of turmeric oleoresin and curcumin in the *Salmonella*/mammalian microsome test. *Mut Res* **105**, 393–396, 1982.
9. Nagabhushan M, Amonkar AJ, and Bhide SV: In vitro antimutagenicity of curcumin against environmental mutagens. *Fd Chem Toxic* **25**, 545–547, 1987.
10. Nagabhushan M and Bhide SV: Nonmutagenicity of curcumin and its antimutagenic action versus chili and capsaicin. *Nutr Cancer* **8**, 201–210, 1986.
11. Jiang TL, Salmon SE, and Liu RM: Activity of camptothecin, harrington, catharidin and curcumae in the human tumor stem cell assay. *Eur J Cancer Clin Oncol* **19**, 263–270, 1983.
12. Mehta RG and Moon RC: Characterization of effective chemopreventive agents in mammary gland in vitro using an initiation-promotion protocol. *Anticancer Res* **11**, 593–596, 1991.
13. Kuttan R, *et al.*: Potential anticancer activity of turmeric (*Curcuma longa*). *Cancer Lett* **29**, 197–202, 1985.
14. Soudamini NK and Kuttan R: Inhibition of chemical carcinogenesis by curcumin. *J Ethnopharmacol* **27**, 227–233, 1989.
15. Azuine M and Bhide S: Chemopreventive effect of turmeric against stomach and skin tumors induced by chemical carcinogens in Swiss mice. *Nutr Cancer* **17**, 77–83, 1992.
16. Nagabhushan N and Bhide SV: Curcumin as an inhibitor of cancer. *J Am Coll Nutr* **11**, 192–198, 1992.
17. Azuine MA, Kayal JJ, and Bhide SV: Protective role of aqueous turmeric extract against mutagenicity of direct-acting carcinogens as well as benzopyrene-induced genotoxicity and carcinogenicity. *J Cancer Res Clin Oncol* **118**, 447–452, 1992.
18. Boone CW, Steele VE, and Kelloff GJ: Screening of chemopreventive (anticarcinogenic) compounds in rodents. *Mutat Res* **267**, 251–255, 1992.
19. Polasa K, *et al.*: Effect of turmeric on urinary mutagens in smokers. *Mutagenesis* **7**, 107–109, 1992.
20. Polasa K, *et al.*: Turmeric (*Curcuma longa*)-induced reduction in urinary mutagens. *Fd Chem Toxic* **29**, 699–706, 1991.
21. Chandra D and Gupta S: Anti-inflammatory and anti-arthritic activity of volatile oil of *Curcuma longa* (Haldi). *Indian J Med Res* **60**, 138–142, 1972.
22. Arora R, *et al.*: Anti-inflammatory studies on *Curcuma longa* (turmeric). *Indian J Med Res* **59**, 1289–1295, 1971.
23. Srimal R and Dhawan B: Pharmacology of diferuloyl methane (curcumin), a non-steroidal anti-inflammatory agent. *J Pharm Pharmacol* **25**, 447–452, 1973.
24. Mukhopadhyay A, *et al.*: Anti-inflammatory and irritant activities of curcumin analogues in rats. *Agents Actions* **12**, 508–515, 1982.
25. Ghatak N and Basu N: Sodium curcuminate as an effective anti-inflammatory agent. *Indian J Exp Biol* **10**, 235–236, 1972.
26. Patacchini R, Maggi CA, and Meli A: Capsaicin-like activity of some natural pungent substances on peripheral ending of visceral primary afferents. *Arch Pharmacol* **342**, 72–77, 1990.

27. Srivastava R and Srimal RC: Modification of certain inflammation-induced biochemical changes by curcumin. *Indian J Med Res* **81**, 215–223, 1985.
28. Srivastava R: Inhibition of neutrophil response by curcumin. *Agents Actions* **28**, 298–303, 1989.
29. Flynn DL and Rafferty MF: Inhibition of 5-hydroxy-eicosatetraenoic acid (5-HETE) formation in intact human neutrophils by naturally-occurring diarylheptanoids: Inhibitory activities of curcuminoids and yakuchinones. *Prostaglandins Leukotrienes Med* **22**, 357–360, 1986.
30. Rao DS, *et al.*: Effect of curcumin on serum and liver cholesterol levels in the rat. *J Nutr* **100**, 1307–1316, 1970.
31. Srinivasan K and Samaiah K: The effect of spices on cholesterol 7 alpha-hydroxylase activity and on serum and hepatic cholesterol levels in the rat. *Int J Vitam Nutr Res* **61**, 364–369, 1991.
32. Srivastava R, *et al.*: Anti-thrombotic effect of curcumin. *Throm Res* **40**, 413–417, 1985.
33. Srivastava R, *et al.*: Effect of curcumin on platelet aggregation and vascular prostacyclin synthesis. *Arzneimittel-Forsch* **36**, 715–717, 1986.
34. Ramprasad C and Sirsi M: *Curcuma longa* and bile secretion—quantitative changes in the bile constituents induced by sodium curcuminate. *J Sci Ind Res* **16C**, 108–110, 1957.
35. Kiso Y, *et al.*: Antihepatotoxic principles of *Curcuma longa* rhizomes. *Planta Medica* **49**, 185–187, 1983.
36. Rafatullah S, *et al.*: Evaluation of turmeric (*Curcuma longa*) for gastric and duodenal antiulcer activity in rats. *J Ethnopharmacol* **29**, 25–34, 1990.
37. Lutomski VJ, Kedzia B, and Debska W: Effect of an alcohol extract and active ingredients from *Curcuma longa* on bacteria and fungi. *Planta Medica* **26**, 17–19, 1974.
38. Huang MT, *et al.*: Inhibitory effect of curcumin, chlorogenic acid, caffeic acid, and ferulic acid tumor promotion in mouse skin by 12-*O*-tetradecanoylphorbol-13-acetate. *Cancer Res* **48**, 5941–5946, 1988.
39. Kuttan R, Sudheeran PC, and Josph CD: Turmeric and curcumin as topical agents in cancer therapy. *Tumori* **73**, 29–31, 1987.
40. Deodhar SD, Sethi R, and Srimal RC: Preliminary studies on antirheumatic activity of curcumin (diferuloyl methane). *Indian J Med Res* **71**, 632–634, 1980.
41. Satoskar RR, Shah SJ, and Shenoy SG: Evaluation of anti-inflammatory property of curcumin (diferuloyl methane) in patients with postoperative inflammation. *Int J Clin Pharmacol Ther Toxicol* **24**, 651–654, 1986.
42. Shankar TNB, *et al.*: Toxicity studies on turmeric (*Curcuma longa*): Acute toxicity studies in rats, guinea pigs and monkeys. *Indian J Exp Biol* **18**, 73–75,1980.
43. Wahlstrom B and Blennow G: A study on the fate of curcumin in the rat. *Acta Pharmacol Toxicol* **43**, 86–92, 1978.
44. Ravindranath V and Chandrasekhara N: Absorption and tissue distribution of curcumin in rats. *Toxicology* **16**, 259–265, 1980.

36

Uva ursi

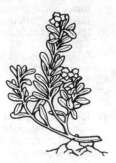

Key uses of uva ursi:

- Urinary tract infections
- As a mild diuretic

General description

Uva ursi (*Arctostaphylos uva ursi*) is a small evergreen shrub found in the northern United States and in Europe. A single long, fibrous main root sends out several prostrate or buried stems 4 to 6 inches high. The bark is dark brown; the leaves are obovate to spatulate, and ½ to 1 inch long; the flowers are pink or white, growing in sparse terminal clusters; and the fruit is a bright red or pink. Uva ursi is also known as bearberry and upland cranberry.

Chemical composition

Uva ursi's most active ingredient is arbutin, which typically composes 7 to 9 percent of the leaves. Other constituents include tannins (6–7 percent), flavonoids (quercetin), allantoin, gallic and ellagic acids, volatile oils, and a resin (urvone).[1,2]

History and folk use

Uva ursi has a long history of use for its diuretic and astringent properties. Conditions for which it was used include bladder and kidney infections, kidney stones, and bronchitis.[1]

Pharmacology

Pharmacological research has focused primarily on arbutin. In fact, at one time arbutin was marketed as a urinary antiseptic and diuretic. The activity of arbutin, however, is less than that of the total plant.[3] Crude plants or their extracts are often much more effective medicinally than the isolated active constituent. This appears to be the case with uva ursi and arbutin.

To be active, arbutin must be converted to another compound, hydroquinonehydroquinone, in the urinary tract.[1,2] The arbutin molecule must be absorbed intact from the intestine. When arbutin is given alone, bacteria in the intestine break down much of the arbutin before it is absorbed. If the whole plant is given, components in the plant prevent this breakdown of arbutin.[3] This allows for improved absorption of the intact arbutin molecule. The net effect is an increase in the amount of arbutin that is converted to hydroquinone if the whole plant or crude extract is given.

The activity of arbutin as an antibiotic in the urinary tract depends on an alkaline urine.[1,2] Again, this suggests another reason why the whole plant is of more value than the isolated compound, as the other components of uva ursi serve to make the urine more alkaline.

Dosage

As a urinary tract disinfectant and mild diuretic in cases of urinary tract infection, uva ursi can be taken in the following dosages three times daily:

- Dried leaves or by infusion (tea): 1.5 to 4 grams
- Tincture (1:5): 4–6 milliliters
- Fluid extract (1:1): 0.5–2.0 milliliters
- Powdered solid extract (20 percent arbutin content): 250–500 milligrams

Toxicity

The toxicity of uva ursi is proportional to the conversion of arbutin to hydroquinone. Hydroquinone has been shown to be toxic at 1 gram (equivalent to approximately 0.5 ounce of the fresh leaves), with signs and symptoms of tinnitus, nausea, vomiting, a sense of suffocation, shortness of breath, cyanosis, convulsions, delirium, and collapse.[2]

References

1. Leung A: *Encyclopedia of Common Natural Ingredients Used in Food, Drugs, and Cosmetics.* John Wiley & Sons, New York, 1980, pp. 316–317.
2. *Merck Index*, 10th ed. Merck & Co, Rahway, NJ, 1983, pp. 796–797 and 4721.
3. Frohne V: Untersuchungen zur Frage der harndesifizierenden Wirkungen von Barentraubenblattextracten. *Planta Medica* **18**, 1–25, 1970.

37
Valerian

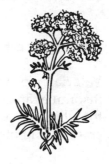

Key uses of valerian:

- Insomnia
- Stress and anxiety

General description

Valerian is a perennial plant native to North America and Europe. The yellow-brown tuberous rootstock produces a flowering stem 2 to 4 feet high. The stem is round, but grooved and hollow, with leaves arranged in pairs. The small, rose-colored flowers are in bloom from June to September. The rootstock is the portion used medicinally.

Chemical composition

The important active compounds of valerian are the valepotriates (iridoid molecules) and valeric acid. These compounds are found exclusively in valerian. Originally it was thought that just the valepotriates were responsible for valerian's sedative effects, but recently an aqueous extract of valerian has also been shown to have a sedative effect. Since the valepotriates are not soluble in water, it was concluded that valeric acid also possesses sedative action and is the chemical factor responsible for the sedative effect noted in human clinical trials with aqueous extracts of valerian.[1]

Also, because the safety of valepotriates was questioned after studies demonstrated mutagenicity, most commercial extracts in use feature water-soluble extracts standardized for valeric acids.[1–3]

Other components of valerian include a volatile oil (0.5–2 percent), choline (3 percent), flavonoids, sterols, and several alkaloids (actinidine, valerianine, valerine, and chatinine).[1]

History and folk use

Valerian's primary traditional use has been as a sedative for the relief of insomnia, anxiety, and conditions associated with pain. Specific conditions for which it was used include migraine, insomnia, hysteria, fatigue, intestinal cramps, and other nervous conditions.

Pharmacology

Valerian demonstrates a number of pharmacological effects, including normalization of the central nervous system (valerian acts as a sedative in states of agitation and as a stimulant in cases of extreme fatigue), lowering of blood pressure, enhancement of the flow of bile (choleretic effect), relaxation of intestinal muscles, and antitumor and antibiotic activity.[4–7] Its prime pharmacological effect, however, is consistent with its historical use as a sedative.

A recent pharmacological study indicated that both valepotriates and valeric acid are capable of binding to the same brain receptors as Valium and other benzodiazepine drugs.[8] However, valerian does not appear to act in a similar fashion, in that side effects such as impaired mental function, morning hangover, and dependency have not been reported with valerian.

Clinical applications

The primary clinical application for valerian is as a sedative in the treatment of insomnia. It can also be used in the treatment of stress and anxiety.

Insomnia

Several recent clinical studies have substantiated valerian's ability to improve sleep quality and relieve insomnia.[9–13]

The first studies were performed on subjects who did not have insomnia. In the first double-blind study involving 128 subjects, an extract of valerian root improved subjective ratings for sleep quality and sleep latency (the time required to go to sleep) but left no "hangover" the next morning.[9]

In another study, valerian's effects on sleep were studied in two groups of healthy, young subjects.[10] One group slept at home, the other in a sleep laboratory. Sleep was evaluated on the basis of questionnaires, self-rating scales, and night-time motor activity. Under home conditions, both doses of valerian extract (450 and 900 milligrams) reduced perceived sleep latency and wake time after sleep onset. Nighttime motor activity was enhanced in the middle third of the night and reduced in the last third. The data suggest a dose-dependent effect. In the sleep laboratory, where only the higher dose of valerian was tested, no significant differences from placebo were obtained. However, the direction of the changes in the subjective and objective measures of sleep latency and wake time after sleep onset, as well as in night-time motor activity, corresponded to that observed under home conditions. There was no evidence of a change in sleep stages and electroencephalogram (EEG) spectra. The results indicate that the aqueous valerian extract exerts a mild sedative effect.

While these two studies demonstrated that valerian could improve sleep quality in normal subjects, they failed to determine whether valerian could improve sleep patterns in people suffering from insomnia. In a follow-up to these two preliminary studies, valerian extract was shown to significantly reduce sleep latency, improve sleep quality, and reduce nighttime awakenings in sufferers of insomnia.[11] This study, performed under strict laboratory conditions, demonstrated that valerian is as effective in reducing sleep latency as small doses of barbiturates or benzodiazepines. However, while these latter compounds also increase morning sleepiness, valerian usually reduces morning sleepiness.

In another study of insomniacs, subjects received either a valerian preparation or placebo.[12] Compared to the placebo, valerian showed a significant effect, with 44 percent reporting perfect sleep and 89 percent reporting improved sleep.

And finally, in another double-blind study of insomniacs, twenty subjects received either a combination of valerian root (160 milligrams) and *Melissa officinalis* (80 milligrams), a benzodiazepine (triazolam, 0.125 milligrams), or placebo.[13] In the insomniac group, the valerian preparation showed an effect comparable to that of the benzodiazopine as well as an increase in deep sleep stages 3 and 4. The valerian preparation did not, however, cause daytime sedation and there was no evidence of diminished concentration based on the Concentration Performance Test or impairment of physical performance.

Dosage

As a mild sedative, valerian may be taken at the following dose 30 to 45 minutes before retiring:

- Dried root (or as tea): 1–2 grams
- Tincture (1:5): 4–6 milliliters (1–1.5 teaspoons)
- Fluid extract (1:1): 1–2 milliliters (0.5–1 teaspoon)
- Valerian extract (0.8 percent valeric acid): 150–300 milligrams

For the rare patient with increased morning sleepiness, reducing the dosage will eliminate the problem. For best results, eliminate dietary factors such as caffeine and alcohol, which disrupt sleep.

Toxicity

Valerian is generally regarded as safe and is approved for food use by the United States Food and Drug Administration.[14]

The safety of the valepotriates has been questioned;[2] until there is better information, your best choice is to use water-soluble extracts standardized for valeric acid content.

References

1. Houghton PJ. The biological activity of valerian and related plants. *J Ethnopharmacol* **22**(2), 121–142, 1988.
2. von der Hude W, Scheutwinkel-Reich M, and Braun R: Bacterial mutagenicity of the tranquilizing constituents of Valerianaceae roots. *Mutat Res* **169**, 23–27, 1986.
3. von der Hude W, *et al.*: In vitro mutagenicity of valepotriates. *Arch Toxicol* **56**, 267–271, 1985.
4. Takeda S, Endo T, and Aburada M: Pharmacological studies on iridoid compounds. III. The choleretic mechanism of iridoid compounds. *J Pharm Dyn* **4**, 612–623, 1981.
5. Hendriks H, *et al.*: Pharmacological screening of valerenal and some other components of essential oil of *Valeriana officinalis*. *Planta Medica* **42**, 62–68, 1981.
6. Hazelhoff B, Malingre TM, and Meijer DK: Antispasmodic effects of *Valeriana* compounds: An in vivo and in vitro study on the guinea pig ileum. *Arch Int Pharmacodyn* **257**, 274–287, 1982.
7. Bounthanh C, *et al.*: Valepotriates, a new class of cytotoxic and antitumor agents. *Planta Medica* **41**, 21–28, 1981.
8. Mennini T, *et al.*: In vitro study on the interaction of extracts and pure compounds from *Valeriana officinalis* roots with GABA, benzodiazepine and barbiturate receptors in rat brain. *Fitoterapia* **54**, 291–300, 1993.
9. Leathwood P, *et al.*: Aqueous extract of valerian root (*Valeriana officinalis* L.) improves sleep quality in man. *Pharmacol Biochem Behav* **17**, 65–71, 1982.
10. Balderer G and Borbely AA. Effect of valerian on human sleep. *Psychopharmacol* **87**, 406–409, 1985.
11. Leathwood PD and Chauffard F: Aqueous extract of valerian reduces latency to fall asleep in man. *Planta Medica* **54**, 144–148, 1985.
12. Lindahl O and Lindwall L: Double blind study of a valerian preparation. *Pharmacol Biochem Behav* **32**(4), 1065–1066, 1989.
13. Dressing H, *et al.*: Insomnia: Are *Valeriana/Melissa* combinations of equal value to benzodiazepine? *Therapiewoche* **42**, 726–736, 1992.
14. Leung A: *Encyclopedia of Common Natural Ingredients Used in Food, Drugs, and Cosmetics.* John Wiley & Sons, New York, 1980.

SECTION III

Recommended herbs for some specific health conditions

Section III features specific herbal recommendations for a number of common health conditions. Although many herbs are effective on their own, they work even better if they are part of a comprehensive natural treatment plan that focuses on diet and lifestyle factors. I have tried to provide a concise description of the health condition, including dietary considerations. For a more complete description, please consult some of my other books, such as the *Encyclopedia of Natural Medicine* (Prima Publishing, Rocklin, CA, 1991), *Natural Alternatives to Over-the-Counter and Prescription Drugs* (Morrow, New York, 1994), or the appropriate *Getting Well Naturally* series (Prima Publishing, 1994).

Before you read on, I want to remind you once again of some important guidelines.

- **Do not self-diagnose** Proper medical care is critical to good health. If you have symptoms suggestive of an illness discussed in this section, please consult a physician, preferably a holistic medical doctor (M.D.), osteopath (D.O.), naturopath (N.D.), chiropractor (D.C.), or other natural health care specialist.

- **Work with your doctor**   If you are currently on a prescription medication, you absolutely must work with your doctor before discontinuing any drug.
- **Educate your doctor**   If you wish to try the natural approach, discuss it with your physician. Since your physician is most likely unaware of the natural alternatives available, you may need to educate him/her. Bring this book along with you to the doctor's office. The herbs recommended here are based on published studies in medical journals. Key references are provided if your physician wants additional information.

Angina

Angina refers to a squeezing or pressure-like pain in the chest. The pain may radiate to the left shoulder blade, left arm, or jaw. The pain typically lasts for only 1–20 minutes. Angina is caused by an insufficient supply of oxygen to the heart muscle. Since physical exertion and stress cause an increased need for oxygen by the heart, they are often preceding factors.

Angina is most often a result of atherosclerosis (hardening of the arteries). The primary lesion of atherosclerosis is the build-up of cholesterol-containing plaque, which progressively narrows and ultimately blocks the coronary artery. This results in a decreased blood and oxygen supply to the heart tissue. When the flow of oxygen to the heart muscle is substantially reduced, or when there is an increased need by the heart, it results in angina. Angina is a serious condition that requires strict medical supervision.

From a natural perspective, there are two primary therapeutic goals in the treatment of angina: improving energy metabolism within the heart and improving the blood supply to the heart. These goals are interrelated, as an increased blood flow means improved energy metabolism and vice versa.

The heart utilizes fats as its major metabolic fuel. It converts free fatty acids to energy much like the way an automobile utilizes gasoline. Defects in the utilization of fats by the heart greatly increase the risk of atherosclerosis, heart attacks, and angina pains. Specifically, impaired utilization of fatty acids by the heart results in accumulation of high concentrations of fatty acids within the heart muscle. This then makes the heart extremely susceptible to cellular damage, which ultimately leads to a heart attack.

Carnitine, coenzyme Q10, and magnesium are essential compounds in normal energy metabolism within the heart. Supplementing the diet with these nutrients is effective in the treatment of angina.[1] Here are the recommended levels:

- Carnitine: 300 milligrams three times daily
- Coenzyme Q10: 150 milligrams one or two times daily
- Magnesium (citrate, aspartate, or Krebs cycle chelate): 250 to 400 milligrams three times daily

Herbal recommendations for angina

Hawthorn extracts are probably the most useful. Follow the dosage recommendations on page 208. *Coleus forskohlii* and *Ginkgo biloba* extracts may also be useful, but I typically use hawthorn in combination with khella (*Ammi visnaga*).

Khella is a medicinal plant native to the Mediterranean region, where it has been used in the treatment of angina and other heart ailments since the time of the pharoahs. Several of its components have demonstrated effects in dilating the coronary arteries. Its mechanism of action appears to be very similar to that of the calcium channel-blocking drugs.

Since the late 1940s, numerous scientific studies have been performed on the clinical effectiveness of khella extracts in the treatment of angina. More specifically, khellin, a derivative of the plant, was shown to be extremely effective in relieving angina symptoms, improving exercise tolerance, and normalizing electrocardiographic tests. This is evident by the concluding statement in a study published in the *New England Journal of Medicine* in 1951: "The high proportion of favorable results, together with the striking degree of improvement frequently observed, has led us to the conclusion that khellin, properly used, is a safe and effective drug for the treatment of angina pectoris."[2]

At higher doses (120–150 milligrams per day), pure khellin was associated with mild side effects such as anorexia, nausea, and dizziness. Although most clinical studies used high dosages, several studies show that as little as 30 milligrams of khellin per day appears to offer as good results with fewer side effects.[3]

Khella extracts standardized for khellin content (typically 12 percent) are preferable to isolated khellin. A daily dose of such an extract would be 250–300 milligrams. Again, khella appears to work very well with hawthorn extracts.

Anxiety

Anxiety is defined as "an unpleasant emotional state ranging from mild unease to intense fear." Anxiety differs from fear, in that while fear is a rational response to a real danger, anxiety usually lacks a clear or realistic cause. Although some anxiety is normal and, in fact, healthy, higher levels of anxiety are not only uncomfortable—they can lead to significant problems.

Anxiety is often accompanied by a variety of symptoms. The most common symptoms relate to the chest, such as heart palpitations (awareness of a more forceful or faster heart beat), throbbing or stabbing pains, a feeling of tightness and inability to take in enough air, and a tendency to sigh or hyperventilate. Tension in the muscles of the back and neck often leads to headaches, back pains, and muscle spasms. Other symptoms can include excessive sweating, dryness of mouth, dizziness, digestive disturbances, and the constant need to urinate or defecate.

The anxious individual usually has a constant feeling that something bad is going to happen. They may fear that they have a chronic or dangerous illness—a belief that is reinforced by the symptoms of anxiety. Their inability to relax may lead to difficulty in getting to sleep and constant waking through the night.

Clinical anxiety, including panic attacks, can be produced by caffeine, certain other drugs, and the infusion of lactate into the blood. The fact that these compounds can produce anxiety and panic attacks can be put to good use in understanding the underlying biochemical features of anxiety.

Perhaps the most significant biochemical disturbance noted in patients with anxiety and panic attacks is an elevated blood lactate level and an increased lactate-to-pyruvate ratio. Lactate (the soluble form of lactic acid) is the final pathway in the breakdown of blood sugar (glucose) when there is a lack of oxygen. Nutrition appears to play a key role in the increased lactate-to-pyruvate ratio seen in patients with anxiety. According to Melvyn Werbach, M.D., author of *Nutritional Influences on Mental Illness: A Sourcebook of Clinical Research*,[1] at least seven nutritional factors may be responsible for elevated lactate or an increased lactate-to-pyruvate ratio:

- Alcohol
- Caffeine
- Sugar
- Deficiency of the B vitamins, niacin, pyridoxine, and thiamin
- Deficiency of calcium or magnesium
- Food allergies

By avoiding alcohol, caffeine, sugar, and food allergies a person with anxiety can go a long way in relieving their symptoms.[1] Simply eliminating coffee can result in complete elimination of symptoms. This recommendation may seem too simple to be true, but substantial clinical evidence indicates that in many cases it is all that is necessary. For example, in one study of four men and two women with generalized anxiety or panic disorder, who were consuming the amount of caffeine in 1.5 to 3.5 cups of coffee per day, avoiding caffeine for 1 week brought about significant relief.[2] The degree of improvement was so noticeable, all patients volunteered to continue abstaining from caffeine. Previously, these patients had been only minimally helped by drug therapy. Follow-up examinations 6 to 18 months afterward indicated that five of the six patients were completely without symptoms; the sixth patient became asymptomatic with a very low dose of benzodiazepine.

Herbal recommendations for anxiety

The best herbs for anxiety are kava and valerian. I would recommend trying kava first, for a period of 4 weeks. If there is little or no benefit, then I would recommend trying valerian.

Arthritis

The three major forms of arthritis are osteoarthritis, rheumatoid arthritis, and gout. Each type has its own unique features. See individual entries.

Asthma and hay fever

Asthma is an allergic disorder characterized by spasm of the bronchial tubes and excessive excretion of a viscous mucus in the lungs that can lead to difficult breathing. It occurs as recurrent attacks, which range from mild wheezing to a life-threatening inability to breathe.

Hay fever (seasonal allergic rhinitis) is an allergic reaction to wind-borne pollens. Ragweed pollen accounts for about 75 percent of the hay fever in the United States. Other significant pollens inducing hay fever include various grass and tree pollens. If the hay fever develops in the spring it is usually due to tree pollens; if it develops in the summer, grass and weed pollens are usually the culprits.

Many studies indicate that food allergies play an important role in asthma and hay fever.[1] Adverse reactions to food may be immediate or delayed. Double-blind food challenges in children have shown that immediate-onset sensitivities are usually due (in decreasing order of frequency) to eggs, fish, shellfish, nuts, and peanuts; while foods most commonly associated with delayed-onset reactions include (in decreasing order of frequency) milk, chocolate, wheat, citrus, and food colorings. Elimination of allergy-inducing foods is usually very successful in treating asthma, particularly in infants and children.

Herbal recommendations for asthma and hay fever

The old-time herbal treatment of asthma and hay fever involves the use of ephedra in combination with herbal expectorants. Expectorants are herbs that modify the quality and quantity of secretions of the respiratory tract, resulting in the expulsion of the secretions and improvement in respiratory tract function. Examples of commonly used expectorants include lobelia (*Lobelia inflata*), licorice (*Glycyrrhiza glabra*), and grindelia (*Grindelia camporum*). When using combination preparations, the dosage should be equivalent to 12.5 to 25 milligrams ephedrine three times daily.

Recent studies on the effects of extracts made from the leaves of *Tylophora asthmatica* have upheld its extensive use in Ayurvedic medicine for asthma and other respiratory tract disorders. Although the exact mode of action of tylophora is unknown, it is thought to be due to the alkaloids, especially tylophorine, which have been reported to possess antihistamine and antispasmodic activity and to inhibit other allergic activities. However, a more central mechanism may be responsible for tylophorine's clinical effects in asthma (several clinical studies have shown positive effects).[2] The dosage for the powdered extract is 40 milligrams daily.

Atherosclerosis

Atherosclerosis refers to the hardening of artery walls, caused by a build-up of plaque-containing cholesterol, fatty material, and cellular debris. If the blood flow through these arteries is restricted or blocked, severe damage or death to the tissue the artery supplies may occur—this results in what is known as a "heart attack" if it occurs in the heart muscle or a "stroke" if it occurs in an artery supplying blood and oxygen to the brain. Atherosclerosis and its complications are the major causes of death in the United States, accounting for nearly 43 percent of all premature deaths.

Foremost in the prevention and treatment of atherosclerosis is the reduction of blood cholesterol levels. The evidence overwhelmingly demonstrates that elevated cholesterol levels greatly increase the risk of death due to heart disease or stroke. Cholesterol is transported in the blood by molecules known as lipoproteins. Cholesterol bound to low-density lipoprotein (LDL) is often referred to as the "bad" cholesterol, whereas cholesterol bound to high-density lipoprotein (HDL) is referred to as the "good" cholesterol. This is because LDL cholesterol increases the risk for heart disease, strokes, and high blood pressure while HDL cholesterol actually protects against heart disease. Research has shown that for every 1 percent drop in the cholesterol level, the risk for a heart attack drops by 2 percent.[1]

Low-density lipoprotein transports cholesterol to the tissues. High-density lipoprotein, on the other hand, transports cholesterol to the liver for metabolism and excretion. Therefore the HDL-to-LDL ratio largely determines whether cholesterol is being broken down or deposited into tissues. The risk for heart disease can be reduced dramatically by lowering LDL cholesterol while simultaneously raising HDL cholesterol levels. This can be done quite easily in just a few weeks by making changes in diet and lifestyle. The dietary changes are simple: eat less saturated fat and cholesterol by reducing or eliminating the amounts of animal products in the diet, increase the consumption of fiber-rich plant foods (fruits, vegetables, grains, and legumes), and lose weight if necessary. The lifestyle changes are equally simple: get regular aerobic exercise, stop smoking, and reduce or eliminate the consumption of coffee (both caffeinated and decaffeinated).

Herbal recommendations for atherosclerosis

Garlic may offer the greatest benefit in the treatment and prevention of atherosclerosis, as it appears to block the development of the cholesterol-containing plaque at every step. As discussed in Chapter 13, garlic lowers LDL cholesterol while raising HDL levels, prevents oxidative damage, promotes fibrinolysis, and inhibits platelet aggregation.

Other herbal recommendations for the prevention and treatment of atherosclerosis are as follows, from most beneficial (in my opinion) to least beneficial:

- Gugulipid
- Curcumin
- Ginger
- Hawthorn
- Grape seed extract

Bladder infections

Bladder infections affect more than 20 percent of women at least once a year. Bladder infections are almost always caused by fecal bacteria, usually *Escherichia coli*, that migrate up the urethra and into the bladder, where they can multiply and cause infection. The most common symptoms of a bladder infection are severe pain with urination and urgency, a constant sensation that one needs to urinate.

Urinary tract infections in men and women are frequently associated with sexual activity. In fact, the condition "honeymoon cystitis" is self-explanatory. However, cystitis is not a sexually transmitted disease. Sexual activity simply facilitates migration of bacteria into the bladder.

If inadequately treated, bladder infections can become chronic or lead to kidney infections—the care of a physician is strongly encouraged. Avoid all simple sugars, refined carbohydrates, and food allergens. Drink large amounts of fluids (at least 3 quarts per day), including at least 16 ounces of unsweetened cranberry juice per day. In addition, the liberal consumption of garlic and onions should be encouraged for their antimicrobial and immune-enhancing effects.

Herbal recommendations for bladder infections

The herb uva ursi or bearberry (*Arctostaphylos uva-ursi*) is probably the single best herb to use for most cases (see pp. 336–338). Berberine-containing plants can also be used (see pp. 162–172).

   The most popular herbal treatment for bladder infections is cranberry juice. It was originally thought that cranberry juice helped by making urine more acidic and less hospitable for the bacteria. However, it is now known that cranberry's primary action is to prevent the bacteria from adhering to the lining of the bladder. To stay in the bladder and cause infection, bacteria must anchor themselves to the cells of the bladder. Components in cranberry prevent this anchoring from taking place.[1]

   In one study, drinking 16 ounces of cranberry juice per day eliminated bladder infections in 73 percent of 44 women and 16 men.[2] In another study published in the *Journal of the American Medical Association* (*JAMA*), the daily ingestion of 8 ounces of cranberry juice led to significant inhibition of the growth of bacteria in the urine.[3]

   In the *JAMA* study, saccharin-sweetened cranberry juice was used because the presence of sugar is thought to nullify some of the effects of cranberry juice. Because most cranberry juice products on the market are loaded with sugar, many herbal practitioners and physicians recommend taking cranberry juice in pill form. Several manufacturers offer cranberry concentrates. If you have symptoms, take the equivalent of 16 ounces of cranberry juice. For prevention, take the equivalent of 8 ounces of cranberry juice.

Boils

A boil is an inflamed, pus-filled area of skin, usually due to a hair follicle (the tiny pit from which a hair grows) infected with the bacteria *Staphylococcus aureus*. A boil will usually start as a painful, red lump. As it swells it fills with pus and becomes rounded, with a yellowish tip (head). Common sites include the back of the neck and moist areas such as the armpits and groin. A more severe and extensive form of a boil is a carbuncle.

   Common measures should be taken to prevent the spread of infection, such as cleaning the affected area, taking showers instead of baths, and washing the face and hands several times a day. Towels, linens, and clothing should be kept away from other family members, to avoid spread to others. Do not burst a boil, as this may spread infection to deeper tissues. A hot compress applied every 2 hours will relieve discomfort and hasten drainage and healing. If the boil is especially large or painful, consult your physician for proper drainage.

Herbal recommendations for boils

The best herbal recommendation for boils is a topical application of tea tree oil. Tea tree oil is active against a wide range of organisms, possesses good penetration, and does not irritate the skin.

Because a boil is an infectious disease, herbs that enhance immune system function (e.g., echinacea and goldenseal) can also be used internally.

Canker sores

Canker sores are single or clustered, shallow, painful ulcers found anywhere in the mouth cavity. The ulcers range from 1 to 15 millimeters in diameter, are surrounded by a reddened border, and are often covered by a white membrane. The ulcers usually resolve in 7 to 21 days, but recur in many people.

Canker sores are often confused with cold sores (see p. 353). However, cold sores most often occur on the borders of the lips and are linked to the herpes virus.

Recurrent canker sores are an extremely common condition; they are estimated to affect 20 percent of the population. While an occasional canker sore may be the result of trauma from your toothbrush, the cause of recurrent canker sores appears, on the basis of studies of initiating factors, to be related to food sensitivities, stress, and/or nutrient deficiency.

Herbal recommendation for canker sores

Deglycyrrhizinated licorice (DGL) in chewable tablets is very effective in the treatment of oral ulcers, just as it is in peptic ulcers (see Chapter 22, p. 235). In one study, DGL was shown to lead to complete healing within 3 days in more than fifteen of twenty patients.[1] One of these patients had recurrent canker sores for over 10 years. He had multiple ulcers on the tongue, lips, inside of the cheek, palate, and back of the throat. By the seventh day of treatment with DGL, the patient was completely free of any mouth ulcers. The patient remained on DGL for 1 year. After battling recurrent canker sores for over

10 years, this patient did not have a single recurrence. I have had similar experiences with my patients. Fortunately, DGL is completely safe and there are no known side effects.

Deglycyrrhizinated licorice is available in tablet form from health food stores. For best results, take two 380-milligram tablets 20 minutes before meals three times daily.

Cold sores

Cold sores are caused by the herpes virus. They are characterized by the appearance of single or multiple clusters of small blisters filled with a clear fluid on a reddened base.

Cold sores are not the same as genital herpes—the strain of virus is different. Cold sores are usually caused by herpes simplex virus type 1 (HSV-1), whereas genital herpes is usually caused by the type 2 virus (HSV-2). Most people, perhaps as many as 90 percent worldwide, are infected with HSV-1. After the initial infection, the virus becomes dormant in the nerve cells in most people. In others, however, it can reactivate, causing recurring outbreaks, usually following minor infections, trauma, stress, and sun exposure.

Herbal recommendations for cold sores

The best herbal treatment for cold sores is a special cream containing a concentrated extract of *Melissa officinalis*. (*Note*: In Germany, the product is named Lomaherpan®. In the United States, the product name is Herpilyn®.)

Melissa officinalis is a member of the mint family that exerts powerful antiviral activity against the herpes virus.[1] The *Melissa* extract in Herpilyn® is a 70:1 concentrate; this means it takes 70 pounds of *Melissa* to produce 1 pound of the extract. Rather than any single antiviral chemical, the *Melissa* extract in this formula contains several components that work together to prevent the virus from infecting human cells.

When Lomaherpan® cream was used in patients with initial herpes infection, results from comprehensive trials from three German hospitals and a dermatology clinic demonstrated that not a single recurrence occurred.[2] In other words, by using the cream not a single patient with a first herpes outbreak developed another cold sore.

Furthermore, it was noted in these studies that Lomaherpan® cream interrupted the infection quickly and promoted healing of the herpes blisters much faster than normal. The control group receiving other topical creams required a healing period of 10 days whereas the group receiving Lomaherpan® healed within 5 days.

Lomaherpan® cream was also studied in patients suffering from recurrent cold sores. Researchers found that if they used Lomaherpan® cream regularly they would either stop having recurrences or they experienced a tremendous reduction in the frequency of recurrences (an average cold sore-free period of greater than 3½ months).

Herpilyn®, the United States version of Lomaherpan® cream, should be applied to the lips two to four times a day during an active recurrence. You can apply a fairly thick layer (1–2 millimeters). Detailed toxicology studies have demonstrated that it is extremely safe and suitable for long-term use.

Herpilyn® is available at most health food stores. If you can't find it, call Enzymatic Therapy (1-800-783-2286) for names of stores or mail order companies in your area.

Another useful topical treatment for cold sores that has some documentation is glycyrrhetinic acid from licorice (see p. 236, Chapter 22—Licorice). Madison Botanicals (Seattle, Washington) offers glycyrrhetinic acid in a gel base with peppermint oil in their product Licromint®. The product may be found at health food stores.

Common cold

The common cold is caused by a wide variety of viruses that are capable of infecting the upper respiratory tract. The symptoms of a cold are well known: general malaise, fever, headache, and upper respiratory tract congestion. Initially, there is a watery nasal discharge and sneezing followed by thicker secretions containing mucus, white blood cells, and dead organisms. The throat may be red, sore, and quite dry.

Although it doesn't always seem this way, it must be kept in mind that a cold is a self-limiting illness. This means that it will run its course. Perhaps the most important thing is to employ some general measures that will give the immune system an opportunity to fight off the infection. Employing some general measures designed to boost immune function will prevent the cold from developing into something more significant. It will also reduce the severity and duration of the symptoms.

General measures

- Rest (bed rest is better)
- Drink large amounts of fluids (preferably diluted vegetable juices, soups, and herb teas)

- Limit simple sugar consumption (including fruit)
- Vitamin C—500 to 1,000 milligrams every 1 to 2 hours (decrease the amount if this produces excess gas or diarrhea)
- Zinc lozenges—one lozenge containing 23 milligrams of elemental zinc every two waking hours for 1 week.

Herbal recommendations for the common cold

Herbal teas are excellent beverage choices at any time, but especially during a cold. Diaphoretic teas such as ginger and peppermint are quite useful during colds. Diaphoretics work to promote perspiration via warming from the inside out. Licorice root teas are also a good choice because of the antiviral activity of licorice.

The most popular herbal treatment of the common cold is echinacea—and for good reason. As detailed in Chapter 8, echinacea is quite effective. Follow the dosage recommendations given on p. 105.

Another useful herb for the common cold is *Astragalus membranaceus*. The Chinese value astragalus as a specific tonic for strengthening the body's resistance to disease. In clinical studies in China, astragalus has been shown to reduce the incidence and shorten the course of the common cold.[1]

While astragalus does exert some antiviral activity, its main effect is to enhance interferon production and secretion. Astragalus can be used at the following dose given three times a day for the common cold:

- Dried root (or as tea): 1 to 4 grams
- Tincture (1:5): 2 to 6 milliliters (1–1½ teaspoons)
- Powdered solid extract (2:1): 250–500 milligrams

Diabetes

Diabetes is divided into two major categories: type I and type II. Type I or insulin-dependent diabetes mellitus (IDDM) occurs most often in children and adolescents. It is associated with complete destruction of pancreatic beta cells, which manufacture the hormone insulin. Type I diabetics require life-long insulin for the control of blood sugar levels; they must learn how to manage their blood sugar levels on a day-by-day basis, modifying insulin types and dosage schedules as necessary, according to the results of regular blood sugar testing. About 10 percent of all diabetics are type I.

Although the exact cause of type I diabetes is unknown, current theory suggests it is due to injury to the insulin-producing beta cells coupled with some defect in tissue regeneration capacity. What ultimately destroys the beta cells are antibodies produced by white blood cells. Antibodies seek out and destroy infecting organisms such as viruses and bacteria. However, in some diseases antibodies develop against the body's own tissues. These disease are referred to as "autoimmune diseases." Type I diabetes appears to have an autoimmune component at its origin, as antibodies for beta cells are present in 75 percent of all type I diabetics compared to 0.5 to 2.0 percent of non-diabetics. It is probable that the antibodies to the beta cells develop in response to cell destruction due to other mechanisms (chemical, free radical, viral, food allergy, etc.). It appears that nondiabetic individuals either do not develop as severe an antibody reaction, or are better able to repair the damage once it occurs.

Type II or non-insulin dependent diabetes mellitus (NIDDM) usually begins after the patient reaches 40 years of age. Up to 90 percent of all diabetics are type II. Insulin levels are typically elevated, indicating a loss of sensitivity to insulin by the cells of the body. Obesity is a major contributing factor to this loss of insulin sensitivity. Approximately 90 percent of individuals with type II diabetes are obese. Achieving ideal body weight in these patients is associated with restoration of normal blood sugar levels in most cases.

In type II diabetes, diet is of primary importance and must be tried diligently before a drug is used. Most cases of type II diabetes can be controlled by diet alone. Despite a high success rate with dietary intervention, eager physicians often use drugs or insulin instead.

Other types of diabetes includes secondary diabetes—a form of diabetes that is secondary to certain conditions and syndromes such as pancreatic disease, hormone disturbances, drugs, and malnutrition; gestational diabetes—a form of glucose intolerance occurring during pregnancy; and impaired glucose tolerance—a condition that includes prediabetic, chemical, latent, borderline, subclinical, and asymptomatic diabetes.

The need for proper monitoring

When employing herbs or other natural methods that improve blood sugar metabolism it is critical that blood glucose levels be monitored carefully, particularly if the patient has relatively uncontrolled diabetes. Careful attention to symptoms, home glucose monitoring, and the glycosylated hemoglobin (Hgb_{A1c}) test are, at this time, the best way to monitor the progress of a diabetic individual. Remember that as the diabetic individual employs herbs as well as diet to improve blood sugar control, drug dosages will have to be altered. A good working relationship with the prescribing doctor is extremely important.

Herbal recommendations for diabetes

Before the advent of insulin, diabetes was treated with plant medicines. In 1980 the World Health Organization urged researchers to examine whether traditional medicines possessed any real medicinal effects. In the last 10–20 years scientific investigation has, in fact, confirmed the efficacy of many of these preparations, some of which are remarkably effective. This discussion is, of necessity, limited to a few plants—those that appear most effective, are relatively nontoxic, and have substantial documentation of efficacy. The following plants are discussed: onions and garlic, bitter melon, *Gymnema sylvestre*, fenugreek, salt bush, and pterocarpus. In addition, three other herbal medicines (bilberry, grape seed, and ginkgo extracts) are discussed because of their important roles in dealing with diabetic complications.

Even though the herbs described here possess blood sugar-lowering effects, proper and effective natural treatment of the diabetic patient requires the careful integration of diet, nutritional supplements, and lifestyle, along with herbal medicine.

Onions (Allium cepa) and garlic (Allium sativum)

Onions and garlic have demonstrated blood sugar lowering action.[1,2] The active principles are believed to be the sulfur-containing compounds allyl propyl disulfide (APDS) and diallyl disulfide oxide (allicin), respectively, although other constituents such as flavonoids may play a role as well. The cardiovascular effects of garlic and onions, that is, cholesterol and blood pressure-lowering actions, further substantiate the liberal intake of garlic and onions by the diabetic patient.

Bitter melon

Bitter melon (*Momordica charantia*), also known as balsam pear, is a tropical fruit widely cultivated in Asia, Africa, and South America. The unripe fruit is eaten as a vegetable. Bitter melon is a green, cucumber-shaped fruit with gourdlike bumps all over it. It looks like an ugly cucumber. In addition to being eaten as a vegetable, unripe bitter melon has been used extensively in folk medicine as a remedy for diabetes. The blood sugar-lowering action of the fresh juice or extract of the unripe fruit has been clearly established in human clinical trials as well as experimental models.[3,4]

Bitter melon is composed of several compounds with confirmed antidiabetic properties. Charantin, extracted by alcohol, is a hypoglycemic agent composed of mixed steroids that is more potent than the oral hypoglycemic drug tolbutamide. *Momordica charantia* also contains an insulin-like polypeptide, polypeptide P, which lowers blood sugar levels when injected subcutaneously into type I diabetics.[5] Since it appears to have fewer side effects than insulin, it has been suggested as a replacement for some patients.

The oral administration of bitter melon preparations has shown good results in clinical trials in patients with type II diabetes.[3,4] In one study, glucose tolerance was improved in 73 percent of type II diabetics given 2 ounces of the juice.[3] The pooled area under the glucose tolerance curves of the patients responding to the bitter melon was 187.0 square centimeters—much lower than the baseline level of 243.6 square centimeters. In another study, 15 grams of the aqueous extract of bitter melon produced a 54 percent decrease in postprandial blood sugar level and a 17 percent reduction in glycosylated hemoglobin in six patients.[4]

Unripe bitter melon is available primarily at Asian grocery stores. Health food stores may have bitter melon extracts, but the fresh juice is probably best, as this was what was used in some of the studies. Bitter melon juice is, in my opinion, very difficult to make palatable. As its name implies, it is quite bitter. If you want the medicinal effects, simply plug your nose and take a 2-ounce shot of the juice. The dosage of other forms should approximate this dose.

Gymnema sylvestre

Gymnema sylvestre is a plant native to the tropical forests of India, and has long been used as a treatment for diabetes. Recent scientific investigation has upheld its effectiveness in both type I and type II diabetes.[6,7] Gymnema is probably the most practical herbal recommendation for improving blood sugar control in diabetics. High-quality gymnema extracts are available in health food stores.

Gymnema sylvestre appeared on the U.S. market a few years ago. Originally it was hyped as a "sugar blocker." Manufacturers erroneously claimed that gymnema could block the absorption of sugar in the gastrointestinal tract and allow the sugar to pass through the intestinal tract unabsorbed. Ridiculous advertisement claims were made, such as "how to cut down on sugar calories without cutting down on sugar." This was, in my opinion, a blatant distortion of the truth.

Gymnema components, such as gymnemic acid, block the sensation of sweetness when applied to the tongue. This has shown some clinical significance. Subjects that had gymnema extracts applied to the tongue consumed fewer calories at a meal compared to subjects not treated with gymnema. It must be stressed that the gymnema extract was applied to the tongues—

subjects did not swallow it in capsule or tablet form, as this would not produce the same effect.

Gymnema extracts enhance glucose control in diabetic dogs and rabbits. Interestingly, in animals that have had their pancreas removed, gymnema possesses no obvious effects. It can therefore be concluded that gymnema enhances the production of endogenous insulin. The results of animal studies suggest that it accomplishes this through regeneration of the insulin-producing beta cells in the pancreas. Studies in humans seem to support this, both in type I and type II diabetes.[6,7]

An extract of the leaves of *Gymnema sylvestre* given to twenty-seven patients with type I diabetes on insulin therapy was shown to reduce insulin requirements and fasting blood sugar levels, and to improve blood sugar control.[6] This study confirmed earlier work in animal studies. In type I diabetes, gymnema appears to work by enhancing the action of insulin. Furthermore, there is some evidence that it may possibly regenerate or revitalize the beta cells of the pancreas.

Gymnema extract has also shown positive results in type II diabetes.[7] In one study, twenty-two type II diabetics were given gymnema extract along with their oral hypoglycemic drugs. All patients demonstrated improved blood sugar control; twenty-one out of the twenty-two were able to reduce their drug dosage considerably; and five subjects were able to discontinue their medication and maintain blood sugar control with the gymnema extract alone.

The dosage for *Gymnema sylvestre* extract is 400 milligrams per day in both type I and type II diabetes. It is interesting to note that gymnema extract is without side effects and exerts its blood sugar-lowering effects only in cases of diabetes. Gymnema extract, when given to healthy volunteers, does not produce any blood sugar lowering or hypoglycemic effects.[7]

Fenugreek (Trigonella foenumgraecum)

Fenugreek seeds have demonstrated significant antidiabetic effects in experimental and clinical studies. The active principle is in the defatted portion of the seed and contains the alkaloid trigonelline, nicotinic acid, and coumarin.

Administration of the defatted seed (in daily doses of 1.5–2 grams per kilogram) to both normal and diabetic dogs reduces fasting and aftermeal blood levels of glucose, glucagon, somatostatin, insulin, total cholesterol, and triglycerides, while increasing high-density lipoprotein (HDL) cholesterol levels.[8]

Human studies confirm these effects. Defatted fenugreek seed powder given twice daily in a 50-gram dose to insulin-dependent diabetics resulted in significant reduction in fasting blood sugar and improved glucose tolerance test results.[9] There was also a 54 percent reduction in 24-hour urinary glucose excretion and significant reductions in low-density lipoprotein (LDL) and very low-density lipoprotein (VLDL) cholesterol and triglyceride values. In noninsulin diabetics the addition of 15 grams of powdered fenugreek seed soaked in water significantly reduced postprandial glucose levels during the meal tolerance test.[10] These results indicate that fenugreek seeds or defatted fenugreek seed powder should be included in the diet of the diabetic.

Salt bush (Atriplex halimus)

Salt bush is a branchy woody shrub native to the Mediterranean, North Africa, and southern Europe. Salt bush is especially common around the Jordan valley in inundated saline depressions and oases. Salt bush is the feeding source of the sand rat. Researchers began investigating the possible therapeutic benefits of atriplex in humans when it was noticed that sand rats switched from a diet rich in atriplex to standard rat chow typically developed severe diabetes. Replacing the atriplex to the diet brought about a quick reversal of the condition.

Human studies conducted in Israel have yielded good results in patients with type II diabetes.[11,12] Blood glucose levels and glucose tolerance were improved. Atriplex is rich in fiber, protein, and numerous trace minerals including chromium. The dosage used in the human studies was 3 grams per day.

Pterocarpus (Pterocarpus marsupium)

Pterocarpus has a long history of use in India as a treatment for diabetes. The flavonoid, (–)-epicatechin, extracted from the bark of this plant, prevents beta cell damage in rats. Further, both epicatechin and a crude alcohol extract of *Pterocarpus marsupium* actually regenerate functional pancreatic beta cells in diabetic animals.[13,14] Epicatechin is also found in green tea (*Camellia sinensis*). As there are no commercial sources of pterocarpus in the United States, green tea may be a suitable alternative. At least two cups of green tea should be consumed per day.

Bilberry (Vaccinium myrtillus), grape seed (Vitis vinifera), and Ginkgo biloba extracts

Bilberry, grape seed, and *Ginkgo biloba* extracts offer significant benefits to diabetics. The active components of these extracts are flavonoids. These flavonoids increase vitamin C levels, decrease the leakiness and breakage of small blood vessels, prevent easy bruising, and exert potent antioxidant effects. These effects are greatly needed in dealing with the microvascular abnormalities of diabetes and preventing diabetic retinopathy.

Although all three of these extracts are of significant benefit, bilberry and grape seed extract are probably best to use in the prevention and treatment of diabetic retinopathy, while *Ginkgo biloba* extract appears most useful in the prevention and treatment of peripheral vascular and nerve disease due to diabetes. Dosages are given in the respective chapters (Chapter 3—Bilberry; Chapter 16—Grape Seed Extract; Chapter 13—*Ginkgo biloba*).

Diarrhea

Diarrhea is a common symptom whose presence usually indicates a mild functional disorder. However, it may also be the first suggestion of a serious underlying disease. Since most acute diarrheal states are self-limited and are due to dietary indiscretions or mild gastrointestinal infections, simple dietary approaches should be used first. If there is no response, then more detailed diagnostic procedures should be used. If significant illness (e.g., fever or debility) accompanies the diarrhea or it lasts for more than a few days, a physician should be consulted.

To help solidify stools, pectin-rich fruits and vegetables such as pears, apples, grapefruit, carrots, potatoes, and beets may offer some benefit. Also, fresh blueberries have a long historical use in diarrhea. Vegetable broths and diluted fruit and vegetable juices should be consumed to maintain electrolyte levels.

Herbal recommendations for diarrhea

Goldenseal and other berberine-containing plants can be used according to the dosages given on p. 170.

Another useful herbal treatment is carob pod powder. It is especially helpful in children and enhances the standard approach to acute diarrhea in children, that is, oral rehydration and rapid refeeding: oral rehydration prevents dehydration and restores normal fluid and electrolyte balance while feeding helps bring about early cessation of diarrhea and minimizes the detrimental consequences of the illness on nutritional well being.

Carob has long been used as both food and medicine by people in the Mediterranean region. Several reports in the medical literature confirm that decoctions (brewed teas) of roasted carob powder are quite effective and without side effect in the treatment of acute-onset diarrhea (see Ref. 1, and references therein).

Infants (3–21 months of age) with acute diarrhea of bacterial and viral origin were treated in a hospital setting with oral rehydration fluid and randomly received for up to 6 days either carob pod powder (1.5 gram per kilogram body weight per day) or an equivalent placebo. The powders were either diluted in oral rehydration solution or in milk. The duration of diarrhea in the carob group was 2 days, whereas it was 3.75 days in the placebo group. Normalizations in defecation, body temperature, and weight and cessation of vomiting were also reached much more quickly in the carob group. No side effects to carob were reported.

Carob is rich in dietary fiber (26 percent) and polyphenols (21 percent). These components are thought to be responsible for the beneficial effects. Carob is efficacious and safe, as proved by this study and by its years of extensive use in many parts of the world; it is quite clear that carob pod powder offers a very useful and low-cost treatment of acute infantile diarrhea.

Eczema

Eczema (atopic dermatitis) is an intensely itchy, allergic disease of the skin. The area of skin affected is usually quite red, thick, and irritated. Eczema is commonly found on the face, wrists, and on the insides of elbows and knees.

The role of food allergy as a major cause in eczema, especially in children, is well established. Control of eczema depends critically on finding and eliminating all, or at least most, food allergens. A recent study conducted at the Middlesex Hospital in London provides additional support to the role of food allergies in childhood eczema.[1] In this study the researchers estimated that simply eliminating cow's milk, eggs, tomatoes, artificial colors, and food preservatives would help up to three-quarters of children with moderate to severe eczema. If eliminating these foods fails to improve the condition, it is likely that another food is the culprit.

In addition to food allergies, dietary oils are also quite important in eczema. Specifically, patients with eczema appear to have an essential fatty acid deficiency. This deficiency results in decreased synthesis of the anti-inflammatory prostaglandins. Increasing the intake of essential fatty acids, in particular omega-3 oils, either by eating more fatty fish (e.g., mackerel, herring, and salmon) or by consumption of nuts, seeds, flaxseed oil, or fish oil supplements, may be quite helpful.

Herbal recommendations for eczema

A number of herbal substances can be used as alternatives to the cortisone-containing creams, lotions, and ointments used for the temporary relief of eczema. Extracts of licorice (glycyrrhetinic acid) and German chamomile are the most active.[2] Natural creams/ointments containing one or both of these herbs can be used in place of cortisone preparations.

Gallstones

Gallstones are extremely common in the United States. This year alone at least 1 million more Americans will develop gallstones and another 300,000 gallbladders will be removed. As is typical of most diseases, gallstones are much easier to prevent than to reverse. Once gallstones have formed, therapeutic intervention involves avoiding aggravating foods and employing measures that increase the solubility of cholesterol in bile. If symptoms persist or worsen, removal of the gallbladder is indicated. However, if no symptoms are apparent surgery should be avoided.

The critical factor in gallstone formation is the solubility of the bile within the gallbladder. Bile solubility is based on the relative concentrations of cholesterol, bile acids, phosphatidylcholine (lecithin), and water.

The belief that the main cause of gallstones is the consumption of fiber-depleted refined foods has considerable research support. Gallstones, like most chronic diseases, are associated with the "Western diet" in population studies. Such a diet, high in refined carbohydrates and fat and low in fiber, leads to a reduction in the synthesis of bile acids by the liver and a lower bile acid concentration in the gallbladder. A diet high in fiber, especially those fibers capable of binding to deoxycholic acid (i.e., predominantly the water-soluble fibers found in vegetables and fruits, pectin, oat bran, and guar gum), is extremely important in the prevention as well as the reversal of most gallstones.

Herbal recommendations for gallstones

Silymarin (see Chapter 24, p. 247) and components of peppermint oil (see Chapter 28, p. 283) are useful in patients with gallstones. Silymarin increases the solubility of the bile while peppermint oil components may actually help dissolve the stones.

Gout

Gout is a common type of arthritis caused by an increased concentration of uric acid in biological fluids. Uric acid is the final breakdown product of purine metabolism. Purines are made in the body and are also ingested in foods. In gout, uric acid crystals are deposited in joints, tendons, kidneys, and other tissues, where they cause considerable inflammation and damage.[1]

Gout is associated with affluence and is often called the "rich man's disease." Throughout history, the sufferer of gout has been depicted as a portly, middle-aged man sitting in a comfortable chair with one foot resting painfully on a soft cushion as he consumes great quantities of meat and wine. In fact, the traditional picture does have some basis in reality, as meats, particularly organ meats, are high-purine foods, while alcohol inhibits uric acid secretion by the kidneys. Furthermore, even today, gout is primarily a disease of adult men; more than 95 percent of gout sufferers are men over the age of 30 years. Approximately 3 adults in 1,000 have gout, and 10–20 percent of the adult population has elevated uric acid levels in the blood.

Several dietary factors are known to cause gout: consumption of alcohol, high-purine foods (organ meats, meat, yeast, poultry, etc.), fats, refined carbohydrates, and overconsumption of calories.[1] The dietary treatment of gout involves the following guidelines:

1. Elimination of alcohol intake
2. Low-purine diet
3. Achievement of ideal body weight
4. Liberal consumption of complex carbohydrates
5. Low fat intake
6. Low protein intake
7. Liberal fluid intake

Herbal recommendations for gout

Consuming the equivalent of one-half pound of fresh cherries per day has been shown to be very effective in lowering uric acid levels and preventing attacks of gout.[1] Cherries, hawthorn berries, blueberries, and other dark red-blue berries are rich sources of anthocyanidin and proanthocyanidin. These flavonoid molecules give the fruits their deep red-blue color, and are remarkable in their ability to prevent collagen destruction. Flavonoid-rich grape seed and hawthorn extracts are the best herbal recommendations for gout.

Hemorrhoids

Hemorrhoids are basically varicose veins of the rectum. They may be near the beginning of the anal canal (internal hemorrhoids) or at the anal opening (external hemorrhoids). Hemorrhoids are extremely common in the United States, as well as other industrialized countries. Estimates indicate that 50 percent of persons over 50 years of age have symptomatic hemorrhoidal disease and up to one-third of the total U.S. population have hemorrhoids to some degree.

Because the venous system supplying the rectal area contains no valves to prevent backflow, factors that increase venous congestion in the region can precipitate hemorrhoid formation. This includes increasing intraabdominal pressure (e.g., defecation, pregnancy, coughing, sneezing, vomiting, physical exertion, and portal hypertension due to cirrhosis), a low-fiber diet-induced increase in straining during defecation, and standing or sitting for prolonged periods of time.

The symptoms most often associated with hemorrhoids include itching, burning, pain, inflammation, irritation, swelling, bleeding, and seepage. Itching is rarely due to hemorrhoids except when there is mucous discharge from prolapsing internal hemorrhoids. The common causes of anal itching include tissue trauma secondary to excessive use of harsh toilet paper, *Candida albicans*, parasitic infections, and allergies.

Natural bulking compounds can be used to reduce fecal straining. These fibrous substances, particularly psyllium seed and guar gum, possess a mild laxative action due to their ability to attract water and form a gelatinous mass. They are generally less irritating than wheat bran and other cellulose fiber products. Several double-blind clinical trials have demonstrated that supplementing the diet with bulk-forming fibers can significantly reduce the symptoms of hemorrhoids (bleeding, pain, pruritis, and prolapse) and improve bowel habits.[1]

Herbal recommendations for hemorrhoids

Many over-the-counter products such as suppositories, ointments, and anorectal pads used for hemorrhoids contain primarily natural ingredients, such as witch hazel (Hamamelis water), shark liver oil, cod liver oil, cocoa butter, Peruvian balsam, zinc oxide, live yeast cell derivative, and allantoin. However, topical therapy will provide only temporary relief in most circumstances. A more comprehensive approach is to use herbs that strengthen the tone of the walls of the vein. These herbs are discussed under Varicose Veins (below).

Hepatitis

In most instances, hepatitis is caused by the hepatitis virus (types A, B, and C are the most common). Hepatitis A occurs sporadically or in epidemics, and is transmitted primarily through fecal contamination. Its incubation period is 2 to 6 weeks, carrier states are unknown, and the death rate is low (0.0–0.2 percent). The rate of hepatitis A in the general population of the United States is surprisingly high. Antibodies to the hepatitis A virus are detected in 10 to 20 percent of children below 10 years of age and increases to 50 to 60 percent of adults by age 50 years. Only 3 to 5 percent of adults were aware that they had had hepatitis A, indicating that the majority of cases are mild or asymptomatic.

Hepatitis B is transmitted through infected blood or blood products, although it is occasionally transmitted through saliva and sexual secretions. It is very common in homosexuals and intravenous drug users. About 5 to 10 percent become carriers. Its incubation period is 6 weeks to 6 months and the fatality rate is moderate (0.3–1.5 percent).

Hepatitis C (formerly known as hepatitis non-A, non-B), is less common, but is becoming more so. Its primary route of transmission is by blood transfusion. In fact, about 10 percent of people receiving blood transfusions develop hepatitis C. Its incubation period is 2 to 20 weeks and the mortality rate is unclear, but higher than for the other forms (1–12 percent).[1,2]

Hepatitis can also be caused by other viruses, including the hepatitis type D virus, Epstein–Barr virus, and cytomegalovirus.[2]

For as yet unknown reasons, 10 percent of hepatitis B cases and 10 to 40 percent of hepatitis non-A, non-B cases develop into chronic forms. The symptomotology varies from an asymptomatic state to chronic fatigue, serious liver damage, and even death.[1]

Acute viral hepatitis is characterized by loss of appetite, nausea, vomiting, fatigue, and other flulike symptoms; fever; an enlarged, tender liver; jaundice (yellowing of the skin the due to the increased level of bilirubin in the blood); dark urine; and elevated liver enzymes in the blood.

Chronic viral hepatitis is most often associated with the type B and C viruses. It may either be an active or latent (silent) infection. Chronic active hepatatis is associated with a significantly increased risk of developing liver cancer.

Herbal recommendations for hepatitis

The single most useful herbal substance in the treatment of hepatitis is silymarin (see Chapter 24). Numerous studies have documented silymarin's benefit in virtually all types of hepatitis.

Another herb that may be of benefit is licorice (see Chapter 22). Still another herb that is showing tremendous promise is bupleuri root or Chinese thoroughwax (*Bupleurum falcatum*). Bupleuri root is the major component of Shosaikoto, one of the most famous Chinese medicines. Clinical studies have shown good results in patients with chronic active hepatitis.[1]

Although all of the components of Shosaikoto exert antiinflammatory actions in animal studies, the main action of the formula is attributed primarily to bupleuri root's steroid-like molecules known as saikosaponins. Saikosaponins may protect the liver and exert antiinflammatory effects.[2]

Herpes

Herpes is often the term used to describe a sexually transmitted disease that produces a painful rash on the genitals; however, herpes simplex virus (HSV) can produce a recurrent viral infection on virtually any area of skin or mucous membrane. The most common sites are around the mouth (cold sores) and the genitals. Cold sores are usually caused by herpes simplex virus type 1 (HSV-1), whereas genital herpes is usually caused by the type 2 virus (HSV-2).

The rash in genital herpes is characterized by the appearance of single or multiple clusters of small blisters filled with a clear fluid on a reddened base. The blisters eventually burst to leave small, painful ulcers that heal within 10 to 21 days.

After the initial infection, the virus becomes dormant in the nerve root near the spine, and tends to reactivate following minor infections, trauma, and stress (emotional, dietary, and environmental). While about 40 percent of people never have a second outbreak, others may suffer four or five attacks a year for several years. Gradually, the attacks become less severe and the intervals between recurrences become longer.

Maintaining a healthy immune system goes a very long way in preventing herpes outbreaks. It is also a good idea to take advantage of the amino acid L-lysine. The herpes virus needs another amino acid—arginine—to reproduce. Because lysine and arginine "look" similar to the virus, the virus can be tricked into trying to use lysine instead of arginine. Because lysine blocks the steps that require arginine, the virus will not reactivate.[1]

The goal in preventing recurrences is to keep lysine levels high and arginine levels low. To accomplish this, you must avoid foods high in arginine, such as chocolate, peanuts, almonds and other nuts, and seeds. High-lysine foods that you should eat regularly include most vegetables, legumes, fish, turkey, and chicken. Along with these dietary recommendations, you must then supplement each meal with 1,000 milligrams of L-lysine.

Several double-blind, placebo-controlled studies have shown that lysine supplementation, along with avoidance of foods high in arginine, can be very effective in preventing recurrences in many cases. In one study, the group receiving L-lysine rated it as 74 percent effective.[2] In contrast, the group receiving the placebo noted a placebo success rate of only 28 percent.

Herbal recommendations for herpes

During an active infection, creams containing *Melissa officinalis* extract (see Cold Sores, p. 353) can be used just as for cold sores.[3] Apply the *Melissa officinalis* cream at the first hint of a lesion. Glycyrrhetinic acid preparations can also be used.

High blood pressure

Each time the heart beats it sends blood coursing through the arteries. The peak reading of the pressure exerted by this contraction is the systolic pressure. Between beats the heart relaxes, and blood pressure drops. The very lowest reading is referred to as the diastolic pressure. A normal blood pressure reading for adults is as follows:

120 (systolic)/80 (diastolic)

Hypertension or high blood pressure is one of the major risk factors for a heart attack or stroke. The number of individuals with hypertension (a blood pressure reading higher than 160/95) in the United States is estimated as 20 percent of white adults and 30 percent of black adults. These values are nearly doubled if a blood pressure reading of 140/90 is considered the upper limit of normal.

Although most physicians rely primarily on drugs to lower blood pressure, most cases of hypertension can be brought under control through changes in diet and lifestyle. Hypertension is another of the many diseases or syndromes associated with the Western diet, and is found almost entirely in developed countries. Many dietary factors have been shown to be linked with high blood pressure, including the following:

- Obesity
- A high sodium-to-potassium ratio
- A diet low in fiber and high in sugar

- A diet high in saturated fats and low in essential fatty acids
- A diet low in calcium and magnesium
- A diet low in vitamin C

Special foods for people with high blood pressure include garlic and onions, nuts and seeds or their oils for their essential fatty acid content, flaxseed oil, green leafy vegetables for their rich source of calcium and magnesium, whole grains and legumes for their fiber, and foods rich in vitamin C such as broccoli and citrus fruits.

Herbal recommendations for high blood pressure

A combination of different herbs may offer the greatest benefit in lowering blood pressure. A high-quality garlic preparation is a must. It can be combined with extracts of hawthorn, *Coleus forskohlii*, or khella (see Angina, p. 345, for a description of khella).

Impotence

The term *impotence* has traditionally been used to signify a male's inability to attain and maintain erection of the penis sufficient to permit satisfactory sexual intercourse. Impotence, in most circumstances, is more precisely referred to as *erectile dysfunction*, as this term differentiates itself from loss of libido, premature ejaculation, or inability to achieve orgasm.

An estimated 10 to 20 million men suffer from erectile dysfunction. This number is expected to increase dramatically as the median age of the population increases. Currently, erectile dysfunction is thought to affect more than 25 percent of men over the age of 50 years.

Although the frequency of erectile dysfunction increases with age, it must be stressed that aging itself is not a cause of impotence. Although the amount and force of the ejaculate as well as the need to ejaculate decrease with age, the capacity for erection is retained. Men are capable of retaining their sexual virility well into their eightieth decade.

Erectile dysfunction may be due to organic or psychogenic factors. In the overwhelming majority of cases the cause is organic, that is, it is due to some physiological reason. In fact, in men over the age of 50 years, organic causes are responsible for erectile dysfunction in more than 90 percent of cases. Atherosclerosis of the penile artery is the primary cause of impotence in nearly half the men over age 50 years that have erectile dysfunction.

Herbal recommendations for impotence

The only Food and Drug Administration (FDA)-approved medicine for impotence is yohimbine—an alkaloid isolated from the bark of the yohimbe tree (*Pausinystalia johimbe*) native to tropical West Africa. Yohimbine hydrochloride increases libido, but its primary action is to increase blood flow to erectile tissue. Contrary to a popular misconception, yohimbine has no effects on testosterone levels.

When used alone, yohimbine is successful in 34–43 percent of cases.[1] However, side effects often make yohimbine very difficult to utilize. Yohimbine can induce anxiety, panic attacks, and hallucinations in some individuals. Other side effects include elevations in blood pressure and heart rate, dizziness, headache, and skin flushing. Yohimbine should not be used by individuals with kidney disease, by women, or by individuals with psychological disturbances.

Because of the yohimbine content of yohimbe bark, the FDA classifies yohimbe as an unsafe herb. I think there is some validity to this classification. I have used yohimbine in my practice and have found that because of side effects it is very difficult to work with. Some men are much more sensitive to yohimbine than others. Because it is such a powerful herb, yohimbe can produce the same kind of side effects as yohimbine (see above). It is my opinion that yohimbe and yohimbine are best used under the supervision of a physician. In addition to the problem of side effects with the use of commercial yohimbe preparations, I am also very suspicious of the quality of yohimbe products that exist in health food stores. To my knowledge there are no commercial sources of yohimbe bark available in health food stores that actually state the level of yohimbine per dose. Without knowing the content of yohimbine, it is virtually impossible to prescribe an effective and consistent dosage.

One of the best herbs to use for erectile dysfunction or lack of libido is potency wood, which is also known as Muira puama (*Ptychopetalum olacoides*). This shrub is native to Brazil and has long been used as a powerful aphrodisiac and nerve stimulant in South American folk medicine. A recent clinical study has validated its safety and effectiveness in improving libido and sexual function in some patients.[2]

At the Institute of Sexology in Paris, France, under the supervision of one of the world's foremost authorities on sexual function, Dr. Jacques Waynberg, a clinical study with 262 patients complaining of lack of sexual desire and the inability to attain or maintain an erection demonstrated Muira puama extract to be effective in many cases. Within 2 weeks, at a daily dose of 1 to 1.5 grams of the extract, 62 percent of patients with loss of libido claimed that the treatment had a dynamic effect, while 51 percent of patients with "erection failures" felt that Muira puama was of benefit.

Presently, the mechanism of action of Muira puama is unknown. From preliminary information, it appears that it works by enhancing both psychological and physical aspects of sexual function. Future research will undoubtedly shed additional light on this extremely promising herb for erectile dysfunction.

Other herbs that may be of benefit include *Ginkgo biloba*, *Panax ginseng*, *Pygeum africanum*, and saw palmetto.

Insomnia

In the course of a year, more than half of the U.S. population will have difficulty falling asleep. About 33 percent of the population experiences insomnia on a regular basis. Many use over-the-counter sedative medications to combat insomnia, while others seek stronger drugs. Each year up to 10 million people in the United States receive prescriptions for drugs to help them go to sleep.

Foremost in the natural approach to insomnia is the elimination of those factors known to disrupt normal sleep patterns, such as sources of caffeine, alcohol, and drugs. Since insomnia is largely due to psychological factors, these should be considered and handled before simply inducing sleep with drugs. Counseling and/or stress reduction techniques such as progressive relaxation and exercise are often very effective.

Herbal recommendations for insomnia

In addition to kava (see pp. 210–219) and valerian (see pp. 339–342), several other herbs can be tried. I would rank these herbs in the following order of effectiveness:

- St. John's wort
- Passion flower (*Passiflora incarnata*)
- Hops (*Humulus lupulus*)
- Oat straw (*Avena sativa*)

Irritable bowel syndrome

Irritable bowel syndrome (IBS) is a very common condition in which the large intestine, or colon, fails to function properly. It is also known as nervous indigestion, spastic colitis, mucous colitis, and intestinal neurosis. Characteristic symptoms of IBS include a combination of any of the following: abdominal pain and distension, more frequent bowel movements with pain, or relief of pain with bowel movements; constipation; diarrhea; excessive production of mucus in the colon; symptoms of indigestion such as flatulence, nausea, or anorexia; and varying degrees of anxiety or depression. Irritable bowel syndrome is an extremely common condition. Estimates suggest that approximately 15 percent of the U.S. population suffers from IBS.[1]

The treatment of IBS by increasing the intake of dietary fiber has a long history. In general, consuming a diet rich in complex carbohydrates and dietary fiber is effective is most cases. Individuals will usually respond better to fiber from sources other than wheat, particularly water-soluble fiber such as that found in vegetables, fruits, oat bran, guar, psyllium, and legumes (beans, peas, etc.). White table sugar or sucrose has a very detrimental effect on bowel function, particularly in patients with IBS. Its use should be limited or, better yet, eliminated.

Food allergies are also a frequent cause of IBS, as the majority of patients with IBS (approximately two-thirds) have at least one food intolerance, and some have multiple intolerances.[1] It is also interesting to note that many IBS patients have other symptoms suggestive of food allergy, such as heart palpitation, hyperventilation, fatigue, excessive sweating, and headaches.[1]

Herbal recommendations for irritable bowel syndrome

The best choice for herbal treatment of IBS is enteric-coated peppermint oil. Other good recommendations are ginger and turmeric, as both of these herbs are excellent carminatives (substances that promote the elimination of intestinal gas) and intestinal spasmolytics (substances that relax and soothe the intestinal tract).

Kidney stones

Kidney stones are extremely common in the United States. Each year nearly 6 percent of the entire U.S. population develops a kidney stone. More than 10 percent of all males and 5 percent of all females experience the pain of a kidney stone during their lifetime. The rate of occurrence of kidney stones has been steadily increasing, paralleling the rise in other chronic diseases associated with the so-called "Western diet."

In the United States, most kidney stones are calcium-containing stones composed of calcium oxalate, calcium oxalate mixed with calcium phosphate, or, very rarely, calcium phosphate alone. The high rate of occurrence of calcium-containing stones in affluent societies is directly associated with the following dietary patterns: low fiber, highly refined carbohydrates, high alcohol consumption, large amounts of animal protein, high fat, high calcium-containing food, high salt, and high vitamin D-enriched food. Some of these factors are discussed more fully below.

Herbal recommendations for kidney stones

Cranberry juice or extracts may be useful, as the consumption of cranberry juice reduces the amount of ionized calcium in the urine by more than 50 percent in patients with recurrent kidney stones.[1] Since high urinary calcium levels greatly increase the risk of developing a kidney stone, it appears that cranberry juice may offer significant benefit. Because most cranberry juice products on the market are loaded with sugar, many herbal practitioners and physicians recommend taking cranberry juice in pill form. Several manufacturers offer cranberry concentrates. To prevent kidney stone formation under high-risk conditions, take the equivalent of 16 ounces of cranberry juice per day.

Macular degeneration

The macula is the portion of the eye responsible for fine vision. Degeneration of the macula is the leading cause of severe visual loss in the United States and Europe in persons aged 55 years or older. The risk factors for macular degeneration include aging, atherosclerosis, and high blood pressure. There is no current medical treatment for the most common form of macular degeneration. Laser surgery is used for those individuals who develop a less common type of macular degeneration (exudative macular degeneration).

The origin of macular degeneration is ultimately related to damage caused by free radicals. As with most diseases related to free radical damage, prevention or treatment at an early stage is more effective than trying to reverse the disease process.

Numerous studies show that individuals consuming more fruits and vegetables are less likely to develop cataracts or macular degeneration compared to individuals who do not regularly consume fruits and vegetables. Fresh fruits and vegetables are rich in a broad range of antioxidant compounds, including vitamin C, carotenes, flavonoids, and glutathione. All of these antioxidants are critically involved in important mechanisms that prevent the development of macular degeneration.

Herbal recommendations for macular degeneration

There are three excellent choices for macular degeneration: *Ginkgo biloba*, bilberry, and grape seed extracts. Use the standardized extract of at least one of these plants at the recommended dosage (Chapter 3—Bilberry; Chapter 13—*Ginkgo biloba*; Chapter 16—Grape Seed Extract).

Menopause

Menopause denotes the cessation of menstruation in women. It usually occurs when a woman reaches the age of 50 years. Six to 12 months without a period is the commonly accepted rule for diagnosing menopause. This time period prior to the official designation of menopause is often referred to as "perimenopausal" while the time period after menopause is referred to as "postmenopausal."

The current medical practice is to view menopause as a disease rather than a normal physiological process. This view contrasts starkly with the view of many cultures that menopause is a natural part of the life process and a positive event in a woman's life. In fact, in many cultures of the world most women do not go through the symptoms associated with menopause. This observation raises some interesting questions about menopause being a sociocultural event.

The current medical view, that menopause has a very negative impact on a woman's life, may reflect a male-dominated medical system. Male doctors may not perceive accurately how women view menopause. Studies of women experiencing natural menopause have found that more women are relieved when menopause occurs than saddened. In other words, more women view menopause as a positive rather than a negative experience.

With the prolongation of life expectancy, the menopausal and post-menopausal periods are becoming more and more significant in a woman's life. In fact, today's average woman can expect to live at least one-third of her life in the postmenopausal phase.

Current medical treatment of menopause primarily involves the use of hormone replacement therapy, featuring the combination of estrogen and progesterone. The obvious question concerns whether hormone replacement therapy is necessary; the interested reader can find more on this topic in *Menopause* (part of the *Getting Well Naturally* series).[1]

Herbal recommendations for menopause

Many plant extracts exhibit a tonic effect on the female glandular system. This tonic effect is thought to result from the action of phytoestrogens, as well as from the plant extract's ability to improve blood flow to the female organs. The herbs work to nourish and tone the female glandular and organ system rather than exert a druglike effect. This nonspecific mode of action makes many herbs useful in a broad range of female conditions.

Phytoestrogens are components of many medicinal herbs historically used to treat conditions now treated with estrogens. Phytoestrogen-containing herbs offer significant advantages over the use of estrogens in the treatment of menopausal symptoms. While both synthetic and natural estrogens may pose significant health risks, including increasing the risk of cancer, gallbladder disease, and thromboembolic disease (strokes, heart attacks, etc.), phytoestrogens have not been associated with these side effects. In fact, experimental studies in animals demonstrated that phytoestrogens are extremely effective in inhibiting mammary tumors, not only because they occupy estrogen receptors, but also because of other, unrelated anti-cancer mechanisms.[2]

Phytoestrogens in herbs are capable of exerting estrogenic effects, although the activity compared to estrogen is only 2 percent as strong as estrogen at the very most.[3] However, because of this low activity, phyto-estrogens exert a balancing action on estrogen effects: if estrogen levels are low, phytoestrogens enhance the estrogen effects; if estrogen levels are high, phytoestrogens reduce the estrogen effects.

Because of the balancing action of phytoestrogens on estrogen effects, it is common to find the same plant recommended for conditions of estrogen excess (such as premenstrual syndrome) as well as conditions of estrogen deficiency (such as menopause, premenstrual syndrome, and menstrual abnormalities). Many of these herbs have been termed "uterine tonics."

The four most useful herbs in the treatment of hot flashes are angelica or Dong quai (*Angelica sinensis*), licorice root (*Glycyrrhiza glabra*), chaste berry (*Vitex agnus-castus*), and black cohosh (*Cimicifuga racemosa*). These herbs have been used historically to lessen a variety of female complaints, including hot flashes.

While these herbs may be effective individually, combining them is thought to produce even greater benefit. Most major suppliers of herbal products feature formulas containing these herbs. Use well-respected brands and follow the dosage instructions on the label. Angelica and licorice are discussed in Section II (Chapter 2—*Angelica* Species; Chapter 22—Licorice); a brief discussion of chaste berry and black cohosh is included here.

Chaste berry

The chaste tree is native to the Mediterranean. Its berries have long been used for female complaints. As its name signifies, chaste berries were used to suppress the libido. Scientific investigation shows that chaste berry has profound effects on pituitary function.[4] Its beneficial effects in menopause may be due primarily to an alteration in pituitary function. The daily dose of chaste berry preparations is an amount equivalent to 30 to 40 milligrams of the seeds.

Black cohosh

Black cohosh was widely used by the American Indians and later by American colonists for the relief of menstrual cramps and menopause. Recent scientific investigation has upheld the use of black cohosh in both dysmenorrhea and menopause. Clinical studies show that extracts of black cohosh relieve not only hot flashes, but also depression and vaginal atrophy.[5] In addition to exerting vascular effects, black cohosh reduces luteinizing hormone (LH) levels, thus implying a significant estrogenic effect. Remifemin®, a commercial formulation, is the most popular natural alternative to estrogen therapy in Germany.

Dose to be taken three times per day:

- Powdered root or as tea: 1 to 2 grams
- Fluid extract (1:1): 4 milliliters (1 teaspoon)
- Solid (dry powdered) extract (4:1): 250 to 500 milligrams
- Remifemin® (containing 1 milligram of 27-deoxyacteine per tablet): Two tablets twice daily

Multiple sclerosis

Multiple sclerosis (MS) is a syndrome of progressive nervous system disturbances occurring early in life. The early symptoms of multiple sclerosis may include:

Muscular symptoms   Feeling of heaviness, weakness, leg dragging, stiffness, tendency to drop things, clumsiness

Sensory symptoms   Tingling, "pins and needles" sensation, numbness, dead feeling, bandlike tightness, electrical sensations

Visual symptoms   Blurring, fogginess, haziness, eyeball pain, blindness, double vision

Vestibular symptoms   Light-headedness, feeling of spinning, sensation of drunkenness, nausea, vomiting

Genitourinary symptoms   Incontinence, loss of bladder sensation, loss of sexual function

Despite considerable research, there are still many questions about MS. Mainstream medicine has become almost obsessed with finding a viral cause for this disease, although most current work suggests immune disturbances cause the disease. In MS, the myelin sheath that surrounds nerves is destroyed. For this reason MS is classified as a "demyelinating" disease. Zones of demyelination (plaques) vary in size and location within the spinal cord. Symptoms correspond in a general way to the distribution of the plaques.

In about two-thirds of cases, the onset is between the ages 20 and 40 years (rarely is the onset after 50 years), and women are affected slightly more often than males (60 percent female : 40 percent male). The definitive cause of MS remains to be determined. Many causative factors have been proposed, including viruses, autoimmune factors, and diet.

Swank[1] has provided convincing evidence that a diet low in saturated fats, maintained for a long period of time (one study lasted more than 34 years), tends to halt the disease process. Swank began treating patients successfully with a low-fat diet in 1948. Swank's diet recommends (1) a saturated fat intake of no more than 10 grams per day, (2) a daily intake of 40 to 50 grams of polyunsaturated oils (margarine, shortening, and hydrogenated oils are not allowed), (3) at least 1 teaspoon of cod liver oil daily, (4) a normal allowance of protein, and (5) the consumption of fish three or more times a week.[1]

Swank's diet was originally thought to help patients with MS by overcoming an essential fatty acid deficiency and reduce the intake of saturated fats. Currently, it is thought that the beneficial effects are probably a result of (1) decreasing platelet aggregation, (2) a decreasing autoimmune response, and (3) normalizing the decreased essential fatty acid levels found in the serum, red blood cells, platelets, and (perhaps most importantly) the cerebrospinal fluid in patients with MS.

In addition to Swank's recommendation, I would suggest taking 2 tablespoons of flaxseed oil, 800 international units (IU) of vitamin E, and 200 micrograms of selenium each day.

Herbal recommendations for multiple sclerosis

Ginkgo biloba extract appears to provide a solution to some of the problems associated with MS. In addition to providing good antioxidant support, *Ginkgo biloba* extract contains several unique terpene molecules, known collectively as ginkgolides, that antagonize platelet activating factor (PAF), a key chemical mediator in many inflammatory and allergic processes including multiple sclerosis. A preliminary study with a pure ginkgolide is a source of hope. In the study,[2] ten patients with multiple sclerosis were treated with a 5-day course of intravenous ginkgolide B, a specific inhibitor of PAF. Eight patients improved their neurological scores, beginning 2 to 6 days after the initiation of therapy. This improvement was sustained in five patients and only transient in three patients.

In addition to *Ginkgo biloba* extract (40 milligrams three times daily), I would recommend bromelain (400–750 milligrams 20 minutes before meals).

Osteoarthritis

Osteoarthritis or degenerative joint disease is the most common form of arthritis. It is seen primarily, but not exclusively, in the elderly. Surveys indicate that more than 40 million Americans have osteoarthritis, including 80 percent of persons over the age of 50 years. Under the age of 45 years, osteoarthritis is much more common in men; after age 45 years it is ten times more common in women than men.[1]

The weight-bearing joints and joints of the hands are most often affected by the degenerative changes associated with osteoarthritis. Specifically, there is much cartilage destruction followed by hardening and the formation of large bone spurs in the joint margins. Pain, deformity, and limitation of motion in the joint result. Inflammation is usually minimal.[1]

The onset of osteoarthritis can be very subtle; morning joint stiffness is often the first symptom. As the disease progresses, there is pain on motion of the involved joint that is made worse by prolonged activity and relieved by rest. There is usually no sign of inflammation.

Perhaps the most important dietary recommendation for individuals suffering from osteoarthritis is that they achieve of normal body weight. Being overweight means increased stress on weight-bearing joints affected with osteoarthritis.

Both in terms of preventing and treating osteoarthritis with diet, it is critical that the diet be rich in whole natural foods, especially raw fruits and vegetables because of their rich source of nutrients critical to joint health, such as vitamin C, carotenes, and flavonoids.

Glucosamine sulfate (a natural constituent of cartilage), at a dosage of 500 milligrams three times daily, has been shown to produce better results than standard drug therapy for osteoarthritis. Unlike the drugs, however, glucosamine sulfate works to address the underlying cause of osteoarthritis by stimulating cartilage repair and is free from side effects.[1]

Herbal recommendations for osteoarthritis

Because of the excellent results achieved with glucosamine sulfate, I recommend herbs for osteoarthritis only rarely. If I do, it is usually a capsaicin-containing cream for topical application or a combination of curcumin and bromelain to reduce inflammation.

Premenstrual syndrome

Premenstrual syndrome (PMS), also called premenstrual tension, is a recurrent condition of women characterized by troublesome, yet often ill-defined, symptoms 7–14 days before menstruation. Typical symptoms include decreased energy, tension, irritability, depression, headache, altered sex drive, breast pain, backache, abdominal bloating, and swelling of the fingers and ankles. The syndrome affects about one-third of women between 30 and 40 years of age, about 10 percent of whom may experience a significantly debilitating form of PMS.

Although the symptoms vary, there are common hormonal patterns in PMS patients when compared to symptom-free control groups. Perhaps the most common pattern is an elevation of plasma estrogen and a decrease in plasma progesterone levels 5–10 days before menses.

Diet appears to play a major role in the development of PMS. Compared to symptom-free women, PMS patients consume 62 percent more refined carbohydrates, 275 percent more refined sugar, 79 percent more dairy products, 78 percent more sodium, 53 percent less iron, 77 percent less manganese, and 52 percent less zinc.[1] The first step in addressing PMS is to limit the consumption of refined sugar and to decrease or eliminate milk and dairy products. This will help eliminate some of the nutritional imbalances produced by eating these foods as well as improve overall nutritional status.

Additional key dietary recommendations for the PMS sufferer include decreasing salt intake, alcohol and tobacco use, and the intake of caffeine-containing foods and beverages such as coffee, tea, and chocolate. Caffeine intake is related to the severity of symptoms in a dose-dependent manner—i.e., the more caffeine consumed, the greater the severity of the symptoms.[2]

Herbal recommendations for premenstrual syndrome

The same herbs used in menopause (see above) are useful in PMS. Again, a combination of the herbs may produce better results than any single herb.

Prostate Enlargement

Nearly 60 percent of men between the ages of 40 and 59 years have an enlarged prostate gland, a condition known in the medical community as benign prostatic hyperplasia (BPH). Symptoms of BPH typically reflect obstruction of the bladder outlet: progressive urinary frequency, urgency and night-time awakening to empty the bladder, and hesitancy and intermittency with reduced force and caliber of urine. The condition, if left untreated, will eventually obstruct the bladder outlet, resulting in the retention of urine in the blood.

Diet appears to play a critical role in the development of BPH. Paramount to an effective BPH prevention and treatment plan is adequate zinc intake and absorption. Zinc has been shown to reduce the size of the prostate—as determined by rectal examination, X-ray, and endoscopy—and to reduce symptoms in the majority of patients.[1] The clinical efficacy of zinc is probably due to its critical involvement in many aspects of hormonal metabolism.[2]

An old folk remedy for BPH is to eat ¼ to ½ cup of pumpkin seeds each day. This appears to be a very sound recommendation, owing to the high zinc and essential fatty acid content of pumpkin seeds.

Herbal recommendations for prostate enlargement

The subject of prostate enlargement was fully detailed in Chapter 32—Saw Palmetto. I would recommend trying saw palmetto; if after 3 months symptoms are not improved, try *Pygeum africanum*. When using saw palmetto, make sure that it is the extract standardized to contain 85 to 95 percent fatty acids and sterols.

Prostatitis

Prostatitis refers to an infection or inflammation of the prostate. Prostatitis is associated with pain during urination, fever, and a discharge from the penis. The standard medical treatment is antibiotics. With antibiotics alone the condition is typically of a chronic nature and difficult to clear. Frequent or chronic prostate infections may be a sign of low zinc levels, as the prostatic fluid contains a powerful zinc-containing antiinfective substance.

Herbal recommendations for prostatitis

The flower pollen extract known as Cernilton has been used to treat prostatitis in Europe for more than 25 years.[1] It has been shown to be quite effective in several double-blind clinical studies in the treatment of prostatitis due to inflammation or infection.[2] The extract has been shown to exert some antiinflammatory action and produce a contractile effect on the bladder while simultaneously relaxing the urethra. Cernilton and similar products are available in health food stores. The standard dosage for Cernilton or similar products is 2 tablets three times daily.

Psoriasis

Psoriasis is an extremely common skin disorder. Its rate of occurrence in the United States is between 2 and 4 percent of the population. Psoriasis affects few blacks, and is rare in Indians and blacks in tropical zones. The condition is caused by a pile-up of skin cells that have replicated too rapidly. The rate at which skin cells divide in psoriasis is roughly 1,000 times greater than in normal skin. This is simply too fast for the cells to be shed, so they accumulate, resulting in the characteristic silvery scale of psoriasis.[1]

A number of dietary factors appear to be responsible for psoriasis, including incomplete protein digestion, alcohol consumption, and excessive consumption of animal fats.

Dietary oils are extremely important in the management of psoriasis. Of particular benefit are the omega-3 oils such as flaxseed oil, and fish oils such as EPA. Several double-blind clinical studies have demonstrated that supplementing the diet with 10–12 grams of EPA results in significant improvement.[1] This would be equivalent to the amount of EPA in a 5-ounce serving of mackerel, salmon, or herring.

Herbal recommendations for psoriasis

As described in Chapter 24, silymarin has been reported to be of value in the treatment of psoriasis. Presumably this is a result of its ability to improve liver function, inhibit inflammation, and reduce excessive cellular proliferation. Sarsaparilla may also be useful.

Topical preparations containing licorice or chamomile extracts can also help. See Eczema (above) for a description.

Rheumatoid arthritis

Rheumatoid arthritis (RA) is a chronic inflammatory condition that affects the entire body but especially the synovial membranes of the joints. It is a classic example of an "autoimmune disease," a condition in which the body's immune system attacks the body's own tissue.

In RA, the joints typically involved are the hands and feet, wrists, ankles, and knees. Somewhere between 1 and 3 percent of the population is affected; female patients outnumber males almost three to one; and the usual age of onset is 20–40 years, although rheumatoid arthritis may begin at any age.

The onset of rheumatoid arthritis is usually gradual, but occasionally it is quite abrupt. Fatigue, low-grade fever, weakness, joint stiffness, and vague joint pain may proceed the appearance of painful, swollen joints by several weeks. Several joints are usually involved in the onset, typically in a symmetrical fashion (i.e., both hands, wrists, or ankles). In about one-third of persons with RA, initial involvement is confined to one or a few joints.

Involved joints will characteristically be quite warm, tender, and swollen. The skin over the joint will take on a ruddy purplish hue. As the disease progresses joint deformities result in the hands and feet. Terms used to describe these deformities include swan neck, boutenniere, and cockup toes.[1]

There is abundant evidence that rheumatoid arthritis is an "autoimmune"reaction, in which antibodies develop against components of joint tissues; yet what triggers this autoimmune reaction remains largely unknown. Speculation and investigation has centered around genetic susceptibility, abnormal bowel permeability, lifestyle and nutritional factors, food allergies, and microorganisms. Rheumatoid arthritis is a classic example of a multifactorial disease in which an interesting assortment of genetic and environmental factors contribute to the disease process.

Herbal recommendations for rheumatoid arthritis

Several herbs discussed in this book should be used at the dosages recommended by individuals with rheumatoid arthritis. All are useful. Their ranking, in order of effectiveness, is as follows:

- Curcumin
- Bromelain
- Ginger
- Capsicum (topical application)

The root of *Tripterygium wilfordi*, a Chinese plant, is showing great promise, but must be used with great caution in children and either men or women of reproductive years, as it may lead to cessation of menstruation or impaired sperm formation. Several components exert antiinflammatory action, but a suppressive effect on the immune system as well. The glycoside extract of the decorticated root is probably better tolerated and less harmful to reproductive function than crude *Tripterygium wilfordi* preparations. Commercial preparations in the United States are not yet available (as of 1994), but will likely be available in the near future.

The following describes the results of three studies. In the first study, a glycoside extract with a code name of T2 was used in a double-blind, controlled, cross-over study to treat seventy patients. T2 (60 milligrams daily) exhibited an overall effectiveness rate of 90 percent in group A and 80 percent in group B after 12 weeks of treatment. Side effects were common. Skin rash and chapped lips occurred in 55.5 percent of patients in group A and 28 percent in group B. Cessation of menstruation occurred in 31 percent of women of child-bearing age in group A and 5.5 percent in group B. Other side effects included gastrointestinal (GI) discomfort, nausea, and mild abdominal pain. Fortunately, these side effects occurred early and disappeared spontaneously after a few days.[1]

In the second study, 144 patients with RA were treated with the glycoside extract. The overall effective rate was 93.3 percent with 17.6 percent having total clinical remission, 37.5 percent having effective treatment, and 37.5 percent noting improvement. The criteria of effectiveness were as follows: "clinical remission" if symptoms disappeared, articular function was recovered, and laboratory findings were normal; "effective" treatment if joint pain was alleviated and there was a complete recovery of function, erythrocyte sedimentation rate (ESR) became normal, and rheumatoid factor (RF) became negative; "improvement" if joint pain was alleviated with increased mobility, and ESR decreased but not to normal; and "no improvement" if symptoms, signs, and laboratory findings remained unchanged. Of 132 patients with severe joint pain before therapy, 124 said the pain was reduced or gone. Most patients noted benefit within the first 2 weeks of therapy. Side effects were common. Poor appetite was reported in 20 percent, dry mouth in 18.7 percent, skin rash in 15.9 percent, hyperpigmentation in 13.2 percent, and nausea in 6.9 percent. Breast development occurred in two males and 23 percent of the women experienced menstrual disturbances.[2]

In the third study, ninety-five patients with rheumatoid arthritis and thirty-eight patients with ankylosing spondylitis were treated with a tincture of *Tripterygium wilfordi* root at a dose of 15–30 milliliters (equivalent to 1.8–3.6 grams of crude root) daily in divided doses from 2 months to 2 years. Relief of joint pain to various degrees was accomplished in 98 percent. Some reduction of joint swelling and improved joint function was noted in 87 percent. Most patients noted benefit within the first 2 weeks of therapy. Side effects were common, but were not serious. In menstruating women, 47 percent experienced amenorrhea or other menstrual disturbance.[3]

As is apparent from these studies, good results can be obtained yet the treatment is associated with some degree of toxicity. Hopefully, further research will clarify the risk versus benefit of this plant in autoimmune disorders.

Ulcers

An ulcer usually refers to a peptic ulcer, a term used to refer to a group of ulcerative disorders of the upper gastrointestinal tract. The major forms of peptic ulcer are chronic duodenal and gastric (stomach) ulcer. Although duodenal and gastric ulcerations occur at different locations, they appear to be the result of similar mechanisms. Specifically, the development of a duodenal or gastric ulcer is generally thought to be the result of pepsin and stomach acids damaging the lining of the duodenum or stomach. Normally there are enough protective factors to prevent the ulcer formation, however, when there is a decrease in the integrity of these protective factors ulceration occurs.

Although symptoms of a peptic ulcer may be absent or quite vague, most often peptic ulcers are associated with abdominal discomfort noted 45–60 minutes after meals or during the night. In the typical case, the pain is described as gnawing, burning, cramplike, or aching, or as "heartburn." Eating or using antacids usually results in great relief.

Note: Individuals with any symptoms of a peptic ulcer need competent medical care. Peptic ulcer complications such as hemorrhage, perforation, and obstruction represent medical emergencies that require immediate hospitalization. Patients with peptic ulcer should be monitored by a physician, even if following the natural approaches discussed below.

The natural approach to peptic ulcers is first to identify, and then eliminate or reduce, all factors that can contribute to the development of peptic ulcers: food allergy, low-fiber diet, cigarette smoking, stress, and drugs such as aspirin and other nonsteroidal analgesics. Once the causative factors have been controlled or eliminated, the focus is directed at healing the ulcers and promoting tissue resistance.

Herbal recommendations for ulcers

The best herbal recommendation is to use deglycyrrhizinated licorice (DGL; see Chapter 22 for discussion). Rather than inhibit the release of acid, licorice stimulates the normal defense mechanisms that prevent ulcer formation. Numerous studies over the years have found DGL to be an effective antiulcer compound. In several head-to-head comparison studies, DGL has been shown to be more effective than either Tagamet, Zantac, or antacids in both short term treatment and maintenance therapy of peptic ulcers. However, while these drugs are associated with significant side effects, DGL is extremely safe and is only a fraction of the cost. The standard dose for DGL is two to four 380-milligram tablets between or 20 minutes before meals. The DGL should be continued for 8 to 16 weeks, depending on the response.

Varicose veins

Varicose veins affect nearly 50 percent of middle-aged adults. The veins just under the skin of the legs are the veins most commonly affected, due to the tremendous strain that standing has on these veins. When an individual stands for long periods of time, the pressure exerted against the vein can increase up to ten times. Hence, individuals with occupations that require long periods of standing are at greatest risk for developing varicose veins.

Women are affected about four times as frequently as men; obese individuals have a much greater risk; and the risk increases with age due to loss of tissue tone, loss of muscle mass, and weakening of the walls of the veins. Pregnancy may also lead to the development of varicose veins, as pregnancy increases venous pressure in the legs.

In general, varicose veins pose little harm if the involved vein is near the surface. These types of varicose veins are, however, cosmetically unappealing. Although significant symptoms are not common, the legs may feel heavy, tight, and tired. A more serious form of varicose vein involves obstruction and valve defects of the deeper veins of the leg.

Herbal recommendations for varicose veins

The best recommendation in my opinion is the triterpenic acid extract of gotu kola (see Chapter 15 for description). Also of benefit are flavonoid-rich extracts of grape seed, bilberry, and *Ginkgo biloba*; and bromelain.

An herb not discussed previously that may also be of benefit is butcher's broom (*Ruscus aculeatus*). This plant is a subshrub of the lily family that grows in the Mediterranean region. The rhizome has a long history of use in treating venous disorders such as hemorrhoids and varicose veins. The active ingredients in butcher's broom are known as ruscogenins. These compounds have demonstrated a wide range of pharmacological actions, including anti-inflammatory and vasoconstrictor effects. The standard dosage of *Ruscus* is based on the ruscogenin content. For best results the dosage of any *Ruscus* preparation should supply 16.5 to 33 milligrams of ruscogenins three times daily.

Most clinical research has employed a *Ruscus* extract standardized for ruscogenin in combination with a flavonoid (trimethyl hesperidine chalcone) and vitamin C. Good results have been obtained in double-blind studies.[1] For example, in one study of forty patients suffering from chronic venous insufficiency of the lower limbs, symptoms of edema, itching, paraesthesia, leg heaviness, and cramps improved significantly in the group given the butcher's broom preparation. No side effects were reported. These results appear to be due to the ruscogenins improving the tone of the venous wall.[2]

References

Angina

1. Cherchi A, *et al.*: Effects of L-carnitine on exercise tolerance in chronic stable angina: A multicenter, double-blind, randomized, placebo controlled crossover study. *Int J Clin Pharm Ther Toxicol* **23**, 569–572, 1985; Kamikawa T, *et al.*: Effects of coenzyme Q10 on exercise tolerance in chronic stable angina pectoris. *Am J Cardiol* **56**, 247, 1985; Altura BM: Ischemic heart disease and magnesium. *Magnesium* **7**, 57–67, 1988.
2. Osher HL, Katz KH, and Wagner DJ: Khellin in the treatment of angina pectoris. *New Engl J Med* **244**, 315–321, 1951.
3. Anrep GV, Kenawy MR, and Barsoum GS: Coronary vasocilator action of khellin. *Am Heart J* **37**, 531–542, 1949; Conn JJ, *et al.*: Treatment of angina pectoris with khellin. *Ann Intern Med* **36**, 1173–1178, 1952.

Anxiety

1. Werbach M: *Nutritional Influences on Mental Illness: A Sourcebook of Clinical Research.* Third Line Press, Tarzana, CA, 1991.
2. Bruce M and Lader M: Caffeine abstention in the management of anxiety disorders. *Psychol Med* **19**, 211–214, 1989.

Asthma and hay fever

1. Gopalakrishnan C, *et al.*: Effect of tylophorine, a major alkaloid of *Tylophora indica*, on immunopathological and inflammatory reactions. *Indian J Med Res* **71**, 940–948, 1980; Haranath PSRK and Shyamalakumari S: Experimental study on mode of action of *Tylophora asthmatica* in bronchial asthma. *Indian J Med Res* **63**, 661–670, 1975.
2. Gupta S, *et al.*: *Tylophora indica* in bronchial asthma—a double blind study. *Indian J Med Res* **69**, 981–989, 1979; Thiruvengadam KV, *et al.*: *Tylophora indica* in bronchial asthma (a controlled comparison with a standard anti-asthmatic drug). *J Indian Med Assoc* **71**, 172–176, 1978; Shivpuri DN, Singhal SC, and Parkash D: Treatment of asthma with an alcoholic extract of *Tylophora indica*: A cross-over, double-blind study. *Ann Allergy* **30**, 407–412, 1972.

Atherosclerosis

1. National Research Council: *Diet and Health. Implications for Reducing Chronic Disease Risk.* National Academy Press, Washington, D.C., 1989.

Bladder infections

1. Sobota AE: Inhibition of bacterial adherence by cranberry juice: Potential use for the treatment of urinary tract infections. *J Urol* **131**, 1013–1016, 1984.
2. Prodromos PN, *et al.*: Cranberry juice in the treatment of urinary tract infections. *Southwestern Med* **47**, 17, 1968.
3. Avorn J, *et al.*: Reduction of bacteriuria and pyuria after ingestion of cranberry juice. *JAMA* **271**, 751–754, 1994.

Canker sores

1. Das SK, *et al.*: Deglycyrrhizinated liquorice in apthous ulcers. *Journal of the Association of Physicians of India (JAPI)* **37**, 647, 1989.

Cold sores

1. Dimitrova Z, *et al.*: Antiherpes effect of *Melissa officinalis* L. extracts. *Acta Microbiol Bulg* **29**, 65–72, 1993; Cohen RA, Kucera LS, and Herrmann EC: Antiviral activity of *Melissa officinalis* (lemon balm) extract. *Proc Soc Exp Biol Med* **117**, 431–434, 1964.
2. Wolbling RH and Milbradt R: Clinical therapy of herpes simplex. *Therapiewoche* **34**, 1193–1200, 1984; Vogt M, *et al.*: *Melissa* extract in herpes simplex. A double-blind placebo-controlled study. *Der Allgemeinarzt* **13**, 832–841, 1991; Wolbling RH and Leonhardt K: Local therapy of herpes simplex with dried extract from *Melissa officinalis*. *Phytomed* **1**, 25–31, 1994.

Common cold

1. Chang HM and But PPH: *Pharmacology and Applications of Chinese Materia Medica*, Vol. 2. World Scientific Publishing, Teaneck, NJ, 1987, pp. 1041–1046.

Diabetes

1. Sheela CG and Augusti KT: Antidiabetic effects of *S*-allyl cysteine sulphoxide isolated from garlic (*Allium sativum* Linn.). *Indian J Exp Biol* **30**, 523–526, 1992.
2. Sharma KK, *et al.*: Antihyperglycemic effect of onion: Effect on fasting blood sugar and induced hyperglycemia in man. *Indian J Med Res* **65**, 422–429, 1977.
3. Welihinda J, *et al.*: Effect of *Momardica charantia* on the glucose tolerance in maturity onset diabetes. *J Ethnopharmacol* **17**, 277–282, 1986.
4. Srivastava Y, *et al.*: Antidiabetic and adaptogenic properties of *Momordica charantia* extract: An experimental and clinical evaluation. *Phytother Res* **7**, 285–289, 1993.
5. Welihinda J, *et al.*: The insulin-releasing activity of the tropical plant *Momordica charantia*. *Acta Biol Med Germ* **41**, 1229–1240, 1982.
6. Shanmugasundaram ERB, *et al.*: Use of *Gymnema sylvestre* leaf extract in the control of blood glucose in insulin-dependent diabetes mellitus. *J Ethnopharmacol* **30**, 281–294, 1990.
7. Baskaran K, *et al.*: Antidiabetic effect of a leaf extract from *Gymnema sylvestre* in non-insulin dependent diabetes mellitus patients. *J Ethnopharmacol* **30**, 295–305, 1990.
8. Ribes G, *et al.*: Effects of fenugreek seeds on endocrine pancreatic secretions in dogs. *Ann Nutr Metab* **28**, 37–43, 1984.
9. Sharma RD, Raghuram TC, and Rao NS: Effect of fenugreek seeds on blood glucose and serum lipids in type I diabetes. *Eur J Clin Nutr* **44**, 301–306, 1990.
10. Mada Z, *et al.*: Glucose-lowering effect of fenugreek in non-insulin dependent diabetics. *Eur J Clin Nutr* **42**, 51–54, 1988.
11. Stern E: Successful use of *Atriplex halimus* in the treatment of type II diabetic patients. A preliminary study. Unpublished study conducted at the Zamenhoff Medical Center, Tel Aviv, Israel, 1989.
12. Earon G, Stern E, and Lavosky H: Succesful use of *Atriplex halimus* in the treatment of type II diabetic patients. Controlled clinical research report on the subject of *Atriplex*. Unpublished study conducted at the Hebrew University of Jerusalem, Jerusalem, Israel, 1989.

13. Chakravarthy BK, et al.: Pancreatic beta-cell regeneration in rats by (–)-epicatechin. Lancet 2, 759–760, 1981.
14. Chakravarthy BK, Gupa S, and Gode KD: Functional beta cell regeneration in the islets of pancreas in alloxan induced diabetic rats by (–)-epicatechin. Life Sci 31, 2693–2697, 1982.

Diarrhea

1. Loeb H, et al.: Tannin-rich carob pod for the treatment of acute-onset diarrhea. J Pediatr Gastroenterol Nutr 8, 480–485, 1989.

Eczema

1. Evans FQ: The rational use of glycyrrhetinic acid in dermatology. Br J Clin Pract 12, 269–279, 1958.
2. Mann C and Staba EJ: The chemistry, pharmacology, and commercial formulations of chamomile. Herbs Spices Med Plants 1, 235–280, 1984.

Gout

1. Blau LW: Cherry diet control for gout and arthritis. Texas Rep Biol Med 8, 309–311, 1950.

Hemorrhoids

1. Webster DJ, Gough DC, and Craven JL: The use of bulk evacuation in patients with hemorrhoids. Br J Surg 65, 291–292, 1978.

Hepatitis

1. Tajiri H, et al.: Effect of sho-saiko-to (xiao-chai-hu-tang) on HBeAg clearance in children with chronic hepatitis B virus infection and with sustained liver disease. Am J Chin Med 19, 121–129, 1991; Okumura M, et al.: A multicenter randomized controlled clinical trial of Sho-saiko-to in chronic active hepatitis. Gastroenterol Jpn 24, 715–719, 1989.
2. Abe H, et al.: Effects of saikosaponin-d on enhanced CCl_4-hepatotoxicity by phenobarbitone. J Pharm Pharmacol 37, 555–559, 1985.

Herpes

1. Griffith R, DeLong D, and Nelson J: Relation of arginine-lysine antagonism to herpes simplex growth in tissue culture. Chemotherapy 27, 209–213, 1981.
2. Griffith RS, et al.: Success of L-lysine therapy in frequently recurrent herpes simplex infection. Dermatologica 175, 183–190, 1987.
3. Wolbling RH and Leonhardt K: Local therapy of herpes simplex with dried extract from Melissa officinalis. Phytomed 1, 25–31, 1994.

Impotence

1. Susset JG, et al.: Effect of yohimbine hydrochloride on erectile impotence: A double-blind study. J Urol 141, 1360–1363, 1989; Morales A, et al.: Is yohimbine effective in the treatment of organic impotence? Results of a controlled trial. J Urol 137, 1168–1172, 1987.
2. Waynberg J: Aphrodisiacs: Contribution to the clinical validation of the traditional use of Ptychopetalum guyanna. Presented at the First International Congress on Ethnopharmacology, Strasbourg, France, June 5–9, 1990.

Irritable bowel syndrome

1. Jones V, et al.: Food intolerance: A major factor in the pathogenesis of irritable bowel syndrome. *Lancet* ii, 1115–1118, 1982; Petitpierre M, Gumowski P, and Girard J: Irritable bowel syndrome and hypersensitivity to food. *Ann Allergy* 54, 538–540, 1985.

Kidney stones

1. Light I, Gursel E, and Zinnser HH: Urinary ionized calcium in urolithiasis. Effect of cranberry juice. *Urology* 1, 67–70, 1973.

Menopause

1. Murray MT: *Menopause.* Prima Publishing, Rocklin, CA, 1994.
2. Kaldas RS and Hughes CL: Reproductive and general metabolic effects of phytoestrogens in mammals. *Reprod Toxicol* 3, 81–89, 1989; Rose DP: Dietary fiber, phytoestrogens, and breast cancer. *Nutrition* 8, 47–51, 1992; Adlercreutz H, et al.: Determination of urinary lignans and phytoestrogen metabolites, potential antiestrogens and anticarcinogens, in urine of women on various habitual diets. *Steroid Biochem* 25, 791–797, 1986.
3. Elghamry MI and Shihata IM: Biological activity of phytoestrogens. *Planta Medica* 13, 352–357, 1965; Tamaya T, et al.: Inhibition by plant herb extracts of steroid bindings in uterus, liver, and serum of the rabbit. *Acta Obstet Gynecol Scand* 65, 839–842, 1986.
4. Commission E Monograph: Agni cast fructus (chaste tree fruits). Translation by the American Botanical Council, Fort Worth, TX, 1992.
5. Duker EM, et al.: Effects of extracts from *Cimicifuga racemosa* on gonatropin release in menopausal women and ovariectomized rats. *Planta Medica* 57, 420–424, 1991.

Multiple sclerosis

1. Swank RL: Multiple sclerosis: Fat-oil relationship. *Nutrition* 7, 368–376, 1991; Swank RL and Pullen MH: *The Multiple Sclerosis Diet Book.* Doubleday, Garden City, NY, 1977.
2. Brochet B, et al.: Pilot study of ginkgolide B, a PAF-acether specific inhibitor in the treatment of acute outbreaks of multiple sclerosis. *Rev Neurol (Paris)* 148, 299–301, 1992.

Osteoarthritis

1. Vaz AL: Double-blind clinical evaluation of the relative efficacy of ibuprofen and glucosamine sulfate in the management of osteoarthrosis of the knee in out-patients. *Curr Med Res Opin* 8, 145–149, 1982; Crolle G and D'este E: Glucosamine sulfate for the management of arthrosis: A controlled clinical investigation. *Curr Med Res Opin* 7, 104–114, 1981; Tapadinhas MJ, Rivera IC, and Bignamini AA: Oral glucosamine sulfate in the management of arthrosis: Report on a multi-centre open investigation in Portugal. *Pharmatherapeutica* 3, 157–168, 1982; D'Ambrosia ED, et al.: Glucosamine sulphate: A controlled clinical investigation in arthrosis. *Pharmatherapeutica* 2, 504–508, 1982.

Premenstrual syndrome

1. Abraham GE: Nutritional factors in the etiology of the premenstrual tension syndromes. *J Repr Med* 28, 446–464, 1983.
2. Boyle CA, et al.: Caffeine consumption and fibrocystic breast disease: A case-control epidemiologic study. *J Natl Cancer Inst* 72, 1015–1019, 1984.

Prostate enlargement

1. Fahim M, *et al.*: Zinc treatment for the reduction of hyperplasia of the prostate. *Fed Proc* **35**, 361, 1976.
2. Wallae AM and Grant JK: Effect of zinc on androgen metabolism in the human hyperplastic prostate. *Biochem Soc Trans* **3**, 540–542, 1975.

Prostatitis

1. Ask-Upmark E: Prostatitis and its treatment. *Acta Med Scand* **181**, 355–357, 1967.
2. Ohkoshi M, Kawamura N, and Nagakubo I: Clinical evaluation of Cernilton in chronic prostatitis. *Jpn J Clin Urol* **21**, 73–85, 1967; Buck AC, Rees RWM, and Ebeling L: Treatment of chronic prostatitis and prostadynia with pollen extract. *Br J Urol* **64**, 496–499, 1989.

Psoriasis

1. Bittiner SB, *et al.*: A double-blind, randomized, placebo-controlled trial of fish oil in psoriasis. *Lancet* **i**, 378–380, 1988; Ziboh VA, *et al.*: Effects of dietary supplementation of fish oil on neutrophil and epidermal fatty acids. *Arch Dermatol* **122**, 1277–1282, 1986.

Rheumatoid arthritis

1. Tao XL, *et al.*: A prospective, controlled, double-blind, cross-over study of *Tripterygium wilfodii* hook F in treatment of rheumatoid arthritis. *Chin Med J* **102**, 327–332, 1989.
2. Deyong Y: Clinical observation of 144 cases of rheumatoid arthritis treated with glycoside of radix *Tripterygium wilfordii*. *J Trad Chin Med* **3**, 125–129, 1983.
3. Deyong Y: *Tripterygium wilfordii* hook F in rheumatoid arthritis and ankylosing spondylitis. *Chin Med J* **7**, 405–412, 1981.

Varicose veins

1. Cappelli R, Nicora M, and Di Perri T: Use of extract of *Ruscus aculeatus* in venous disease in the lower limbs. *Drugs Exp Clin Res* **14**, 277–283, 1988.
2. Rudofsky G: Improving venous tone and capillary sealing. Effect of a combination of *Ruscus* extract and hesperidine methyl chalcone in healthy probands in heat stress. *Forschr Med* **107**(19), 52, 55–58, 1989.

Resources

The following organizations may be useful resources in finding out more information on herbs or an herbal practitioner.

Organizations

American Association of Naturopathic Physicians
P.O. Box 20386
Seattle, WA 98102
(206) 323-7610

The American Association of Naturopathic Physicians (AANP) is the professional organization of licensed naturopathic physicians.

American Botanical Council
P.O. Box 201660
Austin, TX 78720
(512) 331-8868
Fax: (512) 331-1924

A nonprofit organization dedicated to education. Copublishes the *Herbal-Gram* with the Herb Research Foundation. Provides excellent reference materials, including a series of Classic Botanical Reprints.

American Herb Association
P.O. Box 1673
Nevada City, CA 95959
Fax: (916) 265-9552

Membership includes a subscription to the *AHA Quarterly*, which is devoted to providing information on medicinal herbs.

American Herbalist Guild
P.O. Box 1683
Soquel, CA 95073

A nonprofit membership organization. Members receive a quarterly journal and discounts to seminars and workshops.

American Holistic Medical
Association
4101 Lake Boone Trail #201
Raleigh, NC 26707
(919) 787-5146

The American Holistic Medical Association is composed of medical doctors (M.D.s), osteopaths (D.O.s), and naturopaths (N.D.s) who share a common philosophy of encouraging personal responsibility for health and emphasizing the whole person.

American Society of Pharmacognosy
Chicago School of Pharmacy
555 31st St.
Downers Grove, IL 60515

A nonprofit membership organization. Members receive the *Journal of Natural Products*.

The Herb Research Foundation
1007 Pearl St. #200
Boulder, CO 80302
(303) 449-2265
Fax: (303) 443-0949

The foundation provides accurate and reliable information on herbs. Copublisher of the *HerbalGram*. Offers research and educational services.

Naturopathic Medical Schools

Bastyr University
144 N.E. 54th St.
Seattle, WA 98105
(206) 523-9585

National College of Naturopathic Medicine
11231 S.E. Market St.
Portland, OR 97216
(503) 255-4860

Southwest College of Naturopathic Medicine
6535 East Osborn Road
Scottsdale, AZ 85251
(602) 990-7424

Glossary

Abortifacient   A substance that induces abortion.

Abscess   A localized collection of pus and liquefied tissue in a cavity.

Acetylcholine   One of the chemicals that transmits impulses between nerves and between nerves and muscle cells.

Acrid   A pungent biting taste that causes irritation.

Acute   Having a rapid onset, severe symptoms, and a short course; not chronic.

Adaptogen   A substance that is safe, increases resistance to stress, and has a balancing effect on body functions.

Adjuvant   A substance that enhances the effect of the medicinal agent or increases the antigenicity of a cancer cell.

Adrenaline   Hormone secreted by the adrenal gland that produces the "fight or flight" response. Also called epinephrine.

Aldosterone   A hormone secreted by the adrenal gland that causes the retention of sodium and water.

Alkaloids   Naturally occurring amines (nitrogen-containing compounds), arising from heterocyclic and often complex structures, that display pharmacological activity. Their trivial names usually end in -ine. They are usually classified according to the chemical structure of their main nucleus: phenylalkylamines (ephedrine), pyridine (nicotine), tropine (atropine, cocaine), quinoline (quinine), isoquinolone (papaverine), phenanthrene (morphine), purine (caffeine), imidazole (pilocarpine), and indole (physostigmine, yohimbine).

Allopathy   A term that describes the conventional method of medicine, which combats disease by using substances and techniques specifically against the disease.

Alterative   A substance that produces a balancing effect on a particular body function.

Amebiasis   An intestinal infection characterized by severe diarrhea caused by the parasite *Entamoeba histolytica*.

Amino acids   A group of nitrogen-containing chemical compounds that form the basic structural units of proteins.

Analgesic   A substance that reduces the sensation of pain.

Androgen   Hormones that stimulate male charateristics.

Anthelmintic   A substance that causes the elimination of intestinal worms.

Anthocyanidin   A particular class of flavonoids that gives plants, fruits, and flowers colors ranging from red to blue.

Antibody   Proteins manufactured by the body and that bind to an antigen to neutralize, inhibit, or destroy it.

Antidote   A substance that neutralizes or counteracts the effects of a poison.

Antigen   Any substance that, when introduced into the body, causes the formation of antibodies against it.

Antihypertensive   Blood pressure-lowering effect.

Antioxidant   A compound that prevents free radical or oxidative damage.

Aphrodisiac   A substance that increases sexual desire.

Artery   A blood vessel that carries oxygen-rich blood away from the heart.

Atherosclerosis   A process in which fatty substances (cholesterol and triglycerides) are deposited in the walls of medium to large arteries, eventually leading to blockage of the artery.

Atopy   A predisposition to various allergic conditions including eczema and asthma.

Astringent   An agent that causes the contraction of tissue.

Autoimmune   A process in which antibodies develop against the body's own tissues.

Balm   A soothing or healing medicine applied to the skin.

Basal metabolic rate   The rate of metabolism when the body is at rest.

Basophil   A type of white blood cell that is involved in allergic reactions.

Benign   A mild disorder that is usually not fatal.

beta-Carotene   Pro-vitamin A. A plant carotene that can be converted to two vitamin A molecules.

Beta Cell   Pancreatic cells that manufacture insulin.

Bilirubin   The breakdown product of the hemoglobin molecule of red blood cells.

Biopsy   A diagnostic test in which tissue or cells are removed from the body for examination under a microscope.

Bleeding time   The time required for the cessation of bleeding from a small skin puncture as a result of platelet disintegration and blood vessel constriction. Ranges from 1 to 4 minutes.

Blood–brain barrier   A special barrier that prevents the passage of materials from the blood to the brain.

Blood pressure   The force exerted by blood as it presses against and attempts to stretch blood vessels.

Bromelain   The protein-digesting enzyme found in pineapple.

Bursa   A sac or pouch that contains a special fluid that lubricates joints.

Bursitis   Inflammation of a bursa.

Calorie   A unit of heat. A nutritional calorie is the amount of heat necessary to raise 1 kilogram of water 1 degree Celsius.

Candida albicans   A yeast common to the intestinal tract.

Candidiasis   A complex medical syndrome produced by a chronic overgrowth of the yeast *Candida albicans*.

Carbohydrate   Sugars and starches.

Carcinogen   Any agent or substance capable of causing cancer.

Carcinogenesis   The development of cancer caused by the actions of certain chemicals, viruses, and unknown factors on primarily normal cells.

Cardiac output   The volume of blood pumped from the heart in one minute.

Cardiotonic   A compound that tones and strengthens the heart.

Cardiopulmonary   Pertaining to the heart and lungs.

Carminative   A substance that promotes the elimination of intestinal gas.

Carotene   Fat-soluble plant pigments, some of which can be converted into vitamin A by the body.

Cartilage   A type of connective tissue that acts as a shock absorber at joint interfaces.

Cathartic   A substance that stimulates the movement of the bowels; more powerful than a laxative.

Cholagogue   A compound that stimulates the contraction of the gallbladder.

Cholecystitis   Inflammation of the gallbladder.

Choleretic   A compound that promotes the flow of bile.

Cholestasis   The stagnation of bile within the liver.

Cholelithiasis   Gallstones.

Cholinergic   Pertaining to the parasympathetic portion of the autonomic nervous system and the release of acetylcholine as a transmitter substance.

Chronic   Long-term or frequently recurring.

Cirrhosis   A severe disease of the liver characterized by the replacement of liver cells with scar tissue.

Coenzyme   A necessary nonprotein component of an enzyme, usually a vitamin or mineral.

Cold sore   A small skin blister, anywhere around the mouth, caused by the herpes simplex virus.

Colic Severe, spasmodic pain that occurs in waves of increasing intensity, reaches a peak, then abates for a short time before returning.

Collagen The protein that is the main component of connective tissue.

Colitis Colon inflammation that is usually associated with diarrhea with blood and mucus.

Compress A pad of linen applied under pressure to an area of skin and held in place.

Congestive heart failure Chronic disease that results when the heart is not capable of supplying the oxygen demands of the body.

Connective tissue The type of tissue that performs the function of providing support, structure, and cellular cement to the body.

Contagious A disease that can be transferred from one person to another by social contact, such as by sharing the home or workplace.

Coronary artery disease A condition in which the heart receives an inadequate blood and oxygen supply due to atherosclerosis.

Corticosteroid drugs A group of drugs similar to the natural corticosteroid hormones; used predominantly in the treatment of inflammation and to suppress the immune system.

Corticosteroid hormones A group of hormones, produced by the adrenal glands, that control the body's use of nutrients and the excretion of salts and water in the urine.

Cushing's syndrome A condition caused by a hypersecretion of cortisone characterized by spindly legs, "moon face," "buffalo hump," abdominal obesity, flushed facial skin, and poor wound healing.

Cyst An abnormal lump or swelling, filled with fluid or semisolid material, in any body organ or tissue.

Cystitis Inflammation of the inner lining of the bladder. It is is usually caused by a bacterial infection.

Decoctions Teas prepared by boiling the herb with water for a specified period of time, followed by straining or filtering.

Dehydration Excessive loss of water from the body.

Demineralization Loss of minerals from the bone.

Dementia Senility. Loss of mental function.

Demulcent A substance soothing to irritated mucous membranes.

Dermatitis Inflammation of the skin, sometimes due to allergy.

Diastolic The second number in a blood pressure reading. It is the measure of the pressure in the arteries during the relaxation phase of the heart beat.

Disaccharide A sugar composed of two monosaccharide units.

Diuretic A compound that causes increased urination.

Diverticuli Saclike outpouchings of the wall of the colon.

Double-blind study A way of controlling against experimental bias by ensuring that neither the researcher nor the subject know when an active agent or placebo is being used.

Douche Introduction of water and/or a cleansing agent into the vagina, with the aid of a bag with tubing and nozzle attached.

Dysfunction Abnormal function.

Dysplasia Any abnormality of growth.

Edema Accumulation of fluid in tissues (swelling).

Eicosapentaenoic acid (EPA) A fatty acid found primarily in cold-water fish.

Electroencephalogram (EEG) A machine that measures and records brain waves.

Elimination diet A diet that eliminates food allergens.

Emulsify The dispersement of large fat globules into smaller, uniformly distributed particles.

Encephalitis Inflammation of the brain, usually due to viral infection.

Endometrium The mucous membrane lining of the uterus.

Enteric-coated A special way of coating a tablet or capsule so that it does not dissolve in the stomach, thereby ensuring that it reaches the intestinal tract.

Enzyme An organic catalyst that speeds chemical reactions.

Epidemiology The study of the occurrence and distribution of diseases in human populations.

Epithelium The cells that cover the entire surface of the body and that line most of the internal organs.

Epinephrine See *Adrenaline*.

Epstein–Barr virus The virus that causes infectious mononucleosis and is associated with Burkitt's lymphoma and nasopharyngeal cancer.

Essential fatty acid Fatty acids that the body cannot manufacture—linoleic and linolenic acids.

Essential oils Also known as volatile oils, ethereal oils, or essences. They are usually complex mixtures of a wide variety of organic compounds (e.g., alcohols, ketones, phenols, acids, ethers, esters, aldehydes, and oxides) that evaporate when exposed to air. They generally represent the odoriferous principles of plants.

Estrogens Hormones that produce female characteristics.

Excretion The process of elimination of waste products from a cell, tissue, or the entire body.

Extracellular Outside the cell.

Extracts Concentrated forms of natural products obtained by treating crude materials containing these substances with a solvent and then removing the solvent completely or partially from the preparation. The most commonly used extracts are fluid extracts, solid extracts, powdered extracts, tinctures, and native extracts.

Exudate   Fluid or semifluid material that oozes from a body space, and that may contain serum, pus, and cellular debris.

Faruncle   Another name for a boil that involves a hair follicle.

Fibrin   A white insoluble protein formed by the clotting of blood, and that serves as the starting point for wound repair and scar formation.

Fibrinolysis   The dissolution of fibrin or a blood clot by the action of enzymes that convert insoluble fibrin into soluble particles.

Flavonoid   A generic term for a group of flavone-containing compounds found widely in nature. They include many of the compounds that account for plant pigments (anthocyanins, anthoxanthins, apigenins, flavones, flavonols, bioflavonols, etc.). These plant pigments exert a wide variety of physiological effects in the human body.

Fluid extracts   These extracts are typically hydro–alcoholic solutions with a strength of 1 part solvent to 1 part herb. The alcohol content varies with each product. They are in essence concentrated tinctures.

Free radicals   Highly reactive molecules, characterized by an unpaired electron, that can bind to and destroy cellular compounds.

Gerontology   The study of aging.

Giardiasis   An infection of the small intestine caused by the protozoan (single-celled) *Giardia lamblia*.

Gingivitis   Inflammation of the gums.

Glaucoma   A condition in which the pressure of the fluid in the eye is so high it causes damage.

Glucose   A monosaccharide that is found in the blood and is one of the body's primary energy sources.

Gluten   One of the proteins in wheat and certain other grains that gives dough its tough, elastic character.

Glycosides   Sugar-containing compounds composed of a glycone (sugar component) and an aglycone (nonsugar-containing component) that can be cleaved on hydrolysis. The glycone portion may be glucose, rhamnose, xylose, fructose, arabinose or any other sugar. The aglycone portion can be any kind of compound, e.g., sterols, triterpenes, anthraquinones, hydroquinones, tannins, carotenoids, and anthocyanidins.

Goblet cell   A goblet-shaped cell that secretes mucus.

Ground substance   The thick, gellike material in which cell fibers, and blood capillaries of cartilage, bone, and connective tissue, are embedded.

Helper T cell   Lymphocytes that help in the immune response.

Hematocrit   An expression of the percentage of blood occupied by blood cells.

Hemorrhoids   Distended veins in the lining of the anus.

Hepatic   Pertaining to the liver.

Hepatomegaly   Enlargement of the liver.

Holistic medicine   A form of therapy aimed at treating the whole person, not just the part or parts in which symptoms occur.

Hormone   A secretion of an endocrine gland that controls and regulates body functions.

Hyperglycemia   High blood sugar.

Hypersecretion   Excessive secretion.

Hypertension   High blood pressure.

Hypochlorhydria   Insufficient gastric acid output.

Hypoglycemia   Low blood sugar.

Hypolipidemic   Elevations of cholesterol and triglycerides in the blood.

Hypotension   Low blood pressure.

Hypoxia   An inadequate suppy of oxygen.

Iatrogenic   Meaning literally "physician produced," the term can be applied to any medical condition, disease, or other adverse occurrence that results from medical treatment.

Immunoglobulins   Antibodies.

Idiopathic   Of unknown cause.

Incidence   The number of new cases of a disease that occurs during a given period (usually years) in a defined population.

Incontinence   The inability to control urination or defecation.

Infarction   Death of a localized area of tissue due to lack of oxygen supply.

Infusions   Teas produced by steeping an herb in hot water.

Insulin   A hormone, secreted by the pancreas, that lowers blood sugar levels.

Interferon   A potent immune-enhancing substance produced by the body's cells to fight off viral infection and cancer.

In vitro   Outside a living body and in an artificial environment.

In vivo   In the living body of an animal or plant.

Jaundice   A condition caused by elevation of bilirubin in the body and characterized by yellowing of the skin.

Keratin   An insoluble protein found in hair, skin, and nails.

Lactase   An enzyme that breaks down lactose into the monosaccharides glucose and galactose.

Lactose   One of the sugars present in milk. It is a disaccharide.

Laxative   A substance that promotes the evacuation of the bowels.

LD$_{50}$ The dose that will kill 50 percent of the animals taking the substance.

Lesion   Any localized, abnormal change in tissue formation.

Leukocyte   White blood cell.

Lethargy   A feeling of tiredness, drowsiness, or lack of energy.

Leukotrienes   Inflammatory compounds produced when oxygen interacts with polyunsaturated fatty acids.

Lipid   Fats, phospholipids, steroids, and prostaglandins.

Lipotropic   Promoting the flow of lipids to and from the liver.

Lymph   Fluid, contained in lymphatic vessels, that flows through the lymphatic system to be returned to the blood.

Lymphocyte   A type of white blood cell found primarily in lymph nodes.

Malabsorption   Impaired absorption of nutrients most often due to diarrhea.

Malaise   A vague feeling of being sick or of physical discomfort.

Malignant   A term used to describe a condition that tends to worsen and eventually causes death.

Manipulation   As a therapy, the skillful use of the hands to move a part of the body or a specific joint or muscle.

Menorrhagia   Excessive loss of blood during periods.

Menstrums   Solvents used for extraction, e.g., water, alcohol, and acetone.

Mast cell   A cell, found in many tissues of the body, that contributes greatly to allergic and inflammatory processes by secreting histamine and other inflammatory particles.

Metabolism   A collective term for all the chemical processes that take place in the body.

Metabolite   A product of a chemical reaction.

Metalloenzyme   An enzyme that contains a metal at its active site.

Microbe   A popular term for microorganism.

Microflora   The microbial inhabitants of a particular region, e.g., colon.

Mites   Small, eight-legged animals, less than one-twentieth of an inch (1.2 mm) long, similar to tiny spiders.

Molecule   The smallest complete unit of a substance that can exist independently and still retain the characteristic properties of the substance.

Monoclonal antibodies   Genetically engineered antibodies specific for one particular antibody.

Monosaccharide   A simple, one-unit sugar such as fructose and glucose.

Mortality rate   The number of deaths per 100,000 of the population per year.

Mucosa   Another term for mucous membrane.

Mucous membrane   The soft, pink, tissue that lines most of the bodies cavities and tubes in the body, including the respiratory tract, gastrointestinal tract, genitourinary tract, and eyelids. The mucous membranes secrete mucus.

Mucus   The slick, slimy fluid secreted by the mucous membranes and that acts as a lubricant and mechanical protector of the mucous membranes.

Mycotoxins   Toxins from yeast and fungi.

Myelin sheath   A white fatty substance that surrounds nerve cells to aid in nerve impulse transmission.

Neoplasia   A medical term for a tumor formation, characterized by a progressive, abnormal replication of cells.

Neurofibrillary tangles   Clusters of degenerated nerves.

Neurotransmitters   Substances that modify or transmit nerve impulses.

Night blindness   The inability to see well in dim light or at night.

Nocturia   The disturbance of a person's sleep at night by the need to pass urine.

Oleoresins   Primarily mixtures of resins and volatile oils. They either occur naturally or are made by extracting the oily and resinous materials from herbs with organic solvents (e.g., hexane, acetone, ether, and alcohol). The solvent is then removed under vacuum, leaving behind a viscous, semisolid extract that is the oleoresin. Examples of prepared oleoresins are paprika, ginger, and capsicum.

Oligoantigenic diet   See *Elimination diet*.

Otitis media   Acute infection of the middle ear.

Pancreatin   A special extract of pork pancreas.

Papain   The protein-digesting enzyme of papaya.

Parkinson's disease   A slowly progressive, degenerating nervous system disease characterized by resting tremor, pill rolling of the fingers, a masklike facial expression, shuffling gait, and muscle rigidity and weakness.

Pathogen   Any agent, particularly a microorganism, that causes disease.

Pathogenesis   The process by which a disease originates and develops, particularly the cellular and physiological processes.

Peristalsis   Successive muscular contractions of the intestines that move food through the intestinal tract.

Physiology   The study of the functioning of the body, including the physical and chemical processes of its cells, tissues, organs, and systems.

Physostigmine   A drug that blocks the breakdown of acetylcholine.

Phytoestrogen   Plant compounds that exert estrogen effects.

Placebo   An inert or inactive substance used to test the efficacy of another substance.

Polysaccharide   A molecule composed of many sugar molecules linked together.

Powdered extract   A solid extract that has been dried as a powder.

Prostaglandin   Hormone-like compounds manufactured from essential fatty acids.

Psychosomatic   Pertaining to the relationship of the mind and body. Commonly used to refer to those physiological disorders thought to be caused entirely or partly by psychological factors.

Putrefaction   The process of breaking down protein compounds by rotting.

RDA   Recommended Dietary Allowance.

Resins   Complex oxidative products of terpenes that occur naturally as plant exudates, or are prepared by alcohol extraction of herbs that contain resinous principles.

Saccharide   A sugar molecule.

Saponins   Nonnitrogenous glycosides, typically with sterol or triterpenes as the aglycone, that possess the common property of foaming, or making suds, when strongly agitated in aqueous solution.

Satiety   A feeling of fullness or gratification.

Saturated fat   A fat whose carbon atoms are bonded to the maximum number of hydrogen atoms; found in animal products such as meat, milk, milk products, and eggs.

Sclerosis   The process of hardening or scarring.

Senile dementia   Mental deterioration associated with aging.

Slow-reacting substance of anaphylaxis (SRSA)   A potent allergic mediator produced and released by mast cells.

Solid extracts   Extracts that have had all of the residual solvent or liquid removed.

Submucosa   The tissue just below the mucous membrane.

Suppressor T cell   Lymphocytes, controlled by the thymus gland, that suppress the immune response.

Syndrome   A group of signs and symptoms that occur together in a pattern characteristic of a particular disease or abnormal condition.

T cell   A lymphocyte under the control of the thymus gland.

Tincture   Alcoholic or hydro–alcoholic solutions usually containing the active principles of herbs in low concentrations. They are usually prepared by maceration, percolation, or by dilution of their corresponding fluid or native extracts. The strengths of tinctures are typically 1:10 or 1:5. The alcohol content will vary.

Tonic   A substance that exerts a gentle strengthening effect on the body.

trans-**Fatty acid**   The type of fat found in margarine.

Uremia   The retention of urine by the body and the presence of high levels of urine components in the blood.

Urinalysis   The analysis of urine.

Urticaria   Hives.

Vasoconstriction   The constriction of blood vessels.

Vasodilation   The dilation of blood vessels.

Vitamin   An essential compound necessary to act as a catalyst in normal processes of the body.

Western diet   A diet characteristic of Western societies, i.e., a diet high in fat, refined carbohydrate, and processed foods, and low in dietary fiber.

Wheal   The characteristic lesion in hives; a small welt.

Index